Pediatric Oncology

This series provides up-to-date information on important topics in pediatric oncology, from the diagnosis and treatment of particular forms of disease through to, for example, radiation oncology, supportive care, and survivorship. The entire spectrum of clinical management is covered with the aim of equipping readers with the latest knowledge relevant to daily practice. In addition, clinical, methodological, and research issues are addressed. The series benefits from homogeneous design and consistently high quality of illustrations. The volume editors are internationally renowned authorities and contributing authors have been selected for their expertise in the subjects discussed. *Pediatric Oncology* will serve pediatric oncologists, fellows, and residents both as a comprehensive source of information and as a quick reference. The series will also be of interest to pediatricians and general practitioners.

Shahab Asgharzadeh
Frank Westermann
Editors

Neuroblastoma

Discoveries and Challenges

Springer

Editors
Shahab Asgharzadeh
Department of Pediatrics
Children's Hospital Los Angeles
Los Angeles, CA, USA

Frank Westermann
Department of Neuroblastoma Genomics
German Cancer Research Center
Heidelberg, Baden-Württemberg, Germany

ISSN 1613-5318 ISSN 2191-0812 (electronic)
Pediatric Oncology
ISBN 978-3-031-51291-9 ISBN 978-3-031-51292-6 (eBook)
https://doi.org/10.1007/978-3-031-51292-6

This Springer imprint is published by the registered company Springer Nature Switzerland AG
The registered company address is: Gewerbestrasse 11, 6330 Cham, Switzerland

Foreword

Neuroblastoma is one of the most fascinating childhood tumors, due to its variable clinical presentation and unique behavior. Neuroblastomas generally have a more favorable behavior in infants less than 12–18 months old, even if they have metastatic disease, whereas even localized tumors in older patients can be fatal eventually, due in part to intrinsic or acquired drug resistance. A special pattern of metastatic disease in infants called 4S or MS can undergo spontaneous regression, and tumors in older patients can differentiate into a benign ganglioneuroma. Unfortunately, the majority of patients are older with unresectable or metastatic disease, and less than half of these patients can be cured despite aggressive, multimodality therapy. Furthermore, many long-term survivors develop significant toxicities, including deafness, growth retardation, cardiac disease, sterility, and second malignancies. Therefore, more effective and less toxic therapy is needed, especially for high-risk patients.

Genetic and genomic studies have provided considerable insight into identifying subsets of patients with distinct clinical behaviors, and an increasing number of genes have been found that are oncogenic drivers in these subsets. New models of neuroblastoma progression linked to telomere maintenance and cancer pathway mutations have been introduced and improved the existing risk classification systems (Chaps. 2, 4, and 6). Integration of different omics data layers helped to understand the interplay between the tumor genome, transcriptome, epigenome, and proteome (Chaps. 3, 5, and 6). More recently, gene regulatory network analysis and single-cell sequencing approaches have shed light on tumor heterogeneity and plasticity of neuroblastoma cell states (Chap. 5, 6, and 11) and the complex interaction with the tumor microenvironment and the immune system (Chaps. 8, 9, and 12). Molecular comparisons of neuroblastoma subtypes with the normal neural crest development improved our understanding of the cellular origin(s) of neuroblastoma (Chap. 7). Systematic clinical sequencing studies established the infrastructure for novel approaches to therapy with agents targeting specific genes, proteins, and pathways (Chap. 13). Finally, there is considerable interest in harnessing the immune system to selectively target neuroblastoma cells in individual patients. The purpose of this book is to bring all this information together to provide a current snapshot of recent advances in these and other areas, which in turn suggests targeted therapeutic approaches that can be tailored to individual patients.

Genetic predisposition to develop neuroblastoma is very uncommon, and only 1–2% of neuroblastoma patients have a family history of developing this tumor. Two potent predisposition genes have been identified (*ALK, PHOX2B*), but there is increasing evidence that additional genes also play a role. Tumors with amplification of the *MYCN* gene are found in 20–25% of patients with spontaneous neuroblastoma and identify a subset with aggressive clinical behavior and a poor outcome, although multimodality therapy and stem cell transplant have improved this. Older patients frequently have *ATRX* or other mutations affecting telomere formation or maintenance, and although more indolent, these patients also have a very poor outcome overall. Thus, genomic characterization of neuroblastomas at diagnosis has identified distinct subsets, and molecular analysis of tumors both at diagnosis and relapse can identify targets for novel therapeutics.

Although germline activating mutations in the *ALK* tyrosine kinase confer neuroblastoma predisposition, activation of ALK by mutation, duplication, amplification, or other mechanism is also found in 8–10% of high-risk tumors. ALK inhibitors like crizotinib, ceritinib, lorlatinib, or others have been used to treat recurrent neuroblastomas with ALK activation, and they are finding their way into frontline therapy for this patient subset. Activation of the RAS-RAF-MEK-ERK or PI3K-AKT-mTOR pathways can occur in neuroblastoma by a variety of mechanisms, and inhibitors of this pathway (e.g., selumetinib, trametinib, apatinib) are in clinical trials for recurrent/refractory tumors. Additional targeted agents tested in clinical trials are TRK inhibitors (entrectinib, larotrectinib), BCL-2 inhibitors (venetoclax), PARP inhibitors (bortezomib), Aurora kinase inhibitors (alisertib), and others. The downsides of these agents are that, in general, only a small subset of all patients is eligible for treatment, and resistance frequently develops rapidly. In addition, reliable predictive preclinical models allowing efficient translation into the sparse clinical trials are still rare.

Immunotherapy has been an important component of high-risk neuroblastoma treatment for the past 20 years. Monoclonal antibodies targeting the disialoganglioside GD2 (dinutuximab) have been used following stem cell transplant and have been shown to substantially improve long-term survival. With the advent of chimeric antigen receptor T-cell (CAR-T) therapy for B-cell malignancies, there is interest in developing CAR-T-cell therapy for neuroblastomas targeting GD2, the norepinephrine transporter (NET), CD171, or other targets selectively expressed on neuroblastoma cells. Another immunotherapeutic approach is to use checkpoint inhibitors (pembrolizumab, nivolumab, ipilimumab), which are particularly effective against tumors with a high mutational burden. Although most neuroblastomas have a low mutational burden, there is a definite subset for which these checkpoint inhibitors could be useful. Finally, the tumor microenvironment (TME) can prove to be a significant barrier to neuroblastoma therapeutics, especially for immunotherapy. Therefore, understanding the important immunosuppressive cells and factors in the TME and reversing their effects could be important.

Clearly this book is not intended to provide a comprehensive overview of every aspect of relevant neuroblastoma biology and therapy. Current clinical trials and the roles of conventional chemotherapy, radiation therapy, and surgery are not addressed. Also, targeted radiation therapy with radiolabeled meta-iodobenzylguanidine or other carriers are not discussed. Finally, the myriad of late effects of therapy covered by survivorship clinics is not discussed. However, these are areas that are not changing as rapidly, and so the focus areas of this book are on the newer and more dynamic aspects that affect neuroblastoma predisposition, genomic subclassification, single-cell sequencing approaches, therapeutic targets and targeted therapies, and novel immunotherapies. Recent improvements in long-term cure of high-risk neuroblastomas have been modest at best, so the challenge is the development of more effective, less toxic therapies. This is made possible by the identification of individual tumor vulnerabilities also considering emerging new aspects of tumor evolution, incorporation of targeted drugs and targeted drug delivery, and the rapid development of novel immunotherapy. Hopefully these approaches will lead to improved cure rates and fewer problems to address in long-term survivors.

Children's Hospital of Philadelphia
and the University of Pennsylvania,
Philadelphia, PA, USA
brodeur@chop.edu

Garrett M. Brodeur

Department of Pediatric Oncology & Hematology
Charité Universitätsmedizin Berlin,
Berlin, Germany
angelika.eggert@charite.de

Angelika Eggert

Contents

1 **Epidemiology, Presentation, and Evaluation** 1
Rochelle Bagatell and Margaret Macy

2 **Advanced Pathology Classification Toward Precision Stratification of Neuroblastic Tumors** 15
Hiroyuki Shimada and Naohiko Ikegaki

3 **Genetic Predisposition** 33
Apexa Modi, Emily Blauel, and Sharon J. Diskin

4 **Somatic Genomic Alterations in Neuroblastoma** 53
Pauline Depuydt, Gudrun Schleiermacher, and Katleen De Preter

5 **Neuroblastoma Epigenetic Landscape: Drugging Opportunities** 71
Veronica Veschi, Kaat Durinck, Carol J. Thiele, and Frank Speleman

6 **The Genetic Basis of the Divergent Clinical Courses in Neuroblastoma** 97
Carolina Rosswog and Matthias Fischer

7 **Developmental Programs in Neuroblastoma** 111
Selina Jansky and Frank Westermann

8 **Neuroblastoma Tumor Microenvironment: Innate and Adaptive Immunity** 123
Michael Zobel and Shahab Asgharzadeh

9 **Neuroblastoma Tumor Microenvironment: Non-Immune Cells and Exosomes** 143
Lucia Borriello, Laurence Blavier, and Yves A. DeClerck

10 **Metastatic Disease Burden** 155
Araz Marachelian and Meredith S. Irwin

11 **Therapeutically Actionable Genetic Aberrations** 167
Monica Pomaville and Rani E. George

12 **Re-Engaging the Immune System: Immunotherapy for Neuroblastoma** 181
Miho Nakajima and Nai-Kong V. Cheung

13 Future of Clinical Trials and Application of Precision Medicine 197
Theresa Thole and Angelika Eggert

14 Future Aspects of Neuroblastoma Research 217
Frank Westermann and Shahab Asgharzadeh

1 Epidemiology, Presentation, and Evaluation

Rochelle Bagatell and Margaret Macy

1.1 Epidemiology

Neuroblastoma is the most common extracranial solid tumor of childhood and the most common malignancy of infancy [1]. It comprises approximately 10% of all childhood cancers in children in the United States, with an incidence of 10.3 per million children <15 years of age [1]. Neuroblastoma most commonly presents in infancy; median age at diagnosis is approximately 19 months [2]. The incidence of neuroblastoma declines with age and 95% of patients are diagnosed before 10 years of age [3, 4]. Neuroblastoma in adolescents and adults appears to have different biologic and clinical features, following an indolent, but often fatal course [5].

The etiology of neuroblastoma has not yet been elucidated. Environmental exposures including parental occupations, prenatal exposures to drugs or alcohol, chemicals, and radiation exposure have not been consistently linked to the development of neuroblastoma, nor has causation been demonstrated [6–13]. Neuroblastoma has been reported in patients with genetic syndromes affecting the embryonic neural crest (including neurofibromatosis 1 and Hirschsprung's disease), consistent with the concept that neuroblastoma represents a disorder of neural crest development. Increased risk of neuroblastoma has also been reported in the neurochristopathy Congenital Central Hypoventilation Syndrome (CCHS) [14]. Mutations in PHOX2B, a regulator of neural crest development 15], are found in CCHS[16] and have also been reported in familial and sporadic neuroblastoma [16, 17]. Functional differences among mutations in *PHOX2B* may underlie the association between CCHS and neuroblastoma and may provide insights into the genesis of neuroblastoma [18].

1.2 Clinical Presentation

Neuroblastoma most commonly arises in the adrenal gland or along the sympathetic chain. The majority of primary tumors are found in the abdomen. Most occur in the adrenal gland but may also arise in paravertebral ganglia or the organ of Zuckerkandl [19, 20]. Bilateral adrenal tumors are rare, occurring in 2% of patients [21]. Thoracic or cervical primary tumors are more frequently observed in infants than in older children [20]. There are also a small number of

R. Bagatell (✉)
The Children's Hospital of Philadelphia and Perelman School of Medicine, University of Pennsylvania, Philadelphia, PA, USA
e-mail: bagatellr@chop.edu

M. Macy
Children's Hospital Colorado and University of Colorado School of Medicine, Aurora, CO, USA
e-mail: margaret.macy@childrenscolorado.org

S. Asgharzadeh, F. Westermann (eds.), *Neuroblastoma*, Pediatric Oncology,
https://doi.org/10.1007/978-3-031-51292-6_1

patients with metastatic disease in whom a primary tumor cannot be identified.

Patients with localized neuroblastoma may present with an incidental finding of an asymptomatic mass. However, patients usually present with signs and symptoms associated with the location of the primary tumor or metastatic disease. Large primary abdominal tumors may cause distention, pain, constipation, urinary obstruction, hypertension, or renal injury. Compression of large veins in the abdomen can result in venous prominence over the abdomen or lower extremity edema. Liver involvement can lead to respiratory compromise. When metastatic disease in the liver is extensive, coagulopathy may be observed. Tumors in the neck or chest can present with respiratory compromise or distress due to compression of the trachea or bronchi. Superior vena cava syndrome, thoracic outlet obstruction, or Horner's syndrome (ptosis, miosis, anhydrosis) may also be observed in patients with disease in the upper chest and neck. Paravertebral tumors arising from the sympathetic ganglia can invade neural foraminae and impinge on the spinal cord and nerve roots, causing symptoms of spinal cord or nerve root compression.

Constitutional symptoms such as fever, weight loss, failure to thrive, and irritability are usually seen in the metastatic setting and are often nonspecific. The most common sites of metastatic disease in neuroblastoma are bone marrow, cortical bone, liver, and skin. Neuroblastoma has a predilection to metastasize to the bones of the skull and orbits, resulting in proptosis and/or periorbital ecchymosis. External compression of the brain from bony lesions in the calvarium or impingement of the spinal cord or nerve roots due to nearby bony lesions can also be seen. Long bone involvement with tumor can be extensive. These bony lesions as well as bone marrow infiltration can result in marked irritability, limping, and bone pain. Extensive bone marrow involvement can result in clinically significant cytopenias. Lesions in the lung and brain parenchyma are rare at initial presentation of neuroblastoma. Skin metastases (subcutaneous, non-tender, purple, or bluish nodules) are almost exclusively observed in infants with a unique clinical phenotype known as MS disease (previously known as 4S disease). This unique presentation in infants <18 months of age specifically refers to metastatic disease limited to the liver and skin, with only a small amount of bone marrow disease (less than 10%) and no cortical bony involvement.

Specific paraneoplastic syndromes can be associated with neuroblastoma. Opsoclonus myoclonus ataxia syndrome (OMA) occurs in 2–3% of patients with neuroblastoma and is characterized by uncontrolled eye movements, abnormal muscle movements, and ataxia [22, 23]. This disorder is associated with the presence of antineuronal antibodies [24]. While patients with OMA often have tumors with favorable histologic and biologic features [23, 25], they may have long-term neurological and developmental deficits [26–30]. Patients with neuroblastoma can also develop vasoactive intestinal peptide (VIP) syndrome, characterized by abdominal distention, intractable profuse watery diarrhea with associated dehydration and electrolyte abnormalities due to excessive secretion of VIP from the tumor itself [31–33]. Symptoms often improve with resection of the primary tumor. These patients often have low stage tumors with favorable biology [34]. Rarely, patients with neuroblastoma can have symptoms consistent with excessive catecholamine secretion, however this is more common in other sympathetic nervous system tumors, such as pheochromocytoma. Symptoms may include hypertension, tachycardia, irregular heart rate, flushing, and profuse sweating [35, 36].

1.3 Diagnosis and Evaluation

The diagnosis of neuroblastoma is made following a biopsy of the primary tumor or a readily accessible metastatic site. Occasionally, the diagnosis can be made based on detection of neuroblastoma cells in the bone marrow associated with elevated urine catecholamines. However, because molecular diagnostics are important in risk assessment and because bone marrow may not provide sufficient tumor material for all nec-

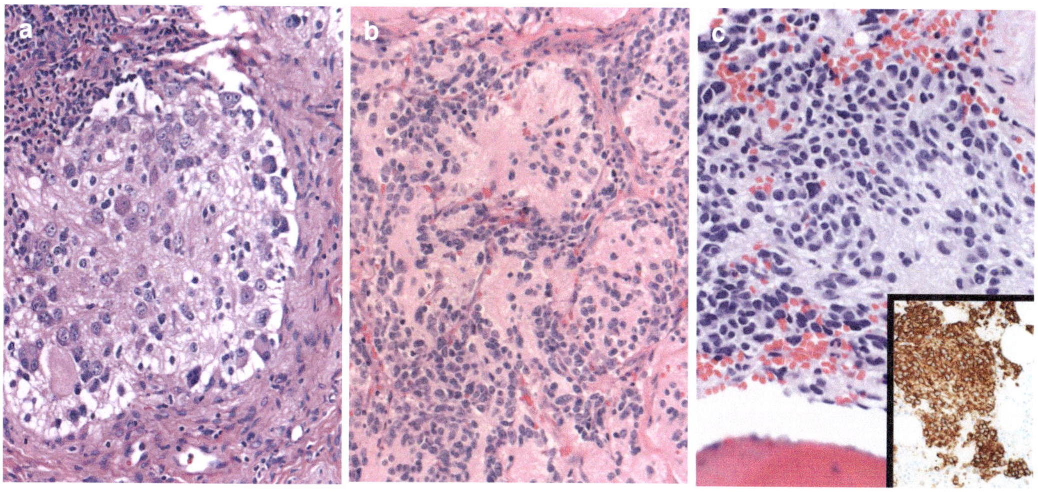

Fig. 1.1 (**a**) Hematoxylin and eosin staining (20× magnification) of a ganglioneuroblastoma, intermixed subtype. The tumor is composed of >50% mature Schwannian stroma with scattered microscopic foci of neuroblastic cells in association with neuropil. (**b**) Hematoxylin and eosin staining (20× magnification) of a neuroblastoma (Schwannian stroma-poor), poorly-differentiated subtype. Nests of primitive-appearing neuroblasts are set in fibrillary neuropil. (**c**) Bone marrow biopsy (40× magnification) showing extensive infiltration with neuroblastoma cells. Inset shows neuron-specific enolase (NSE) staining) of the neuroblastoma population. Images courtesy of Dr. Tricia Bhatti (Department of Pathology, The Children's Hospital of Philadelphia) and Dr. Xiayuan Liang (Department of Pathology, Children's Hospital Colorado)

essary studies, biopsy of an accessible soft tissue site is strongly encouraged. Neuroblastoma is classified histologically as a peripheral neuroblastic tumor. The benign counterpart of neuroblastoma, ganglioneuroma, is composed of cells that show maturation, with neuronal differentiation to ganglion cells. In contrast, neuroblastoma is predominantly composed of immature small round cells with limited or no evidence of differentiation. Ganglioneuroblastoma is a mixture of these components, containing both immature cells and cells with neuronal differentiation (Fig. 1.1). The International Neuroblastoma Pathology Committee (INPC) has provided a detailed framework for classification of neuroblastic tumors based upon the extent of Schwannian development (stroma poor, stroma rich, stroma dominant), degree of differentiation (differentiating, poorly differentiated, undifferentiated), and an index of mitosis and karyorrhexis (MKI) [37]. The presence or absence of macroscopically visible nodules and the appearance of the tumor cells within the nodules is also evaluated [38].

Imaging studies in newly diagnosed patients should facilitate anatomic definition of the primary site and assessment of metastatic disease. Computerized tomography (CT) or magnetic resonance imaging (MRI) scans should be performed to evaluate the primary site and the extent of loco-regional disease, with specific attention paid to effects of the tumor on normal structures (Fig. 1.2a). Ultrasound is often used for follow-up of abdominal disease in low risk patients but does not provide adequate anatomic detail for risk assessment at the time of diagnosis. MRI should be used to assess paraspinal tumors, as it is superior for assessment of extension into neural foraminae as well as spinal cord or nerve root compression.

To evaluate the primary tumor and metastatic bone and soft tissue disease, ^{123}I-Metaiodobenzylguanidine scintigraphy (MIBG) scans are used. Approximately 90% of neuroblastomas selectively take up MIBG, a norepinephrine analog. Two scoring methods (Curie and SIOPEN) are widely used to evaluate disease burden using MIBG scans [39, 40]. These scoring systems

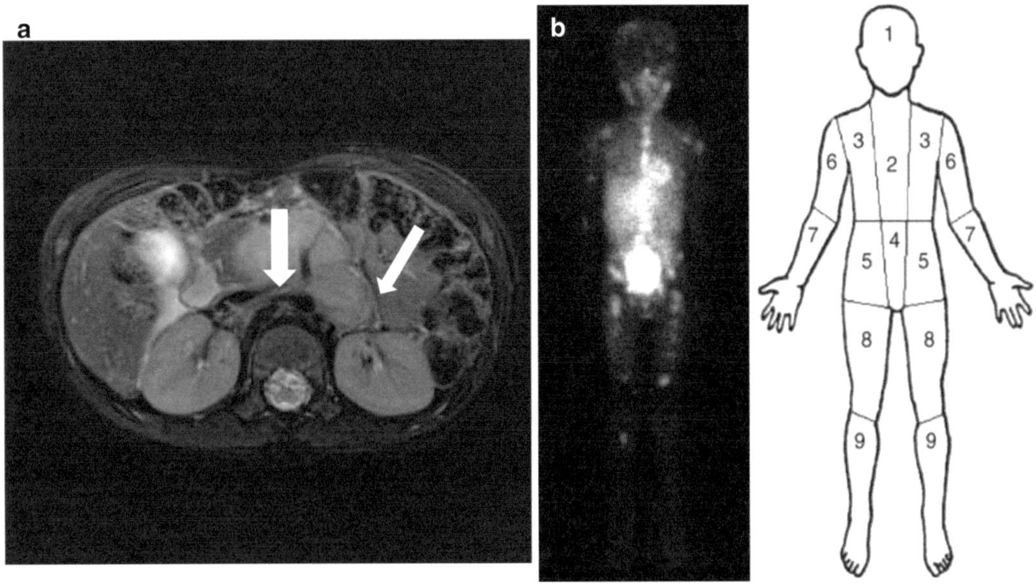

Fig. 1.2 (**a**) Axial image of an abdominal primary tumor with multiple imaging defined risk factors, including encasement of the inferior vena cava, aorta, left renal artery, right renal vein. (**b**) Left panel: MIBG scan in a patient with widespread osteomedullary disease involving the skull, shoulders, spine, pelvis, and long bones of all extremities; overall Curie score for this scan is 23. Right panel: regions for scoring used in the Curie system. Images courtesy of Dr. Lisa States (Department of Radiology, The Children's Hospital of Philadelphia). *Diagram of Curie score regions was originally published in *JNM*. Yanik GA, Parisi MT, Shulkin BL, Naranjo A, Kreissman SG, London WB, Villablanca JG, Maris JM, Park JR, Cohn SL, McGrady P, Matthay KK. Semiquantitative mIBG scoring as a prognostic indicator in patients with stage 4 neuroblastoma: a report from the Children's Oncology Group. *J Nucl Med.* 2013; 54(4):541-8. © by the Society of Nuclear Medicine and Molecular Imaging, Inc

divide the skeleton into 9 (Curie) or 12 regions (SIOPEN) (Fig. 1.2b), with Curie scoring adding one region for soft tissue disease. Scores from each region (0–3) are summed to determine a cumulative score, which can be tracked throughout therapy. Relative MIBG scores (absolute score divided by the corresponding baseline/pretreatment score) are also used in response assessment. For neuroblastomas that are MIBG-non-avid, fluorodeoxyglucose positron emission tomography (FDG-PET) scan can be used for staging. Historically, ^{99}mTc-diphosphonate scintigraphy (^{99}Tc bone scan) was used to detect bony metastases, however MIBG and PET scans have replaced bone scans as standard of care [41]. Bone marrow disease should be assessed with bilateral bone marrow aspirates and trephine biopsies. Samples should be evaluated via both hematoxylin and eosin staining and immunohistochemistry (Fig. 1.1) [42].

Metabolites of catecholamines secreted by neuroblastomas can be detected in urine in approximately 90% of patients with neuroblastoma [43]. DOPA, dopamine, norepinephrine, and epinephrine produced by tumor cells are converted by catechol-O-methyl transferase and monamine oxidase to the metabolites homovanillic acid (HVA) and vanillylmandelic acid (VMA), respectively. HVA and VMA levels must be normalized for age and urine creatinine concentration and may aid in the diagnosis of neuroblastoma. Although changes in levels of HVA and VMA were previously included in the International Neuroblastoma Response Criteria (INRC) [44], assessment of these metabolites is no longer included in response assessment [45].

1.4 Risk Assessment

Treatment for children with neuroblastoma is determined based on risk for disease recurrence, as assessed by evaluation of clinical and tumor biologic factors. Risk stratification systems have evolved as our understanding of neuroblastoma biology has expanded and as prognostic risk factors have been critically evaluated. To create a uniform, international pre-treatment classification algorithm, the International Neuroblastoma Risk Group (INRG) Task Force analyzed data regarding 36 prognostic factors in more than 8800 patients [46]. The factors found to be most important for risk assignment included clinical features (age at diagnosis and disease stage) and tumor-related factors (histology, *MYCN* amplification status, segmental chromosomal aberration status, and DNA content) [46].

1.4.1 Stage

Several different staging systems have been used to describe extent of disease in children with neuroblastoma. In 2009, the International Risk Group Staging System was adopted worldwide [47]. Localized tumors are classified based on whether the tumor involves vital structures, as indicated by the presence of image-defined risk factors (IDRFs; Table 1.1) [47]. Examples of IDRFs include encasement of major vascular

Table 1.1 Image-defined risk factors

Cervical	Carotid and/or vertebral artery and/or internal jugular vein	Encasement[a]
Cervical	Base of skull	Extension of tumor to site
Cervical	Trachea	Encasement or compression[b]
Cervico-thoracic	Brachial plexus roots	Encasement
Cervico-thoracic	Subclavian and/or vertebral and/or carotid artery	Encasement
Cervico-thoracic	Trachea	Encasement or compression
Thoracic	Aorta and/or major branches	Encasement
Thoracic	Trachea and/or principal bronchi	Encasement or compression
Thoraco-abdominal	Aorta and/or vena cava	Encasement
Abdominal and/or pelvic	Porta hepatis and/or hepatoduodenal ligament	Infiltration[c]
Abdominal and/or pelvic	Branches of the superior mesenteric artery at mesenteric root	Encasement
Abdominal and/or pelvic	Origin of celiac axis and/or superior or inferior mesenteric artery	Encasement
Abdominal and/or pelvic	One or both renal pedicles	Infiltration or encasement
Abdominal and/or pelvic	Aorta and/or vena cava	Encasement
Abdominal and/or pelvic	Iliac vessels	Encasement
Pelvic	Sciatic notch	Extension of tumor through site
Any	Neural foramina	Extension of tumor through site with symptoms of cord compression or abnormal spinal cord signal
Any	Neural foramina	Extension of tumor through site with tumor invading >1/3 of spinal canal in axial plane
Any	Adjacent organs including pericardium, diaphragm, kidney, liver, duodeno-pancreatic block, mesentery, etc.	Infiltration
Any	Contiguous ipsilateral extension across multiple body compartments (e.g., neck and chest, chest and abdomen)	

[a] Encasement: tumor surrounds a structure with >50% circumferential contact or a vein is completely flattened by tumor with no visible lumen

[b] Compression: refers only to airways and requires a narrowing due to tumor effects (deviation without compression is not an IDRF)

[c] Infiltration: Tumor extends into or deviates a vital structure and the margin between tumor and structure on imaging is absent or ill-defined

structures (Fig. 1.2a), infiltration/invasion of adjacent organs, or extensive involvement of the spinal canal [47, 48]. Patients with localized tumors confined to one body compartment and not associated with an IDRF are considered to have L1 disease, while those with tumors that have one or more IDRFs are designated as having L2 neuroblastoma. Patients with tumors that extend ipsilaterally into another body compartment may still be considered to have L1 disease, provided that no additional IDRF is seen. In contrast to older staging systems, extent of resection and the relationship of tumor to midline are not used in the INRG system. Patients with metastatic disease are categorized as having Stage M or MS disease. The latter includes children <18 months of age at diagnosis who have metastases confined to liver, skin, and bone marrow (with <10% of nucleated cells in the marrow being tumor cells). In MS patients with MIBG-avid primary tumors, there can be no MIBG uptake suggestive of osteomedullary disease. Despite presenting with metastatic disease, patients with MS neuroblastoma and favorable biologic features have a good prognosis and often require minimal therapy. Patients with metastatic disease not included in the definition of MS disease are considered to have Stage M neuroblastoma.

1.4.2 Age

The relationship between age at diagnosis and clinical outcome was described in 1971 [49], and is thought to reflect aspects of tumor biology that are still not well understood. Age is a continuous variable [2], with younger age associated with a more favorable outcome in child. Based upon practical considerations, however, an age cutoff of 18 months (547 days) has been adopted for use in risk classification [46]. While much is known about the mutational landscape of neuroblastoma [50, 51], genomic markers alone do not fully explain the relationship between age and outcome. Mutations in the SWI/SNF chromatin remodeling ATP-dependent helicase *ATRX* were detected in tumors from >40% of patients >14 years of age in one study [52], but tumors from a substantial portion of older patients do not harbor *ATRX* aberrations. Biomarkers that may further explain the correlation between age and outcome are being evaluated [53, 54].

1.4.3 Tumor Histology

INPC criteria are currently used to categorize neuroblastic tumors based upon features detected by routine microscopy [37, 38]. In addition, the INPC system takes the age of the patient into account as tumors are designated as favorable or unfavorable [38]. Tumors classified as ganglioneuroma and ganglioneuroblastoma intermixed are designated as favorable histology subtypes, as are differentiating and poorly differentiating neuroblastomas with low MKI in young children. Undifferentiated neuroblastomas are considered to have unfavorable histology regardless of age or MKI, as are poorly differentiated tumors in patients >18 months of age and poorly differentiated tumors with an MKI >4% in patients of any age [38]. While the INPC approach remains widely used in clinical practice, the INRG classification system incorporates tumor differentiation and histologic category (ganglioneuroma, ganglioneuroblastoma, neuroblastoma) in risk stratification rather than the overall INPC categories (favorable/unfavorable). Further analyses of outcome based on the components of tumor histology are in progress, and future risk assessment systems may make use of select variables rather than all of those historically used in histologic classification.

1.4.4 *MYCN* Amplification Status

The relationship between *MYCN* copy number status and prognosis in children with neuroblastoma was described more than 30 years ago [55, 56], and *MYCN* remains a powerful independent prognostic marker in this disease. *MYCN* amplification occurs in approximately 16% of neuroblastoma tumors overall but is more common among patients with metastatic disease and those with other unfavorable genomic features [57].

MYCN status is particularly important for risk assessment in patients who would not necessarily be considered to be at high risk for recurrence based only on age and stage. For example, young infants with MS neuroblastoma whose tumors are found to be *MYCN* amplified would generally be considered to have high-risk disease and would be treated with multi-modality therapy, while those whose tumors do not have *MYCN* amplification may be candidates for observation alone. *MYCN* amplification status has historically been determined based on the results of interphase fluorescence in situ hybridization (FISH) testing [58]. Using this method, *MYCN* amplification is defined as greater than fourfold increase in *MYCN* signal compared to a chromosome 2 reference probe [59]. As next generation sequencing becomes more widely used for genomic profiling at diagnosis, it may be more routinely used to determine *MYCN* status. Careful attention to the percentage of neuroblastoma cells and the heterogeneity within the tumor specimen will be required for accurate determination of *MYCN* copy number using this approach.

1.4.5 Segmental Chromosomal Aberration Status

While numerical chromosomal abnormalities (whole chromosome gains and losses) are associated with a favorable prognosis in children with neuroblastoma, gains, and losses of portions of chromosomes (referred to as segmental chromosomal aberrations or SCAs) are associated with unfavorable outcomes [60]. Alterations in chromosomes 1p, 11q, and 17q were the first to be linked with poor prognosis in children with neuroblastoma [61–64], however segmental alterations in several other chromosomes have been linked to lower survival [60]. The presence of any SCA has been associated with an increased risk of relapse [60], and the accumulation of SCAs reflects genomic instability and is associated with a very poor outcome [65]. The presence of any SCA appears be particularly important for risk assessment in patients with localized or MS disease whose tumors are *MYCN* non-amplified [66]. Although earlier studies focused on individual chromosome loci, the need to assess the genome as a whole has led to the use of multilocus genomic approaches. Array-based comparative genomic hybridization and multiplex ligation probe amplification have been successfully used to assess SCA status in the context of a large, multi-center trial in Europe [67], and an array-based method is being used in a current North American study. Next-generation genomic techniques are currently being adopted by various international groups.

1.4.6 DNA Content/Ploidy

The ploidy (DNA index) of neuroblastoma primary tumors has become a significant predictor of patient outcome and is a main component of the current INRG classification system [16]. Diploid tumors (DNA index 51) occur in approximately 33% of patients, whereas 66% of neuroblastoma tumors are hyperdiploid (DNA index >1) [15]. Tumor ploidy is one of the most significant prognostic markers for children younger than 18 months, and infants with hyperdiploid tumors have significantly increased survival. Tumor DNA content was identified as a predictor of response to chemotherapy in children with neuroblastoma in 1984, [68] and found to have prognostic significance in the 1990s [69]. Ploidy can be readily assessed using flow cytometry, and there is a general consensus that a DNA index >1.0 should be considered hyperdiploidy, while a DNA index of 1.0 represents diploidy [59]. While tumor cell ploidy does not have independent prognostic value in patients >18 months of age and in those with *MYCN* amplified tumors, ploidy does have significant prognostic utility in young infants with tumors that have otherwise favorable features, including those with metastatic disease [46]. Ploidy was also found to be a significant prognostic variable in a multi-center study of reduced therapy for patients with intermediate risk disease [70] and remains in use in current risk stratification systems. Further study of the prognostic significance of ploidy in rare subsets of patients (such as 12–18-month old toddlers with metastatic disease [71] and children with low stage, *MYCN* amplified disease [72]) treated with current-era therapy is needed, particularly since SCA status is now being incorporated into risk assessment. The prognostic variables discussed above have been integrated into comprehensive risk assessment systems. The INRG approach to pretreatment risk stratification has been used for nearly a decade (Table 1.2) [46]. However, as more data become available regarding the prognostic factors included in this system and as approaches to treatment evolve, risk stratification systems will also evolve. It is expected that as new biomarkers are validated and more advanced techniques for whole genome analysis become standardized and widely adopted, they will be incorporated into revised risk assessment tools.

Table 1.2 International neuroblastoma risk group pretreatment risk classification schema

INRG stage	Age	Histologic category	Grade of tumor differentiation	MYCN	11q aberration	Ploidy	Pre-treatment risk group
L1/L2		GN maturing; GNB intermixed					Very low
L1		Any, except GN maturing or GNB intermixed		NA			Very low
				Amp			High
L2	<18	Any, except GN maturing or GNB intermixed		NA	No		Low
					Yes		Intermediate
	≥18	GNB nodular; neuroblastoma	Differentiating	NA	No		Low
					Yes		Intermediate
			Poorly differentiated	NA			
				Amp			High
M	<18			NA		Hyperdiploid	Low
	<12			NA		Diploid	Intermediate
	12 to <18			NA		Diploid	Intermediate
	<18			Amp			High
	≥18						High
MS	<18			NA	No		Low
					Yes		High
				Amp			High

GN ganglioneuroma, *GNB* ganglioneuroblastoma, *Amp* amplified, *NA* not amplified, *L1* localized tumor confined to one body compartment and with absence of image-defined risk factors (IDRFs), *L2* locoregional tumor with presence of one or more IDRFs, *M* distant metastatic disease (except stage MS), *MS* metastatic disease confined to skin, liver and/or bone marrow in children <18 months of age

Modified and reproduced with permission from *The Journal of Clinical Onco*logy. Originally published by Cohn et al, 27 (2): 289–297, 2009

1.5 Response Evaluation

In 2017, revisions to the International Neuroblastoma Response Criteria (INRC) were adopted worldwide [45]. These response criteria eliminate the use of less sensitive and specific methods for disease assessment (including ^{99}Tc bone scans and urinary catecholamines) and include the use of current technology for quantitation of marrow disease and tumor imaging. The INRC provides guidance regarding the assessment of components of response, including primary site, metastatic bone and soft tissue disease, and bone marrow, as well as integration of findings into an overall response designation.

The primary site is defined as a measurable lesion ≥10 mm in diameter as assessed by cross sectional imaging (CT or MRI scan). Serial primary tumor assessments are made by measuring the single longest diameter in the same orthogonal plane. A primary site complete response (CR) is defined as <10 mm residual soft tissue, with complete resolution of uptake on the appropriate functional imaging study. A partial response (PR) is defined as a ≥30% decrease in longest diameter, similar to the definition used in RECIST [73]. Likewise, the definition of progressive disease (PD) mirrors RECIST, as a >20% increase in longest diameter is considered progression [73], provided there is a minimum absolute increase of 5 mm in longest dimension. Primary site stable disease (SD) is defined as insufficient shrinkage to qualify as PR and insufficient progression to qualify as PD. While assessment of volume was required in previous iterations of the INRC, the use of serial 3-dimensional measurements did not improve the ability of primary site assessment to predict overall outcome in high-risk patients [74]. Therefore, the revised INRC require measurement in only a single dimension. In patients with bilateral adrenal tumors, response is based on the sum of the longest dimensions of both lesions, provided that both have been histologically proven to be neuroblastoma. In patients with multi-focal non-adrenal masses, the largest tumor is considered the primary tumor [45].

Response in metastatic bone and soft tissue disease is assessed using anatomic (CT/MRI) and functional (^{123}I-MIBG and FDG-PET) imaging. Measurable metastatic lymph nodes ≥15 mm in short axis are followed per Response Evaluation Criteria In Solid Tumors (RECIST) [73]. However, if the short axis of a discreet node cannot be identified, a nodal conglomerate can be measured using the longest diameter of the composite lesion [45]. The status of metastatic soft tissue and bony disease is followed using ^{123}I-MIBG scans in patients with MIBG-avid disease. In patients with MIBG non-avid disease, FDG-PET is used. A CR in metastatic sites is defined as a decrease in size of soft tissue lesions as per RECIST guidelines, as well as resolution of abnormal tracer uptake. A PR is defined as ≥30% decrease in sum of diameters of measurable lesions without new lesions or growth in small, non-measurable lesions. In addition, a ≥50% reduction in MIBG absolute bone score (relative MIBG bone score ≥0.1 to ≤0.5) or ≥50% reduction in number of FDG-PET avid bone lesions is required [45]. PD is defined as the presence of a new bone or soft tissue lesion that is tracer-avid or histologically proven to be tumor, a relative MIBG score ≥1.2, or a >20% increase in the sum of longest diameters of soft tissue lesions, provided the absolute increase in this sum is ≥5 mm. If neither the definition of PR nor SD is met, a patient is considered to have SD at metastatic soft tissue and bone sites.

Revisions to the INRC bone marrow criteria have focused on increasing accuracy and reproducibility of testing. Bilateral marrow aspirates and biopsies are required due to the patchy nature of marrow disease in patients with neuroblastoma. Whereas bone marrow involvement was previously assessed using only morphological evaluation of marrow specimens, immunohistochemical staining of bone marrow biopsy samples is now recommended to permit more accurate estimation of the percentage of tumor involvement. The number of tumor cells detected is divided by the number of mononuclear cells seen; the highest percentage is used for response determination [42]. A CR is defined as complete resolution of marrow disease, while PD is defined as marrow previously without tumor that contains >5% tumor upon reassessment, or bone marrow infiltration that increases by greater than twofold and has ≥20% tumor involvement upon repeat evaluation. A new minimal disease (MD) category was added due to concerns regarding the sampling issues inherent in marrow assessment in neuroblastoma. Patients with MD are those with no detectable marrow disease or ≤5% tumor involvement at baseline who continue to have detectable tumor cells in the marrow but have ≤5% tumor upon reassessment. Also included are those with more extensive tumor involvement at baseline who upon reassessment continue to have tumor cells that comprise ≤5% of the mononuclear cell population. Patients with >5% marrow involvement on initial evaluation who continue to have tumor infiltration will be considered to have SD in the marrow if requirements for PD and MD are not met. The use of highly sensitive methods of detection and quantification of marrow disease (such as reverse transcriptase quantitative polymerase chain reaction; RTqPCR) has not been incorporated into the revised INRC to date, however these methods are likely be included in future revisions.

Accurate designation of overall response requires that all components be evaluated. A CR in all components is required for an overall response of CR. PD in any component results in an overall response of PD. PR is designated when there is a PR in at least one component, with other components in CR, PR (soft tissue or bone) or MD (bone marrow). A minor response (MR) has been achieved when there is CR or PR in at least one component but SD in others.

Newer imaging modalities and laboratory techniques will undoubtedly emerge within the next several years, and it will be important to consider modifying the INRC as the clinical utility of these techniques becomes clear. Fortunately, the framework for international consensus around response assessment is in place, and there is resounding agreement regarding the need for uniformity in disease evaluation and response assessment around the world.

References

1. Howlader N, Noone A, Krapcho M, et al. SEER cancer statistics review, 1975-2014. Bethesda: National Cancer Institute; 2017.
2. London WB, Castleberry RP, Matthay KK, et al. Evidence for an age cutoff greater than 365 days for neuroblastoma risk group stratification in the Children's Oncology Group. J Clin Oncol. 2005;23(27):6459–65.
3. Esiashvili N, Goodman M, Ward K, Marcus RB Jr, Johnstone PA. Neuroblastoma in adults: incidence and survival analysis based on SEER data. Pediatr Blood Cancer. 2007;49(1):41–6.
4. Brodeur G, Hogarty MD, Bagatell R, Mosse YP, Maris JM. Neuroblastoma. In: Pizzo PA, Poplack DG, editors. Principles and practice of pediatric oncology. 7th ed. Alphen aan den Rijn: Wolters Kluwer; 2015. p. 772–97.
5. Mosse YP, Deyell RJ, Berthold F, et al. Neuroblastoma in older children, adolescents and young adults: a report from the International Neuroblastoma Risk Group project. Pediatr Blood Cancer. 2014;61(4):627–35.
6. Bluhm EC, Daniels J, Pollock BH, Olshan AF, Children's Oncology Group. Maternal use of recreational drugs and neuroblastoma in offspring: a report from the Children's Oncology Group (United States). Cancer Causes Control. 2006;17(5):663–9.
7. Chow EJ, Friedman DL, Mueller BA. Maternal and perinatal characteristics in relation to neuroblastoma. Cancer. 2007;109(5):983–92.
8. Cook MN, Olshan AF, Guess HA, et al. Maternal medication use and neuroblastoma in offspring. Am J Epidemiol. 2004;159(8):721–31.
9. De Roos AJ, Teschke K, Savitz DA, et al. Parental occupational exposures to electromagnetic fields and radiation and the incidence of neuroblastoma in offspring. Epidemiology. 2001;12(5):508–17.
10. Heck JE, Ritz B, Hung RJ, Hashibe M, Boffetta P. The epidemiology of neuroblastoma: a review. Paediatr Perinat Epidemiol. 2009;23(2):125–43.
11. McCall EE, Olshan AF, Daniels JL. Maternal hair dye use and risk of neuroblastoma in offspring. Cancer Causes Control. 2005;16(6):743–8.
12. Olshan AF, De Roos AJ, Teschke K, et al. Neuroblastoma and parental occupation. Cancer Causes Control. 1999;10(6):539–49.
13. Olshan AF, Smith J, Cook MN, et al. Hormone and fertility drug use and the risk of neuroblastoma: a report from the Children's Cancer Group and the Pediatric Oncology Group. Am J Epidemiol. 1999;150(9):930–8.
14. Trochet D, O'Brien LM, Gozal D, et al. PHOX2B genotype allows for prediction of tumor risk in congenital central hypoventilation syndrome. Am J Hum Genet. 2005;76(3):421–6.

15. Pattyn A, Morin X, Cremer H, Goridis C, Brunet JF. The homeobox gene Phox2b is essential for the development of autonomic neural crest derivatives. Nature. 1999;399(6734):366–70.
16. Trochet D, Bourdeaut F, Janoueix-Lerosey I, et al. Germline mutations of the paired-like homeobox 2B (PHOX2B) gene in neuroblastoma. Am J Hum Genet. 2004;74(4):761–4.
17. van Limpt V, Schramm A, van Lakeman A, et al. The Phox2B homeobox gene is mutated in sporadic neuroblastomas. Oncogene. 2004;23(57):9280–8.
18. Di Lascio S, Benfante R, Di Zanni E, et al. Structural and functional differences in phox2b frameshift mutations underlie isolated or syndromic congenital central hypoventilation syndrome. Hum Mutat. 2017;39(2):219–36.
19. Berdon WE, Stylianos S, Ruzal-Shapiro C, Hoffer F, Cohen M. Neuroblastoma arising from the organ of Zuckerkandl. an unusual site with a favorable biologic outcome. Pediatr Radiol. 1999;29(7):497–502.
20. Vo KT, Matthay KK, Neuhaus J, et al. Clinical, biologic, and prognostic differences on the basis of primary tumor site in neuroblastoma: a report from the international neuroblastoma risk group project. J Clin Oncol. 2014;32(28):3169–76.
21. Dinh T, Truong B, Matthay KK, DuBois SG. Comparison of clinical features and outcomes in patients with bilateral versus unilateral adrenal neuroblastoma. J Pediatr Hematol Oncol. 2017;39(2):108–13.
22. Pranzatelli MR. The neurobiology of the opsoclonus-myoclonus syndrome. Clin Neuropharmacol. 1992;15(3):186–228.
23. Rudnick E, Khakoo Y, Antunes NL, et al. Opsoclonus-myoclonus-ataxia syndrome in neuroblastoma: clinical outcome and antineuronal antibodies-a report from the Children's Cancer Group Study. Med Pediatr Oncol. 2001;36(6):612–22.
24. Antunes NL, Khakoo Y, Matthay KK, et al. Antineuronal antibodies in patients with neuroblastoma and paraneoplastic opsoclonus-myoclonus. J Pediatr Hematol Oncol. 2000;22(4):315–20.
25. Mitchell WG, Davalos-Gonzalez Y, Brumm VL, et al. Opsoclonus-ataxia caused by childhood neuroblastoma: developmental and neurologic sequelae. Pediatrics. 2002;109(1):86–98.
26. Altman AJ, Baehner RL. Favorable prognosis for survival in children with coincident opso-myoclonus and neuroblastoma. Cancer. 1976;37(2):846–52.
27. Cooper R, Khakoo Y, Matthay KK, et al. Opsoclonus-myoclonus-ataxia syndrome in neuroblastoma: histopathologic features-a report from the Children's Cancer Group. Med Pediatr Oncol. 2001;36(6):623–9.
28. Hayward K, Jeremy RJ, Jenkins S, et al. Long-term neurobehavioral outcomes in children with neuroblastoma and opsoclonus-myoclonus-ataxia syndrome: relationship to MRI findings and anti-neuronal antibodies. J Pediatr. 2001;139(4):552–9.
29. De Grandis E, Parodi S, Conte M, et al. Long-term follow-up of neuroblastoma-associated opsoclonus-myoclonus-ataxia syndrome. Neuropediatrics. 2009;40(3):103–11.
30. De Alarcon P, Matthay KK, London WB, et al. Intravenous immunoglobulin with prednisone and risk-adapted chemotherapy for children with opsoclonus myoclonus ataxia syndrome associated with neuroblastoma (ANBL00P3): a randomised, open-label, phase 3 trial. Lancet Child Adolesc Health. 2018;2(1):25–34.
31. Cooney DR, Voorhess ML, Fisher JE, Brecher M, Karp MP, Jewett TC. Vasoactive intestinal peptide producing neuroblastoma. J Pediatr Surg. 1982;17(6):821–5.
32. El Shafie M, Samuel D, Klippel CH, Robinson MG, Cullen BJ. Intractable diarrhea in children with VIP-secreting ganglioneuroblastomas. J Pediatr Surg. 1983;18(1):34–6.
33. Scheibel E, Rechnitzer C, Fahrenkrug J, Hertz H. Vasoactive intestinal polypeptide (VIP) in children with neural crest tumours. Acta Paediatr Scand. 1982;71(5):721–5.
34. Qualman SJ, O'Dorisio MS, Fleshman DJ, Shimada H, O'Dorisio TM. Neuroblastoma. Correlation of neuropeptide expression in tumor tissue with other prognostic factors. Cancer. 1992;70(7):2005–12.
35. Wolff JE, Bauch HJ, Roessner A, et al. Development of hypertension in neuroblastoma during therapy: a case report. Med Pediatr Oncol. 1993;21(6):460–4.
36. Seefelder C, Sparks JW, Chirnomas D, Diller L, Shamberger RC. Perioperative management of a child with severe hypertension from a catecholamine secreting neuroblastoma. Paediatr Anaesth. 2005;15(7):606–10.
37. Shimada H, Umehara S, Monobe Y, et al. International neuroblastoma pathology classification for prognostic evaluation of patients with peripheral neuroblastic tumors: a report from the Children's Cancer Group. Cancer. 2001;92(9):2451–61.
38. Peuchmaur M, d'Amore ES, Joshi VV, et al. Revision of the International Neuroblastoma Pathology Classification: confirmation of favorable and unfavorable prognostic subsets in ganglioneuroblastoma, nodular. Cancer. 2003;98(10):2274–81.
39. Matthay KK, Edeline V, Lumbroso J, et al. Correlation of early metastatic response by 123I-metaiodobenzylguanidine scintigraphy with overall response and event-free survival in stage IV neuroblastoma. J Clin Oncol. 2003;21(13):2486–91.
40. Lewington V, Lambert B, Poetschger U, et al. (123) I-mIBG scintigraphy in neuroblastoma: development of a SIOPEN semi-quantitative reporting, method by an international panel. Eur J Nucl Med Mol Imaging. 2017;44(2):234–41.
41. Gauguet JM, Pace-Emerson T, Grant FD, et al. Evaluation of the utility of (99m) Tc-MDP bone scintigraphy versus MIBG scintigraphy and cross-sectional imaging for staging patients with neuroblastoma. Pediatr Blood Cancer. 2017;64:11.
42. Burchill SA, Beiske K, Shimada H, et al. Recommendations for the standardization of bone

marrow disease assessment and reporting in children with neuroblastoma on behalf of the International Neuroblastoma Response Criteria Bone Marrow Working Group. Cancer. 2017;123(7):1095–105.
43. Laug WE, Siegel SE, Shaw KN, Landing B, Baptista J, Gutenstein M. Initial urinary catecholamine metabolite concentrations and prognosis in neuroblastoma. Pediatrics. 1978;62(1):77–83.
44. Brodeur GM, Pritchard J, Berthold F, et al. Revisions of the international criteria for neuroblastoma diagnosis, staging, and response to treatment. J Clin Oncol. 1993;11(8):1466–77.
45. Park JR, Bagatell R, Cohn SL, et al. Revisions to the international neuroblastoma response criteria: a consensus statement from the National Cancer Institute Clinical Trials Planning Meeting. J Clin Oncol. 2017;35(22):2580–7.
46. Cohn SL, Pearson AD, London WB, et al. The International Neuroblastoma Risk Group (INRG) classification system: an INRG Task Force report. J Clin Oncol. 2009;27(2):289–97.
47. Monclair T, Brodeur GM, Ambros PF, et al. The International Neuroblastoma Risk Group (INRG) staging system: an INRG Task Force report. J Clin Oncol. 2009;27(2):298–303.
48. Brisse HJ, McCarville MB, Granata C, et al. Guidelines for imaging and staging of neuroblastic tumors: consensus report from the International Neuroblastoma Risk Group Project. Radiology. 2011;261(1):243–57.
49. Breslow N, McCann B. Statistical estimation of prognosis for children with neuroblastoma. Cancer Res. 1971;31(12):2098–103.
50. Pugh TJ, Morozova O, Attiyeh EF, et al. The genetic landscape of high-risk neuroblastoma. Nat Genet. 2013;45(3):279–84.
51. Molenaar JJ, Koster J, Zwijnenburg DA, et al. Sequencing of neuroblastoma identifies chromothripsis and defects in neuritogenesis genes. Nature. 2012;483(7391):589–93.
52. Cheung NK, Zhang J, Lu C, et al. Association of age at diagnosis and genetic mutations in patients with neuroblastoma. JAMA. 2012;307(10):1062–71.
53. Asgharzadeh S, Pique-Regi R, Sposto R, et al. Prognostic significance of gene expression profiles of metastatic neuroblastomas lacking MYCN gene amplification. J Natl Cancer Inst. 2006;98(17):1193–203.
54. Asgharzadeh S, Salo JA, Ji L, et al. Clinical significance of tumor-associated inflammatory cells in metastatic neuroblastoma. J Clin Oncol. 2012;30(28):3525–32.
55. Brodeur GM, Seeger RC, Schwab M, Varmus HE, Bishop JM. Amplification of N-myc in untreated human neuroblastomas correlates with advanced disease stage. Science. 1984;224(4653):1121–4.
56. Seeger RC, Brodeur GM, Sather H, et al. Association of multiple copies of the N-myc oncogene with rapid progression of neuroblastomas. N Engl J Med. 1985;313(18):1111–6.
57. Thompson D, Vo KT, London WB, et al. Identification of patient subgroups with markedly disparate rates of MYCN amplification in neuroblastoma: a report from the International Neuroblastoma Risk Group project. Cancer. 2016;122(6):935–45.
58. Shapiro DN, Valentine MB, Rowe ST, et al. Detection of N-myc gene amplification by fluorescence in situ hybridization. Diagnostic utility for neuroblastoma. Am J Pathol. 1993;142(5):1339–46.
59. Ambros PF, Ambros IM, Brodeur GM, et al. International consensus for neuroblastoma molecular diagnostics: report from the International Neuroblastoma Risk Group (INRG) Biology Committee. Br J Cancer. 2009;100(9):1471–82.
60. Janoueix-Lerosey I, Schleiermacher G, Michels E, et al. Overall genomic pattern is a predictor of outcome in neuroblastoma. J Clin Oncol. 2009;27(7):1026–33.
61. Caron H, van Sluis P, de Kraker J, et al. Allelic loss of chromosome 1p as a predictor of unfavorable outcome in patients with neuroblastoma. N Engl J Med. 1996;334(4):225–30.
62. Rubie H, Delattre O, Hartmann O, et al. Loss of chromosome 1p may have a prognostic value in localised neuroblastoma: results of the French NBL 90 Study. Neuroblastoma Study Group of the Societe Francaise d'Oncologie Pediatrique (SFOP). Eur J Cancer. 1997;33(12):1917–22.
63. Bown N, Cotterill S, Lastowska M, et al. Gain of chromosome arm 17q and adverse outcome in patients with neuroblastoma. N Engl J Med. 1999;340(25):1954–61.
64. Attiyeh EF, London WB, Mosse YP, et al. Chromosome 1p and 11q deletions and outcome in neuroblastoma. N Engl J Med. 2005;353(21):2243–53.
65. Schleiermacher G, Janoueix-Lerosey I, Ribeiro A, et al. Accumulation of segmental alterations determines progression in neuroblastoma. J Clin Oncol. 2010;28(19):3122–30.
66. Schleiermacher G, Michon J, Ribeiro A, et al. Segmental chromosomal alterations lead to a higher risk of relapse in infants with MYCN-non-amplified localised unresectable/disseminated neuroblastoma (a SIOPEN collaborative study). Br J Cancer. 2011;105(12):1940–8.
67. Defferrari R, Mazzocco K, Ambros IM, et al. Influence of segmental chromosome abnormalities on survival in children over the age of 12 months with unresectable localised peripheral neuroblastic tumours without MYCN amplification. Br J Cancer. 2015;112(2):290–5.
68. Look AT, Hayes FA, Nitschke R, McWilliams NB, Green AA. Cellular DNA content as a predictor of response to chemotherapy in infants with unresectable neuroblastoma. N Engl J Med. 1984;311(4):231–5.

69. Look AT, Hayes FA, Shuster JJ, et al. Clinical relevance of tumor cell ploidy and N-myc gene amplification in childhood neuroblastoma: a Pediatric Oncology Group study. J Clin Oncol. 1991;9(4):581–91.
70. Baker DL, Schmidt ML, Cohn SL, et al. Outcome after reduced chemotherapy for intermediate-risk neuroblastoma. N Engl J Med. 2010;363(14):1313–23.
71. George RE, London WB, Cohn SL, et al. Hyperdiploidy plus nonamplified MYCN confers a favorable prognosis in children 12 to 18 months old with disseminated neuroblastoma: a Pediatric Oncology Group study. J Clin Oncol. 2005;23(27):6466–73.
72. Bagatell R, Beck-Popovic M, London WB, et al. Significance of MYCN amplification in international neuroblastoma staging system stage 1 and 2 neuroblastoma: a report from the International Neuroblastoma Risk Group database. J Clin Oncol. 2009;27(3):365–70.
73. Eisenhauer EA, Therasse P, Bogaerts J, et al. New response evaluation criteria in solid tumours: revised RECIST guideline (version 1.1). Eur J Cancer. 2009;45(2):228–47.
74. Bagatell R, McHugh K, Naranjo A, et al. Assessment of primary site response in children with high-risk neuroblastoma: an international multicenter study. J Clin Oncol. 2016;34(7):740–6.

2 Advanced Pathology Classification Toward Precision Stratification of Neuroblastic Tumors

Hiroyuki Shimada and Naohiko Ikegaki

2.1 Introduction

Neuroblastoma, as well defined by Willis [1], is an embryonal tumor of neural crest origin. Tumors of neuroblastoma group include neuroblastoma, ganglioneuroblastoma, and ganglioneuroma. We believe that all ganglioneuromas were once neuroblastomas in their early stage of tumor development. They are collected under the name of peripheral neuroblastic tumors and well known to present with a wide range of clinical behaviors, such as spontaneous regression, tumor maturation, and aggressive progression refractory to intensive treatment. Recent advances in research indicate that molecular/genomic properties of the individual tumors are closely associated with their unique clinical behaviors [2–4]. In this chapter, we briefly outline the International Neuroblastoma Pathology Classification, and present recent progress in pathology research contributing to precise pathway-targeting medicine for personalized treatment options for the patients with this disease.

H. Shimada (✉)
Department of Pathology and Pediatrics, Lucile Packard Children's Hospital, Stanford University, Stanford, CA, USA
e-mail: hshimada@stanford.edu

N. Ikegaki
Department of Anatomy and Cell Biology, College of Medicine, University of Illinois at Chicago, Chicago, IL, USA
e-mail: ikegaki@uic.edu

2.2 International Neuroblastoma Pathology Classification

The International Neuroblastoma Pathology Classification (INPC) is applicable only to tumor specimens obtained before chemotherapy and/or irradiation therapy and classifies individual cases into Favorable Histology Group or Unfavorable Histology Group [5, 6]. Based on our experience, histological/cytological changes after chemotherapy, especially those representing acute chemotherapy effects, are often unreliable in predicting the clinical behavior of individual cases. Those acute chemotherapy effects frequently observed in biologically unfavorable neuroblastomas include the presence of large areas of necrosis, extensive hemorrhage and hemosiderin deposition. Even neuroblastic differentiation and focal Schwannian stromal development could be observed in some biologically unfavorable neuroblastomas after chemotherapy.

2.2.1 Histological Categories and Subtypes

According to the recommendation by the International Neuroblastoma Pathology Committee, four categories are distinguished in this group of tumors. The first three categories: i.e., "Neuroblastoma (Schwannian stroma-poor),"

S. Asgharzadeh, F. Westermann (eds.), *Neuroblastoma*, Pediatric Oncology,
https://doi.org/10.1007/978-3-031-51292-6_2

"Ganglioneuroblastoma, Intermixed (Schwannian stroma-rich)," and "Ganglioneuroma (Schwannian stroma-dominant)," represent the morphologically defined maturational sequences indicated by the grade of neuroblastic differentiation and the degree of Schwannian stromal development [5–7]. Tumor maturation is prompted by the "cross-talk" supported by critical signaling pathways, such as trkA/NGF signaling and Nrg1/ErbB signaling [8–10], between neuroblasts and Schwannian stromal cells. The fourth category is "Ganglioneuroblastoma Nodular (composite, Schwannian stroma-rich/stroma-dominant and stroma-poor)," which is defined as multi-clonal tumor composed of either "Ganglioneuroblastoma, Intermixed" or "Ganglioneuroma" co-existing with "Neuroblastoma." Tumors in the "Neuroblastoma" category include undifferentiated, poorly differentiated, and differentiating subtype, and those in the "Ganglioneuroma" category include maturing and mature subtype.

2.2.2 Prognostic Grouping (Favorable Histology Vs. Unfavorable Histology)

Favorable Histology (FH) Group and Unfavorable Histology (UH) Group distinguished by the INPC are summarized in Table 2.1 [5–7, 11]. First, category ("Neuroblastoma," "Ganglioneuroblastoma, Intermixed," "Ganglioneuroma," or "Ganglio-

Table 2.1 International neuroblastoma pathology classification

Category and subtype	Favorable histology group	Unfavorable histology group
Neuroblastoma (Schwannian stroma-poor)		
Undifferentiated subtype		Any age with any MKI
Poorly differentiated subtype	<1.5 years at Dx. with low/ intermediate MKI	Any age with high MKI ≥1.5 years at Dx. with any MKI
Differentiating subtype	<1.5 years at Dx. with low/ intermediate MKI <5 years at Dx. with low MKI	Any age with high MKI ≥1.5 years at Dx. with intermediate MKI ≥5 years at Dx. with any MKI
Ganglioneuroblastoma, intermixed (Schwannian stroma-rich)	Any age[a]	
Ganglioneuroma (Schwannian stroma-dominant) Maturing subtype Mature subtype	Any age[a]	
Ganglioneuroblastoma, nodular (composite, Schwannian stroma-rich stroma-dominant and stroma-poor)	Based on Neuroblastoma Nodule[b]	Based on Neuroblastoma Nodule[b]

Dx.= Diagnosis; MKI=Mitosis-Karyorrhexis Index.

* Ganglioneuroblastoma, Intermixed and Ganglioneuroma are diagnosed in older children, adolescents, and even adults.

** Favorable Histology or Unfavorable Histology in Ganglioneuroblastoma, Nodular is determined by age-dependent evaluation of histologic features of Neuroblastoma Nodules.

neuroblastoma, Nodular") of each tumor is determined. All tumors in the "Ganglioneuroblastoma, Intermixed" and "Ganglioneuroma," which are usually diagnosed in older children, adolescents, and even in adults, are classified into the FH Group. Those tumors in the "Neuroblastoma" category are classified into FH Group or UH Group, based on the age-depending evaluation of grade of neuroblastic differentiation and MKI (mitosis-karyorrhexis index). Neuroblastoma with undifferentiated subtype and that with High MKI (>200/5000 cells) are classified into the UH Group regardless of the age at diagnosis. Neuroblastoma with poorly differentiated subtype with either Low (<100/5000 cells) or Intermediate MKI (100–200/5000 cells) diagnosed less than 1.5 years of age; Neuroblastoma with differentiating subtype and Low or Intermediate MKI diagnosed less than 1.5 years of age; and Neuroblastoma with differentiating subtype with Low MKI diagnosed less than 5 years of age are classified into the FH Group. All Neuroblastoma with poorly differentiated subtype diagnosed over 1.5 years of age; all Neuroblastoma with differentiating subtype and Intermediate MKI diagnosed over 1.5 years of age; and all Neuroblastoma with differentiating subtype diagnosed over 5 years of age are classified into the UH Group. As for the classification of "Ganglioneuroblastoma, Nodular" tumors, distinction of FH and UH is determined based on the evaluation of "Neuroblastoma" component using the same age-dependent criteria of grade of neuroblastic differentiation and MKI.

Peripheral neuroblastic tumors in the FH Group have a potential of differentiation/maturation through the "cross-talk" between tumor cells and Schwannian stromal cells. In order to observe tumor differentiation/maturation, however, a certain period of time, i.e., in vivo latent period or age-appropriate framework seems to be required. As described above, the INPC defines two critical time points: up to 1.5 years from "Neuroblastoma, poorly differentiated subtype" to "Neuroblastoma, differentiating subtype," and up to 5 years from "Neuroblastoma, differentiating subtype" to "Ganglioneuroblastoma, Intermixed" or "Ganglioneuroma." In contrast, peripheral neuroblastic tumors in the UH Group have no or limited potential of differentiation/maturation and they are outside the age-appropriate framework. Prognostic effects of mitotic and karyorrhectic activities are also age-dependent, and High MKI in any age group, Intermediate MKI ≥1.5 years of age at diagnosis, and Low MKI ≥5 years of age at diagnosis indicate that we are dealing with neuroblastomas in the UH Group [12]. A significant correlation between *MYCN* amplification and High MKI has been reported in neuroblastoma tumors [13, 14].

2.3 Toward Precision Medicine for Therapy Resistant and Refractory Neuroblastomas

As stated above, FH and UH Groups of peripheral neuroblastic tumors are defined based on the INPC. Importantly, survival rate of FH group is estimated to around or over 90%, whereas that of UH group has remained at 40–50% or less [5, 11, 15]. This indicates that at least one in two UH group patients is expected to have tumor progression with often fatal outcome from the disease despite the current high intensity multimodal therapy. New innovative therapeutic approaches are thus needed for those in the UH group. To address this problem, we and others have sought and identified the expression of potentially "drug-targetable" proteins responsible for the aggressive behavior of certain neuroblastomas in the UH group.

MYCN oncogene, whose amplification is detected in approximately 20% of all neuroblastoma tumors [16, 17], is considered as a major oncogenic driver. The vast majority of *MYCN*-amplified tumors overexpress MYCN protein. In addition, about 10% of undifferentiated and poorly differentiated neuroblastomas are found to over-express MYC (aka C-Myc) protein [18] (Fig. 2.1a). Notably, UH tumors with either MYCN or MYC expression show ~45% 3-year event-free survival. These tumors have been defined as "MYC-driven neuroblastoma" [18] (Fig. 2.1b). In non-MYC family driven unfavorable neuroblastoma, recent Next-Generation Sequencing (NSG) analysis has further provided

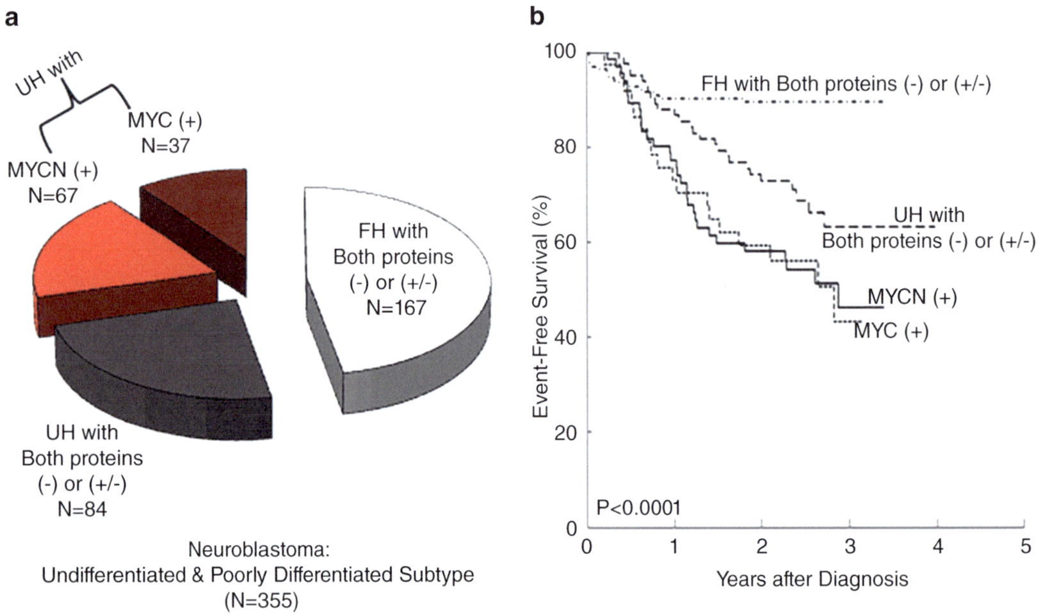

Fig. 2.1 Case distribution and survival by MYC-family protein expression and International Neuroblastoma Pathology Classification. (**a**) Distribution of 355 neuroblastomas of undifferentiated/poorly differentiated subtypes. (**b**) Even-free survivals for the four groups based on MYCN/MYC-family protein expression and Histopathology. Patients with MYCN protein overexpressing tumor have a similar and significantly low survival rate compared with those with MYC protein overexpressing tumor. *FH* favorable histology, *UH* unfavorable histology according to the International Neuroblastoma Pathology Classification. MYCN (+) indicates MYCN protein overexpression and MYC (+) indicates MYC protein overexpression. [Figure 3 of [18] with minor modifications]

a clue as to the possible additional drivers of tumor aggressiveness [19–21]. Those include loss of function mutations of *ATRX* (alpha-thalassemia/mental retardation syndrome X-linked), leading to ATRX loss and ALT (Alternative Lengthening of Telomere) phenotype and TERT (telomerase reverse transcriptase) overexpression due to *TRET* gene rearrangements. Both mechanisms prevent tumor cells from replication senescence/cell death due to telomere erosion and provide them with infinite proliferating capability.

2.3.1 Proposed Subgrouping of Unfavorable Histology Neuroblastomas

As we are gaining additional knowledge about the potential molecular targets that underlay the therapy resistant phenotype associated with UH neuroblastomas, we are ready to incorporate such information into the INPC towards "precision prognosis and therapy stratification." We can refine the UH neuroblastoma stratification using an immunohistopathological analysis shown in Table 2.2. An immunohistochemical staining of tumors with anti-pan-MYC antibody (or anti-MYCN and anti-MYC), anti-TERT antibody, and anti-ATRX antibody will allow classifying UH neuroblastomas into four subgroups. Based on the proposed subgrouping of UH neuroblastomas, it is expected that tumors unlikely to respond to the current high intensity multimodal therapy (MYC, TERT, and ATL subgroups) will be identified and separated from the responder (Null subgroup) with a high probability prior to the initiation of therapy.

2.3.1.1 MYC Subgroup

MYC-driven neuroblastoma shows augmented expression of either MYCN protein or MYC protein [18]. As augmented MYC-family protein

Table 2.2 Proposed subgroups of unfavorable histology neuroblastoma

	Subgroups	Immunohistochemistry (IHC) markers			Histologic markers	Predicted survival based on current therapy
		Pan-MYC or (MYCN/MYC)	TERT	ATRX		
MYC family protein-driven neuroblastomas	MYC (MYCN/MYC)	Overexpression	Overexpression or no overexpression	Retention	Nucleolar hypertrophy (including large cell neuroblastoma)	Dismal
Non-MYC family protein-driven neuroblastomas	TERT	No overexpression	Overexpression	Retention	Salt-and-pepper nuclei Conventional neuroblastoma	Dismal
	ALT	No overexpression	No overexpression	Loss	Salt-and-pepper nuclei Conventional neuroblastoma	Dismal
	Null	No overexpression	No overexpression	Retention	Salt-and-pepper nuclei Conventional neuroblastoma	Better response

TERT telomerase reversed transcriptase, *ALT* alternative lengthening of telomere, *ATRX* alpha-thalassemia/mental retardation syndrome X-linked

MYC subgroup is characterized by augmented MYC-family protein expression and exhibits prominent nucleolar formation and hypertrophic cell morphology. It is also expected that a considerable number of MYC family-driven neuroblastomas are associated with TERT overexpression, because *TERT* is a direct gene target of MYC-family proteins, and others have little to no TERT over expression. **TERT subgroup**: Higher levels of TERT expression are observed in this group with little to low level expression of MYC or MYCN protein. The activation of TERT expression in this case is likely due to *TERR* genomic rearrangements. *TERT* promoter hypermethylation might also be its activating mechanism. **ALT subgroup** is characterized by ATRX loss, which results in the ALT phenotype. ATRX is rarely mutated in the MYC subgroup and TERT subgroup. Because one of the normal ATRX functions is to insert the variant histone H3, namely H3.3, into chromatin to maintain transcriptionally active euchromatin, the absence of ATRX may result into a more heterochromatic state globally. Thus, the histological appearance of the ALT subgroup could be conventional with the "salt-and-pepper" nuclei. **Null subgroup:** There are still UH neuroblastomas without MYCN/MYC overexpression, no TERT overexpression, and no ATRX loss. Unless otherwise any other aggravated factors are found, the patients in the Null subgroup would hopefully respond to the current high-risk treatment regimens expression stimulates rRNA synthesis and protein translation, neuroblastic cells in this subgroup often exhibit prominent nucleolar formation (nucleolar hypertrophy) and hypertrophic cell morphology [18, 22]. Because of the presence of one to a few prominent nucleoli, MYC-driven neuroblastoma is cytologically distinguishable from the conventional "small round blue cell" neuroblastoma with "salt-and-pepper" nuclei (Fig. 2.2a, b). MYC-driven neuroblastoma tumors, comprising more than 50% of high-risk neuroblastomas, include rare tumors named "Large cell neuroblastoma" that are often characterized by the "bull's eye" appearance of enlarged and uniquely open "euchromatin-rich" nuclei containing highly conspicuous nucleoli (Fig. 2.2c) [23]. Most "Large cell neuroblastomas" overexpress higher levels of MYCN protein or MYC protein than other MYC-driven neuroblastomas (Fig. 2.2d–g). Their "euchromatin-rich" open nuclei also suggest the stem cell-like nature of the tumor cells [24]. A considerable number of MYC-driven neuroblastomas are also associated with TERT overexpression, since *TERT* is a direct gene target of MYC-family proteins, and TERT can also stabilize MYC protein

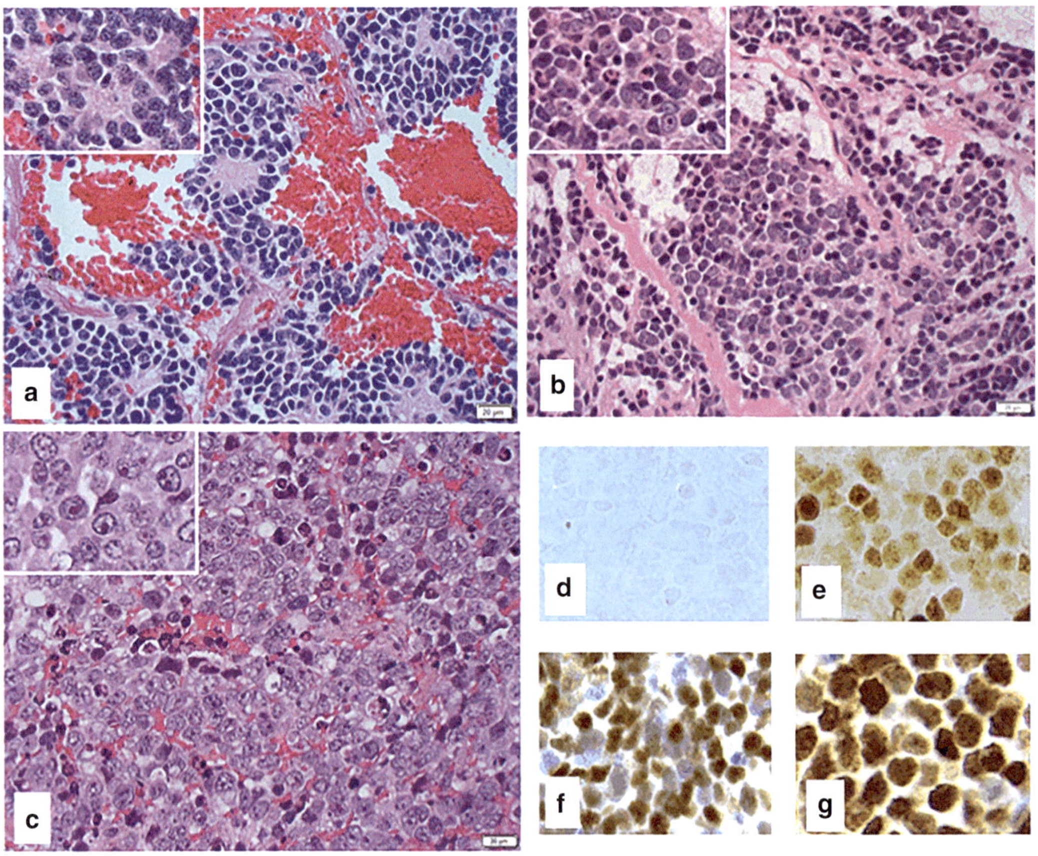

Fig. 2.2 H&E staining of Neuroblastoma, poorly differentiated subtype: (**a**) without *MYCN* oncogene amplification and the protein overexpression (Note: Neuroblastic cells show typical salt-and pepper nuclei), (**b**) with *MYCN* oncogene amplification and the protein overexpression (Note: Neuroblastic cells demonstrate nucleolar hypertrophy with prominent nucleolar formation), and (**c**) with MYC protein overexpression (Note: This is an example of large cell neuroblastoma with characteristically vesicular nuclei containing one to a few very prominent nucleoli). Immunostaining of neuroblastoma, poorly differentiated subtype: (**d**) without MYCN/MYC protein overexpression, (**e**) with MYCN protein overexpression, (**f**) with MYC protein overexpression, and (**g**) of large cell type with a higher level of MYC protein overexpression

via its non-canonical enzymatic function, creating a positive feed-back loop between MYCN/MYC and TERT expression [25, 26].

2.3.1.2 TERT Subgroup (Fig. 2.3a, b)

TERT is the protein component of telomerase, which also includes TERC (telomere RNA component). TERT overexpression is likely due to long-range genomic rearrangements but not to promote mutations in neuroblastoma [27]. *TERT* promoter hypermethylation may also be involved in its overexpression [28, 29]. Higher levels of TERT expression are also observed in neuroblastomas without MYCN/MYC protein overexpression (see Sect. 2.3.1.2).

2.3.1.3 ALT Subgroup (Fig. 2.3c, d)

ATRX loss results in the ALT phenotype. ATRX mutation is rarely observed in the Sects. 2.3.1.2 and 2.3.1.3, and loss of ATRX is exclusively seen in the older neuroblastoma children over 5 years of age. Because one of the normal ATRX functions is to insert the variant histone H3, namely H3.3, in concert with DAXX into chromatin to maintain transcriptionally active euchromatin [30], the ATRX loss may result into a more transcriptionally inactive heterochromatic state. Thus, the histological/cytological appearance of the Sect. 2.3.1.3 could be the conventional type with salt-and-pepper nuclei rather than that with nucleolar hypertrophy or bull's eye type in the Sect. 2.3.1.1.

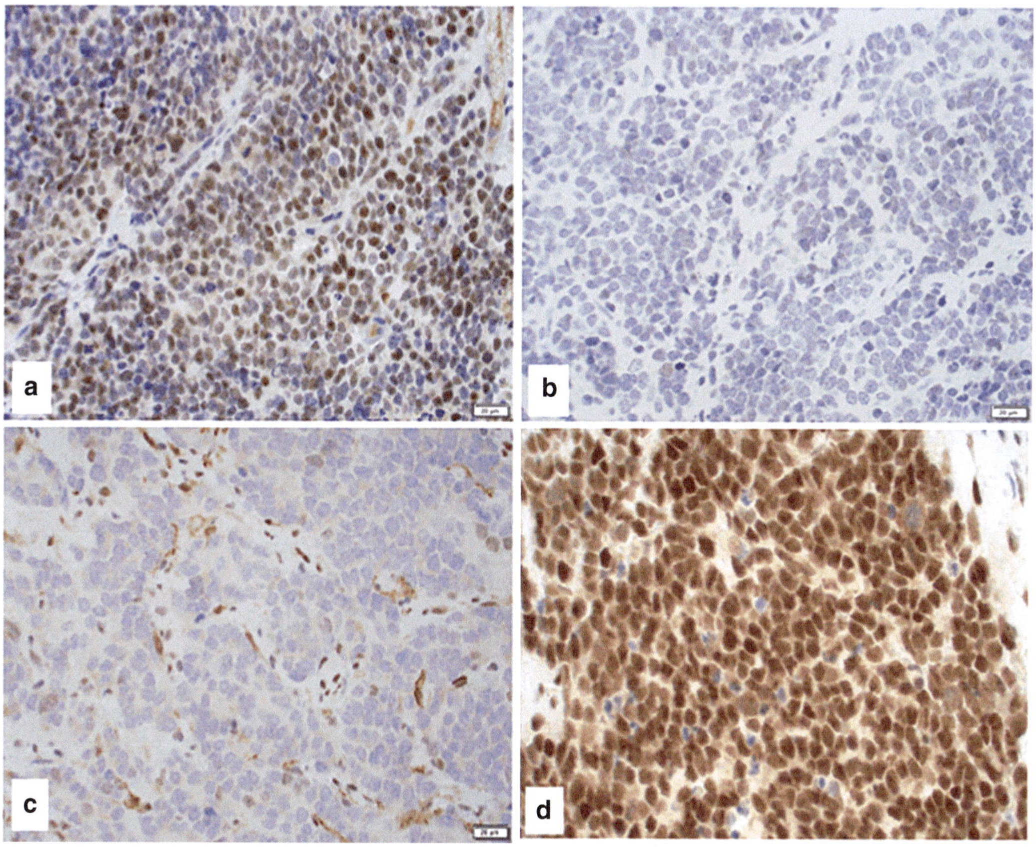

Fig. 2.3 Immunostaining of neuroblastoma (**a**) with TERT overexpression and (**b**) without TERT overexpression. Immunostaining of neuroblastoma with (**c**) ATRX loss (Note: Endothelial cells are positively stained) and (**d**) ATRX retained. Please note that current immunostainings for TERT (positive) and ATRX (negative) do not seem to identify efficiently all neuroblastoma tumors with abnormal maintenance of telomeres

2.3.1.4 Null Subgroup

There are still UH neuroblastomas without MYC-family protein overexpression, TERT overexpression, and ATRX loss. As long as any other aggravated factors are found, the patients in the **Null subgroup** would hopefully respond to the current high-risk treatment regimens.

2.3.2 Therapeutic Targeting in Unfavorable Histology Neuroblastomas

In this section, we discuss the contribution of pathology to the identification of new therapeutic options that could be available to patients with tumors in the non-responder subgroups.

2.3.2.1 MYC-Family Protein Overexpression

Direct Targeting Approaches

MYC-family proteins heterodimerize with the partner, MAX, and become functional molecular complexes as transcription factors. They bind to E-Box sequences throughout the genome and globally modulate cellular transcriptional activity. However, MYC-family proteins being transcriptional factors are notoriously "undruggable" [31]. Nonetheless, attempts have been made to address this problem. One such approach is to inhibit the interaction between MYC-family proteins and MAX protein via small molecules. Berg et al. published the first study on MYC/MAX dimerization inhibitors in 2002 [32] and several others followed the study since then [33–36]. Although the efficacy of these small molecules have been improving, it appears that further refinements are still needed for MYC/MAX dimerization inhibitors before they are given further consideration for human clinical trials.

Indirect Targeting Approaches

Given the current status of direct MYC-family protein inhibitors, many have sought indirect approaches to down regulate MYC-family protein expression in cancer cells. The strategies under current consideration include, but are not limited to, (1) transcriptional repression of *MYC* and *MYCN* genes by G-quadruplex (G4) stabilizers [37, 38], by BET (Bromo- and Extra-Terminal)-inhibitors [39, 40], and by inhibitors of a transcriptional cyclin-dependent kinase 7 (CDK7) [41, 42], (2) destabilization of MYCN by Aurora kinase A inhibitors [43] and destabilization of MYC and MYCN proteins by RAS signaling pathway inhibitors [44, 45], and (3) translational blockade of *MYC* mRNA by eIF4F inhibition and stabilization of RNA G4 by RNA G4 ligands [46, 47]. These approaches are discussed below.

DNA G-Quadruplex Stabilizers

Nucleic acid (DNA and RNA) sequences rich in guanine can form four-stranded structures, called G-quadruplexes (G4) that inhibit transcription. Siddiqui-Jain et al. in 2002 first showed that a G4 structure is present in a promoter region of *MYC* and could be targeted with small stabilizer molecules to repress *MYC* transcription [48]. Interestingly, *MYCN* promoter also possesses G4 sequences [37], suggesting that G4 stabilizers can target both *MYC* and *MYCN*. To date, several more potent G4 stabilizers have been reported [49–51] (http://www.g4ldb.org/ci2/index.php), including the synthetic fluoroquinolone, Quarfloxin (CX-3543), which was developed for its ability to interact with the *MYC* G-quadruplex [38]. However, it turns out that CX-3543 is preferentially concentrated in the nucleoli of cancer cells and inhibits rRNA transcription by RNA Pol I, not at *MYC* locus [52]. This selective inhibition of Pol I is likely due to the binding of CX-3543 to G-quadruplexes in the rDNA as the study identified 14 putative G4-forming sequences on the non-template strand of rDNA [52]. Based on these findings, CX-3543 went into human cancer clinical trials (NCT00955292). Conversely, another fluoroquinolone, CX-5461, which was originally developed as an rRNA synthesis inhibitor (see below), has recently been shown to exhibit a G4-stabilizing activity [53]. APTO-253 is another small molecule tested in a Phase 1 clinical trial (NCT02267863), and both monomeric APTO-253 and a ferrous complex $Fe(253)_3$ stabilize G4 structures present in telomeres, *MYC* and *KIT* promoters [54].

BET (Bromo- and Extra-Terminal)-Inhibitors

BET family proteins include BRD2, BRD3, BRD4, and BRDT. These proteins bind to acetylated lysine residues of target proteins via their bromodomains. In particular, BRD4 has been shown to accumulate at super-enhancer regions through its binding to acetylated histones [55]. BRD4 co-localizes with an active enhancer marker, histone H3K27Ac, suggesting that BRD4 could directly interacts with H3K27Ac [56]. BRD4 also interacts with the multi-component scaffold protein MEDIATOR and the positive transcription elongation complex P-TEFb [57] to activate gene transcription elongation. Notably, the expression of *MYC* and *MYCN* is under the control of super-enhancers [42, 56], and the MYC super-enhancers appear to be essential for MYC-dependent tumorigenesis [58]. The involvement of BRD4 in super-enhancer driven transcriptional overdrive of *MYC* and *MYCN* expression suggests that BRD4 inhibition with small molecules can be an effective way to down-regulate *MYC* and *MYCN* transcription. Delmore et al. reported in 2011 the first of its kind, called JQ1, and the treatment of MYC-driven cancer cells with JQ1 resulted in rapid down-regulation of MYC protein and its transcriptional network [39]. Subsequently, it has also been shown that JQ1 is effective in down-regulating *MYCN* [40]. Clinically more relevant BET inhibitors have been tested in several clinical trials of adult cancers [NCT02391480 (Drug: ABBV-075), NCT03068351 (Drug: RO6870810), NCT02158858 (Drug: CPI-0610), NCT02419417 (Drug: BMS-986158)], and OTX015 (NCT02698189), which has been shown to be effective against mouse and human MYCN-driven tumor models [59].

Inhibitors of Cyclin-Dependent Kinases 7

The active involvement of super-enhancers of the over-driven *MYCN* expression in *MYCN* amplified neuroblastoma came to light through the study of a covalent CDK7 inhibitor, THZ1 [42]. CDK7 complexes with cyclin H and MAT1 and forms a Cdk-activating kinase (CAK). CAK is a component of the transcription factor TFIIH, which is involved in transcription initiation [60]. TFIIH is a component of general transcription factors and recruits RNA Pol II to the promoters of genes to complete the formation of the transcription pre-initiation complex (PIC) [61]. Phosphorylation by CDK7 of the C-terminal domain (CTD) of serine at position 5 (S5) of RNA Pol II initiates gene transcription [61]. Subsequently, Pol II advances to the pause site, where it is stabilized by pausing factors, such as negative elongation factor (NELF) and DRB-sensitivity-inducing factor (DSIF). P-TEFb is the main factor required to release paused Pol II from the promoter-proximal region. P-TEFb is composed of CDK9 and cyclin T. P-TEFb phosphorylates the CTD of serine at position 2 (S2). Phosphorylation of the CTD at S2 position fully activates transcription elongation [62]. Super-enhancers together with gene specific transcription factors, BRD4 and the MEDIATOR complex help assemble PIC more efficiently and initiate transcription via TFIIH/CAK (the CDK7 complex) at the transcriptional start site. Super-enhancer bound BRD4 and the super elongation complex (SEC) then recruit P-TEFb to release paused Pol II via phosphorylation of the CTD at S5 [62]. Because of the hyper-activated super-enhancer driven transcription of *MYCN*, the CDK7inhibitor, THZ1, preferentially suppresses *MYCN* transcription. A similar finding was made for *MYC* in response to THZ1 in *MYC* amplified SCLC (small cell lung cancer) cells [41]. Surprisingly, inhibition of CDK9 by a small molecule inhibitor, i-CDK9, enhances MYC expression, and only simultaneous inhibition of CDK9 and BRD4 can efficiently induce growth arrest and apoptosis in cancer cells [63]. More clinically suitable CDK7 inhibiting drugs, SY-1365 and CT7001, are currently tested in Phase I clinical trials for advanced solid tumors (NCT03134638 and NCT03363893, respectively).

Destabilization of MYCN by Aurora Kinase A Inhibitors

Otto et al. revealed in 2009 that Aurora A binds to and stabilizes MYCN by preventing it from FBXW7 E3 ubiquitin ligase-mediated proteasomal degradation [64]. This activity is independent of Aurora A catalytic activity. Gustafson et al. have further shown that inhibitors disrupting the native conformation of Aurora kinase A cause the degradation of MYCN protein [43]. Alisertib (MNL8237), an investigational inhibitor of Aurora kinase A developed by Takeda Inc., being tested in several adult cancer clinical trials, binds to the catalytic domain of Aurora kinase A and causes an allosteric change in the protein structure. This in turn releases MYCN from Aurora kinase A and causes proteasome-mediated MYCN degradation [64]. Alisertib had been tested in a Phase I trial by COG [65], and is now tested in combination with Irinotecan and Temozolomide (NCT01601535). However, Takeda terminated an Alisertib Phase 3 trial relapsed or refractory peripheral T-cell lymphoma in adult, and its future in pediatric cancer trials is uncertain [66].

Destabilization of MYC/MYCN by Inhibitors of RAS Signaling Pathways

Two arms of RAS signaling pathways regulate the stability of MYC-family proteins through phosphorylations at T58 and S62 of MYC or equivalent residues of other MYC-family members. The phosphorylation at S62 by ERK of the MEK/ERK arm of RAS pathways enhances MYC protein stability; this phosphorylation subsequently allows T58 phosphorylation by active (non-phosphorylated) GSK3β, whereas the PI3K/PDK1/AKT arm of RAS pathways inactivates GSK3β by phosphorylation; when MYC proteins are doubly phosphorylated at T58 and S62, the proteins are recognized by the protein phosphatase PP2A, which keeps GSK3β active and dephosphorylates S62; T58 monophosphorylated MYC proteins are then recognized by FBWX7 E3 ubiquitin ligase, which polyubiquitinates MYC proteins for proteasomal degradation. Therefore, inhibition of either arm of the RAS signaling pathways results in destabilization of MYC family proteins. Over the years, potent and selective inhibitors of the RAS signaling pathways have been developed and on human clinical trials [67–69]. Some of the RAS pathway inhibitors are tested in The Pediatric MATCH Screening Trial (NCT03155620).

Translational Initiation Blockade of *MYC* mRNA by eIF4F Inhibition

One of the components of the eukaryotic translation initiation complex (EIF) is eIF4A, which functions as an ATP-dependent DEAD-box RNA helicase to remove secondary structures from 5′UTR of mRNA. Ribosome-profiling assay experiments have shown that eIF4A regulates mRNA translation of transcripts with 5′UTRs containing G4-forming CGG motifs. Among the most eIF4A-sensitive mRNAs there are several oncogenes and transcription factors (e.g., *MYC*, *MYB*, *NOTCH*, *CDK6*, *BCL2*) [47]. These RNA G4 sequences may be selectively targeted by RNA G4 specific ligands [70]. These observations suggest that inhibition of eIF4A and/or stabilization of RNA G4 at 5''UTR of mRNA can suppress translation of the eIF4A-sensitive mRNAs. In fact, an inhibitor of eIF4A, Silvestrol, causes marked down-regulation of MYC, MYB, NOTCH, CDK6, and BCL2 proteins [47]. Silvestrol has been tested in preclinical studies, but clinically relevant inhibitors of eIF4A have not been reported. Conversely, other translational initiation inhibitors have been tested in clinical trials, including ribavirin (e.g., NCT02073838) and eFT508 (e.g., NCT02605083). Ribavirin, a broad-spectrum antiviral drug mimics the m^7G cap structure, whereas eFT508 is an inhibitor of mitogen-activated protein kinase interacting kinase 1 and 2. Both drugs target eIF4E to inhibit translation initiation.

Targeting MYC-Driven Hypertrophic Nucleoli

Other indirect strategies to down-regulate MYC-family protein expression have been explored in neuroblastoma. Since MYC family-driven neuroblastomas are characterized by prominent nucleolar formation, inhibition of rRNA gene transcription and protein translation by small molecule inhibitors could be a potential therapeutic approach for this subset of biologically unfavorable neuroblastomas [71]. In fact, small molecule inhibitors of rRNA synthesis and protein translation are available, such as CX-5461 and Halofuginone, respectively, and are currently examined for their efficacy in various human diseases in clinical trials [72, 73]. CX-5461 disrupts the binding of the SL1 transcription factor to the rDNA promoter and prevents the initiation of rRNA synthesis by RNA Pol I [74]. Consequently, ribosomal assembly will be halted, leading to the accumulation of unassembled ribosomal proteins. Free ribosomal proteins will then promote cancer-specific activation of p53 [72]. Interestingly, a similar set of free ribosomal proteins could also down-regulate MYC protein by distinct mechanisms [75, 76]. Halofuginone, on the other hand, specifically inhibits glutamyl-prolyl tRNA synthetase (EPRS) [77], resulting in the accumulation of uncharged prolyl tRNAs, which then leads to suppression of protein translation via the induction of amino acid starvation response [78]. In addition, inhibition of EPRS may also liberate one of the cofactors from the human multi-tRNA-synthetase complex (i.e., AIMP2—Aminoacyl TRNA Synthetase Complex Interacting Multifunctional Protein 2). Freed AIMP2 could then migrate into the nucleus and inhibit FBP (FUBP1), which otherwise functions as the transcriptional activator of *MYC* [79, 80]. Consequently, Halofuginone could induce down regulation of MYC-family proteins through both global translational suppression and transcriptional inhibition. We have in fact shown that treatment of MYC-driven neuroblastoma cells with CX-5461 and Halofuginone causes down-regulation of MYC and MYCN proteins and growth suppression [71]. As stated above, the effect of CX-5461 on MYC-family protein expression may also be due to its direct effect on transcription of *MYC* and *MYCN* through the binding to DNA G-quadruplexes in their promoter regions.

2.3.2.2 Telomere Maintenance and Elongation

TERT Inhibitors

For those patients with TERT overexpressing neuroblastoma, clinical trials with telomerase inhibitors can be considered. Imetelstat (GRN163L; JNJ-63935937) (http://www.geron.com/r-d/imetelstat/) is a potent and specific inhibitor of telomerase that binds with high affinity to TERC. Imetelstat is administered by intravenous infusion and it has been tested in human clinical Phase 2 and 2/3 trials (http://www.geron.com/r-d/imetelstat/). These trials are currently on going. An interesting note to the Imetelstat efficacy is that Sorafenib and UC2288 have been shown to synergize with Imetelstat to inhibit growth of mouse xenografts of human cancer. Sorafenib is a FDA-approved kinase inhibitor that is tested in combination with topotecan and cyclophosphamide in patients with relapsed neuroblastoma by the New Approaches to Neuroblastoma Therapy (NANT) consortium (NCT02298348) [81]. Sorafenib inhibits several tyrosine protein kinases such as VEGFR, PDGFR, and Raf family kinases. Interestingly, it has been shown that Sorafenib also attenuates the expression of p21 induced by chemotherapy [82]. Moreover, UC2288, a more selective p21 inhibitor based Sorafenib with minimal kinase inhibitory activity, similarly synergizes with Imetelstat to inhibit growth of mouse xenografts of human cancer [83], suggesting that the ability of Sorafenib to synergize with Imetelstat is due to its p21 attenuating activity. Based on these observations, a combination of Imetelstat and Sorafenib may prove more efficacious than Imetelstat alone to those neuroblastomas with elevated telomerase activity.

Inhibitors for ALT Phenotype

ALT inhibition could also be considered in the clinical trials for those patients with neuroblastoma having loss of ATRX. However, because ATRX loss is due to structural alterations in *ATRX* gene, including in-frame deletions, missense, nonsense, and frame-shift single-nucleotide variations (SNVs) [84], it would be difficult to regain the expression of ATRX in neuroblastoma.

One of the ATRX activities includes repression of the telomeric repeat-containing RNA (TERRA) expression. Hence, loss of ATRX compromises the decline of TERRA in G2/M phase, leading to persistent association of replication protein A (RPA) with telomeres after DNA replication. This results in the persistent formation of a recombinogenic nucleoprotein structure (RPA-ssDNA) at telomeres. In non-ALT cells, RPA at telomeres will be replaced by POT1 (protection of telomeres 1) due to the decline of TERRA during G2/M via the hNRNPA1-mediated mechanism. POT1 recruitment at telomeres at G2/M is to inhibit ATR (Ataxia Telangiectasia and Rad3-related protein) activation by RPA-ssDNA. In ALT cells, in contrast, RPA persists at telomeres through cell cycle. This RPA-ssDNA at telomeres will then be recognized by ATR along with a partner protein called ATRIP (ATR Interacting Protein) as replication errors of DNA. This activates the ATR-medicated DNA damage response, leading to the activation of CHK1 (Checkpoint Kinase 1). The CHK1 activation in turn results in phosphorylation and nuclear import of RAD51 recombinase. ALT is known to be mediated by sister chromatid homologous recombination. RAD51 recombinase plays a central role in homologous recombinational repair of DNA; RAD51 catalyzes strand transfer between a broken sequence and its undamaged homologue to allow re-synthesis of the damaged region. BRCA2 (Breast Cancer 2) is also involved in this process to remove RPA from ssDNA and replace it with RAD51. In ALT cells, this mechanism appears to be used to maintain telomeres [85].

In essence, ATR is a key regulator of ALT. Inhibition of ATR thus disrupts ALT and triggers chromosome fragmentation and apoptosis in ALT cells. Importantly, the cell death induced by ATR inhibitors appears highly selective for ALT cells. AZD6738 is an orally bioactive and selective ATR kinase inhibitor with IC50 of 1 nM and currently tested in Phase I clinical trials in adults (https://openinnovation.astrazeneca.com/azd6738.html). Because CHK1 comes downstream of ATR and facilitates Homologous recombination repair (HRR), CHK1 inhibitors, such as MK8776/SCH900776 [86] could also be selectively efficacious against ATL cells. It should be mentioned that in neuroblastoma, the expression of *ATR*, *CHK1*, *BRCA2*, and *RAD51* is significantly associated with adverse outcome of the patients (NI, unpublished observations).

Induction of Telomere Erosion

Xu et al. have discovered that CX-5461 (and related CX-3543) binded and stabilized G-quadruplex (G4) DNA structures in vitro, inhibited the progression of DNA replication complexes, and resulted in increased in vivo G4 structures. They further investigated the effect of CX-5461 on the integrity of telomeres, which are enriched with G4 structures. Telomere FISH results showed an increased frequency of telomere defects in both $BRCA2^{+/+}$ and $BRCA2^{-/-}$ HCT116 cells after exposure to CX-5461, and this defect was more prominent in $BRCA2^{-/-}$ cells. Collectively, these data suggest that CX-5461 is a G4 stabilizer and induces genome instability specifically at G-quadruplex sequences [53]. These observations suggest that CX-5461 is preferentially efficacious against neuroblastoma cells with telomere maintenance and elongation aberrations. In addition, it has been reported that ATR inhibitors can synergize with CX-5461 to show more robust cancer cell killing of leukemia cells [87]. Thus, a combination of ATR inhibitors and CX-5461 may be a better option for the treatment of ALT neuroblastomas.

2.3.2.3 An Emerging Common Strategy for Therapy Resistant or Refractory UH Neuroblastoma

Based on the discussion above, one common strategy to treat therapy resistant or refractory UH neuroblastomas appears to be DNA G4 stabilizers, such as CX-5461. This drug can target MYC family-driven, TERT-overexpressing, and ALT-phenotype neuroblastomas and it may be considered the core agent in a cocktail of drugs to treat the aggressive UH neuroblastomas.

2.4 Conclusion

Pathology classification of neuroblastic tumors has made a pivotal contribution to prognosis and therapy stratification of peripheral neuroblastic tumors for the last 40 years. Unlike most adult cancer pathology classifications, the Shimada neuroblastoma pathology classification system and the subsequent INPC incorporated age as the determining factor of the classification systems, taking into account the age-distribution of the patients and development of the peripheral nervous system during the period of disease occurrence. To date, INPC can clearly define Favorable and Unfavorable Histology categories of neuroblastic tumors, having over 90% and below 50% overall survival probabilities, respectively. This makes the INPC the most significant prognostic indicator among the prognostic factors used in the current COG risk classification scheme for neuroblastic tumors. However, this also leaves one important unsolved issue that at least one in two patients with UH tumors succumbs to the disease despite receiving multimodal and high-intensity therapy regiments. The proposed subclassification of UH neuroblastomas into therapy-responsive "Null" and therapy-resistant/refractory "Extremely Unfavorable Histology" (EUH) groups constitutes a first step forward to precision medicine approaches to treat EUH neuroblastic tumors effectively [88].

The molecular target-defined subclassification of UH tumors has a significant merit because one can selectively target the drivers of the disease by specific therapeutics. As we have discussed in this chapter, vigorous attempts have been made to develop such therapeutics, and the idea of "undruggable" targets by small molecules may be fading away. We hope that in near future, such therapeutics become available for the effective treatment of EUH neuroblastic tumors to save the children without severe late side effects.

References

1. Willis R. Neuroblastoma and ganglioneuroma. In: Pathology of tumours. New York: Appleton-Century-Crofts; 1967.
2. Brodeur GM, Hogarty MD, Moose YP, Maris JM. Neuroblastoma. In: Pizzo PA, Poplack DG, editors. Principles and practice of pediatric oncology. Philadelphia: Lippincott Williams & Wilkins; 2011. p. 886–922.
3. Bosse KR, Maris JM. Advances in the translational genomics of neuroblastoma: From improving risk stratification and revealing novel biology to identifying actionable genomic alterations. Cancer. 2016;122(1):20–33. https://doi.org/10.1002/cncr.29706.
4. Matthay KK, Maris JM, Schleiermacher G, Nakagawara A, Mackall CL, Diller L, Weiss WA. Neuroblastoma. Nat Rev Dis Primers. 2016;2:16078. https://doi.org/10.1038/nrdp.2016.78.
5. Shimada H, Ambros IM, Dehner LP, Hata J, Joshi VV, Roald B, Stram DO, Gerbing RB, Lukens JN, Matthay KK, Castleberry RP. The International Neuroblastoma Pathology Classification (the Shimada system). Cancer. 1999;86(2):364–72. https://doi.org/10.1002/(SICI)1097-0142(19990715)86:2<364::AID-CNCR21>3.0.CO;2-7.
6. Shimada H, Ambros IM, Dehner LP, Hata J, Joshi VV, Roald B. Terminology and morphologic criteria of neuroblastic tumors: recommendations by the International Neuroblastoma Pathology Committee. Cancer. 1999;86(2):349–63.
7. Peuchmaur M, d'Amore ES, Joshi VV, Hata J, Roald B, Dehner LP, Gerbing RB, Stram DO, Lukens JN, Matthay KK, Shimada H. Revision of the International Neuroblastoma Pathology Classification: confirmation of favorable and unfavorable prognostic subsets in ganglioneuroblastoma, nodular. Cancer. 2003;98(10):2274–81. https://doi.org/10.1002/cncr.11773.
8. Liu S, Tian Y, Chlenski A, Yang Q, Zage P, Salwen HR, Crawford SE, Cohn SL. Cross-talk between Schwann cells and neuroblasts influences the biology of neuroblastoma xenografts. Am J Pathol. 2005;166(3):891–900. https://doi.org/10.1016/S0002-9440(10)62309-7.
9. Brodeur GM, Minturn JE, Ho R, Simpson AM, Iyer R, Varela CR, Light JE, Kolla V, Evans AE. Trk receptor expression and inhibition in neuroblastomas. Clin Cancer Res. 2009;15(10):3244–50. https://doi.org/10.1158/1078-0432.CCR-08-1815.
10. Pajtler KW, Mahlow E, Odersky A, Lindner S, Stephan H, Bendix I, Eggert A, Schramm A, Schulte JH. Neuroblastoma in dialog with its stroma: NTRK1 is a regulator of cellular cross-talk with Schwann cells. Oncotarget. 2014;5(22):11180–92. https://doi.org/10.18632/oncotarget.2611.
11. Shimada H, Umehara S, Monobe Y, Hachitanda Y, Nakagawa A, Goto S, Gerbing RB, Stram DO, Lukens JN, Matthay KK. International neuroblastoma pathology classification for prognostic evaluation of patients with peripheral neuroblastic tumors: a report from the Children's Cancer Group. Cancer. 2001;92(9):2451–61. https://doi.org/10.1002/1097-0142(20011101)92:9<2451::AID-CNCR1595>3.0.CO;2-S.
12. Teshiba R, Kawano S, Wang LL, He L, Naranjo A, London WB, Seeger RC, Gastier-Foster JM, Look AT, Hogarty MD, Cohn SL, Maris JM, Park JR, Shimada H. Age-dependent prognostic effect by Mitosis-Karyorrhexis Index in neuroblastoma: a report from the Children's Oncology Group. Pediatr Dev Pathol. 2014;17(6):441–9. https://doi.org/10.2350/14-06-1505-OA.1.

13. Shimada H, Stram DO, Chatten J, Joshi VV, Hachitanda Y, Brodeur GM, Lukens JN, Matthay KK, Seeger RC. Identification of subsets of neuroblastomas by combined histopathologic and N-myc analysis. J Natl Cancer Inst. 1995;87(19):1470–6.
14. Goto S, Umehara S, Gerbing RB, Stram DO, Brodeur GM, Seeger RC, Lukens JN, Matthay KK, Shimada H. Histopathology (International Neuroblastoma Pathology Classification) and MYCN status in patients with peripheral neuroblastic tumors: a report from the Children's Cancer Group. Cancer. 2001;92(10):2699–708.
15. Sano H, Bonadio J, Gerbing RB, London WB, Matthay KK, Lukens JN, Shimada H. International neuroblastoma pathology classification adds independent prognostic information beyond the prognostic contribution of age. Eur J Cancer. 2006;42(8):1113–9. https://doi.org/10.1016/j.ejca.2005.11.031.
16. Spitz R, Hero B, Skowron M, Ernestus K, Berthold F. MYCN-status in neuroblastoma: characteristics of tumours showing amplification, gain, and non-amplification. Eur J Cancer. 2004;40(18):2753–9. https://doi.org/10.1016/j.ejca.2004.05.002.
17. Campbell K, Gastier-Foster JM, Mann M, Naranjo AH, Van Ryn C, Bagatell R, Matthay KK, London WB, Irwin MS, Shimada H, Granger MM, Hogarty MD, Park JR, DuBois SG. Association of MYCN copy number with clinical features, tumor biology, and outcomes in neuroblastoma: a report from the Children's Oncology Group. Cancer. 2017;123(21):4224–35. https://doi.org/10.1002/cncr.30873.
18. Wang LL, Teshiba R, Ikegaki N, Tang XX, Naranjo A, London WB, Hogarty MD, Gastier-Foster JM, Look AT, Park JR, Maris JM, Cohn SL, Seeger RC, Asgharzadeh S, Shimada H. Augmented expression of MYC and/or MYCN protein defines highly aggressive MYC-driven neuroblastoma: a Children's Oncology Group study. Br J Cancer. 2015;113(1):57–63. https://doi.org/10.1038/bjc.2015.188.
19. Cheung NK, Zhang J, Lu C, Parker M, Bahrami A, Tickoo SK, Heguy A, Pappo AS, Federico S, Dalton J, Cheung IY, Ding L, Fulton R, Wang J, Chen X, Becksfort J, Wu J, Billups CA, Ellison D, Mardis ER, Wilson RK, Downing JR, Dyer MA, St Jude Children's Research Hospital-Washington University Pediatric Cancer Genome P. Association of age at diagnosis and genetic mutations in patients with neuroblastoma. JAMA. 2012;307(10):1062–71. https://doi.org/10.1001/jama.2012.228.
20. Valentijn LJ, Koster J, Zwijnenburg DA, Hasselt NE, van Sluis P, Volckmann R, van Noesel MM, George RE, Tytgat GA, Molenaar JJ, Versteeg R. TERT rearrangements are frequent in neuroblastoma and identify aggressive tumors. Nat Genet. 2015;47(12):1411–4. https://doi.org/10.1038/ng.3438.
21. Peifer M, Hertwig F, Roels F, Dreidax D, Gartlgruber M, Menon R, Kramer A, Roncaioli JL, Sand F, Heuckmann JM, Ikram F, Schmidt R, Ackermann S, Engesser A, Kahlert Y, Vogel W, Altmuller J, Nurnberg P, Thierry-Mieg J, Thierry-Mieg D, Mariappan A, Heynck S, Mariotti E, Henrich KO, Gloeckner C, Bosco G, Leuschner I, Schweiger MR, Savelyeva L, Watkins SC, Shao C, Bell E, Hofer T, Achter V, Lang U, Theissen J, Volland R, Saadati M, Eggert A, de Wilde B, Berthold F, Peng Z, Zhao C, Shi L, Ortmann M, Buttner R, Perner S, Hero B, Schramm A, Schulte JH, Herrmann C, O'Sullivan RJ, Westermann F, Thomas RK, Fischer M. Telomerase activation by genomic rearrangements in high-risk neuroblastoma. Nature. 2015;526(7575):700–4. https://doi.org/10.1038/nature14980.
22. Wang LL, Suganuma R, Ikegaki N, Tang X, Naranjo A, McGrady P, London WB, Hogarty MD, Gastier-Foster JM, Look AT, Park JR, Maris JM, Cohn SL, Seeger RC, Shimada H. Neuroblastoma of undifferentiated subtype, prognostic significance of prominent nucleolar formation, and MYC/MYCN protein expression: a report from the Children's Oncology Group. Cancer. 2013;119(20):3718–26. https://doi.org/10.1002/cncr.28251.
23. Tornoczky T, Kalman E, Kajtar PG, Nyari T, Pearson AD, Tweddle DA, Board J, Shimada H. Large cell neuroblastoma: a distinct phenotype of neuroblastoma with aggressive clinical behavior. Cancer. 2004;100(2):390–7. https://doi.org/10.1002/cncr.20005.
24. Ikegaki N, Shimada H, Fox AM, Regan PL, Jacobs JR, Hicks SL, Rappaport EF, Tang XX. Transient treatment with epigenetic modifiers yields stable neuroblastoma stem cells resembling aggressive large-cell neuroblastomas. Proc Natl Acad Sci U S A. 2013;110(15):6097–102. https://doi.org/10.1073/pnas.1118262110.
25. Koh CM, Khattar E, Leow SC, Liu CY, Muller J, Ang WX, Li Y, Franzoso G, Li S, Guccione E, Tergaonkar V. Telomerase regulates MYC-driven oncogenesis independent of its reverse transcriptase activity. J Clin Invest. 2015;125(5):2109–22. https://doi.org/10.1172/JCI79134.
26. Wu KJ, Grandori C, Amacker M, Simon-Vermot N, Polack A, Lingner J, Dalla-Favera R. Direct activation of TERT transcription by c-MYC. Nat Genet. 1999;21(2):220–4. https://doi.org/10.1038/6010.
27. Lindner S, Bachmann HS, Odersky A, Schaefers S, Klein-Hitpass L, Hero B, Fischer M, Eggert A, Schramm A, Schulte JH. Absence of telomerase reverse transcriptase promoter mutations in neuroblastoma. Biomed Rep. 2015;3(4):443–6. https://doi.org/10.3892/br.2015.463.
28. Lindsey JC, Schwalbe EC, Potluri S, Bailey S, Williamson D, Clifford SC. TERT promoter mutation and aberrant hypermethylation are associated with elevated expression in medulloblastoma and characterise the majority of non-infant SHH subgroup tumours. Acta Neuropathol. 2014;127(2):307–9. https://doi.org/10.1007/s00401-013-1225-3.
29. Lee S, Borah S, Bahrami A. Detection of aberrant TERT promoter methylation by combined bisulfite restriction enzyme analysis for cancer diagno-

sis. J Mol Diagn. 2017;19(3):378–86. https://doi.org/10.1016/j.jmoldx.2017.01.003.
30. Salomoni P. The PML-interacting protein DAXX: histone loading gets into the picture. Front Oncol. 2013;3:152. https://doi.org/10.3389/fonc.2013.00152.
31. Darnell JE Jr. Transcription factors as targets for cancer therapy. Nat Rev Cancer. 2002;2(10):740–9. https://doi.org/10.1038/nrc906.
32. Berg T, Cohen SB, Desharnais J, Sonderegger C, Maslyar DJ, Goldberg J, Boger DL, Vogt PK. Small-molecule antagonists of Myc/Max dimerization inhibit Myc-induced transformation of chicken embryo fibroblasts. Proc Natl Acad Sci U S A. 2002;99(6):3830–5. https://doi.org/10.1073/pnas.062036999.
33. Muller I, Larsson K, Frenzel A, Oliynyk G, Zirath H, Prochownik EV, Westwood NJ, Henriksson MA. Targeting of the MYCN protein with small molecule c-MYC inhibitors. PLoS One. 2014;9(5):e97285. https://doi.org/10.1371/journal.pone.0097285.
34. Chauhan J, Wang H, Yap JL, Sabato PE, Hu A, Prochownik EV, Fletcher S. Discovery of methyl 4′-methyl-5-(7-nitrobenzo [c][1, 2, 5] oxadiazol-4-yl)-[1, 1′-biphenyl]-3-carboxylate, an improved small-molecule inhibitor of c-Myc–Max dimerization. ChemMedChem. 2014;9(10):2274–85.
35. Wang H, Hammoudeh DI, Follis AV, Reese BE, Lazo JS, Metallo SJ, Prochownik EV. Improved low molecular weight Myc-Max inhibitors. Mol Cancer Ther. 2007;6(9):2399–408. https://doi.org/10.1158/1535-7163.MCT-07-0005.
36. Perini G, Diolaiti D, Porro A, Della Valle G. In vivo transcriptional regulation of N-Myc target genes is controlled by E-box methylation. Proc Natl Acad Sci U S A. 2005;102(34):12117–22.
37. Benabou S, Ferreira R, Avino A, Gonzalez C, Lyonnais S, Sola M, Eritja R, Jaumot J, Gargallo R. Solution equilibria of cytosine- and guanine-rich sequences near the promoter region of the n-myc gene that contain stable hairpins within lateral loops. Biochim Biophys Acta. 2014;1840(1):41–52. https://doi.org/10.1016/j.bbagen.2013.08.028.
38. Brooks TA, Hurley LH. Targeting MYC expression through G-quadruplexes. Genes Cancer. 2010;1(6):641–9. https://doi.org/10.1177/1947601910377493.
39. Delmore JE, Issa GC, Lemieux ME, Rahl PB, Shi J, Jacobs HM, Kastritis E, Gilpatrick T, Paranal RM, Qi J, Chesi M, Schinzel AC, McKeown MR, Heffernan TP, Vakoc CR, Bergsagel PL, Ghobrial IM, Richardson PG, Young RA, Hahn WC, Anderson KC, Kung AL, Bradner JE, Mitsiades CS. BET bromodomain inhibition as a therapeutic strategy to target c-Myc. Cell. 2011;146(6):904–17. https://doi.org/10.1016/j.cell.2011.08.017.
40. Puissant A, Frumm SM, Alexe G, Bassil CF, Qi J, Chanthery YH, Nekritz EA, Zeid R, Gustafson WC, Greninger P, Garnett MJ, McDermott U, Benes CH, Kung AL, Weiss WA, Bradner JE, Stegmaier K. Targeting MYCN in neuroblastoma by BET bromodomain inhibition. Cancer Discov. 2013;3(3):308–23. https://doi.org/10.1158/2159-8290.CD-12-0418.
41. Christensen CL, Kwiatkowski N, Abraham BJ, Carretero J, Al-Shahrour F, Zhang T, Chipumuro E, Herter-Sprie GS, Akbay EA, Altabef A, Zhang J, Shimamura T, Capelletti M, Reibel JB, Cavanaugh JD, Gao P, Liu Y, Michaelsen SR, Poulsen HS, Aref AR, Barbie DA, Bradner JE, George RE, Gray NS, Young RA, Wong KK. Targeting transcriptional addictions in small cell lung cancer with a covalent CDK7 inhibitor. Cancer Cell. 2014;26(6):909–22. https://doi.org/10.1016/j.ccell.2014.10.019.
42. Chipumuro E, Marco E, Christensen CL, Kwiatkowski N, Zhang T, Hatheway CM, Abraham BJ, Sharma B, Yeung C, Altabef A, Perez-Atayde A, Wong KK, Yuan GC, Gray NS, Young RA, George RE. CDK7 inhibition suppresses super-enhancer-linked oncogenic transcription in MYCN-driven cancer. Cell. 2014;159(5):1126–39. https://doi.org/10.1016/j.cell.2014.10.024.
43. Gustafson WC, Meyerowitz JG, Nekritz EA, Chen J, Benes C, Charron E, Simonds EF, Seeger R, Matthay KK, Hertz NT, Eilers M, Shokat KM, Weiss WA. Drugging MYCN through an allosteric transition in Aurora kinase A. Cancer Cell. 2014;26(3):414–27. https://doi.org/10.1016/j.ccr.2014.07.015.
44. Burotto M, Chiou VL, Lee JM, Kohn EC. The MAPK pathway across different malignancies: a new perspective. Cancer. 2014;120(22):3446–56. https://doi.org/10.1002/cncr.28864.
45. Manning BD, Toker A. AKT/PKB signaling: navigating the network. Cell. 2017;169(3):381–405. https://doi.org/10.1016/j.cell.2017.04.001.
46. Cammas A, Millevoi S. RNA G-quadruplexes: emerging mechanisms in disease. Nucleic Acids Res. 2017;45(4):1584–95. https://doi.org/10.1093/nar/gkw1280.
47. Wolfe AL, Singh K, Zhong Y, Drewe P, Rajasekhar VK, Sanghvi VR, Mavrakis KJ, Jiang M, Roderick JE, Van der Meulen J. RNA G-quadruplexes cause eIF4A-dependent oncogene translation in cancer. Nature. 2014;513(7516):65.
48. Siddiqui-Jain A, Grand CL, Bearss DJ, Hurley LH. Direct evidence for a G-quadruplex in a promoter region and its targeting with a small molecule to repress c-MYC transcription. Proc Natl Acad Sci U S A. 2002;99(18):11593–8. https://doi.org/10.1073/pnas.182256799.
49. Sun D, Liu WJ, Guo K, Rusche JJ, Ebbinghaus S, Gokhale V, Hurley LH. The proximal promoter region of the human vascular endothelial growth factor gene has a G-quadruplex structure that can be targeted by G-quadruplex-interactive agents. Mol Cancer Ther. 2008;7(4):880–9. https://doi.org/10.1158/1535-7163.MCT-07-2119.
50. Ruggiero E, Richter SN. G-quadruplexes and G-quadruplex ligands: targets and tools in antiviral therapy. Nucleic Acids Res. 2018;46(7):3270–83. https://doi.org/10.1093/nar/gky187.

51. Pagano B, Amato J, Iaccarino N, Cingolani C, Zizza P, Biroccio A, Novellino E, Randazzo A. Looking for efficient G-quadruplex ligands: evidence for selective stabilizing properties and telomere damage by drug-like molecules. ChemMedChem. 2015;10(4):640–9. https://doi.org/10.1002/cmdc.201402552.
52. Drygin D, Siddiqui-Jain A, O'Brien S, Schwaebe M, Lin A, Bliesath J, Ho CB, Proffitt C, Trent K, Whitten JP, Lim JK, Von Hoff D, Anderes K, Rice WG. Anticancer activity of CX-3543: a direct inhibitor of rRNA biogenesis. Cancer Res. 2009;69(19):7653–61. https://doi.org/10.1158/0008-5472.CAN-09-1304.
53. Xu H, Di Antonio M, McKinney S, Mathew V, Ho B, O'Neil NJ, Santos ND, Silvester J, Wei V, Garcia J, Kabeer F, Lai D, Soriano P, Banath J, Chiu DS, Yap D, Le DD, Ye FB, Zhang A, Thu K, Soong J, Lin SC, Tsai AH, Osako T, Algara T, Saunders DN, Wong J, Xian J, Bally MB, Brenton JD, Brown GW, Shah SP, Cescon D, Mak TW, Caldas C, Stirling PC, Hieter P, Balasubramanian S, Aparicio S. CX-5461 is a DNA G-quadruplex stabilizer with selective lethality in BRCA1/2 deficient tumours. Nat Commun. 2017;8:14432. https://doi.org/10.1038/ncomms14432.
54. Local A, Zhang H, Benbatoul KD, Folger P, Sheng X, Tsai C-Y, Howell SB, Rice WG. APTO-253 stabilizes G-quadruplex DNA, inhibits MYC expression and induces DNA damage in acute myeloid leukemia cells. Mol Cancer Ther. 2018;17(6):1177–86.
55. Zippo A, Serafini R, Rocchigiani M, Pennacchini S, Krepelova A, Oliviero S. Histone crosstalk between H3S10ph and H4K16ac generates a histone code that mediates transcription elongation. Cell. 2009;138(6):1122–36.
56. Chapuy B, McKeown MR, Lin CY, Monti S, Roemer MG, Qi J, Rahl PB, Sun HH, Yeda KT, Doench JG. Discovery and characterization of super-enhancer-associated dependencies in diffuse large B cell lymphoma. Cancer Cell. 2013;24(6):777–90.
57. Yang Z, Yik JH, Chen R, He N, Jang MK, Ozato K, Zhou Q. Recruitment of P-TEFb for stimulation of transcriptional elongation by the bromodomain protein Brd4. Mol Cell. 2005;19(4):535–45.
58. Dave K, Sur I, Yan J, Zhang J, Kaasinen E, Zhong F, Blaas L, Li X, Kharazi S, Gustafsson C. Mice deficient of Myc super-enhancer region reveal differential control mechanism between normal and pathological growth. elife. 2017;6:e23382.
59. Henssen A, Althoff K, Odersky A, Beckers A, Koche R, Speleman F, Schäfers S, Bell E, Nortmeyer M, Westermann F. Targeting MYCN-driven transcription by BET-bromodomain inhibition. Clin Cancer Res. 2015;22(10):2470–81.
60. Larochelle S, Chen J, Knights R, Pandur J, Morcillo P, Erdjument-Bromage H, Tempst P, Suter B, Fisher RP. T-loop phosphorylation stabilizes the CDK7–cyclin H–MAT1 complex in vivo and regulates its CTD kinase activity. EMBO J. 2001;20(14):3749–59.
61. Compe E, Egly J-M. TFIIH: when transcription met DNA repair. Nat Rev Mol Cell Biol. 2012;13(6):343.
62. Jonkers I, Lis JT. Getting up to speed with transcription elongation by RNA polymerase II. Nat Rev Mol Cell Biol. 2015;16(3):167.
63. Lu H, Xue Y, Yu GK, Arias C, Lin J, Fong S, Faure M, Weisburd B, Ji X, Mercier A, Sutton J, Luo K, Gao Z, Zhou Q. Compensatory induction of MYC expression by sustained CDK9 inhibition via a BRD4-dependent mechanism. elife. 2015;4:e06535. https://doi.org/10.7554/eLife.06535.
64. Richards MW, Burgess SG, Poon E, Carstensen A, Eilers M, Chesler L, Bayliss R. Structural basis of N-Myc binding by Aurora-A and its destabilization by kinase inhibitors. Proc Natl Acad Sci. 2016;113(48):13726–31.
65. Mossé YP, Lipsitz E, Fox E, Teachey DT, Maris JM, Weigel B, Adamson PC, Ingle MA, Ahern CH, Blaney SM. Pediatric phase I trial and pharmacokinetic study of MLN8237, an investigational oral selective small-molecule inhibitor of Aurora kinase A: a Children's Oncology Group Phase I Consortium study. Clin Cancer Res. 2012;18(21):6058–64.
66. Takeda. Takeda announces termination of alisertib phase 3 trial in relapsed or refractory peripheral T-cell lymphoma. News Releases. 2015. https://www.takeda.com/newsroom/newsreleases/2015/takeda-announces-termination-of-alisertib-phase-2013-trial-in-relapsed-or-refractory-peripheral-t-cell--lymphoma/.
67. Nissan MH, Rosen N, Solit DB. ERK pathway inhibitors: how low should we go? Cancer Discov. 2013;3(7):719–21.
68. Janku F, Yap TA, Meric-Bernstam F. Targeting the PI3K pathway in cancer: are we making headway? Nat Rev Clin Oncol. 2018;15(5):273–91.
69. Tasian SK, Teachey DT, Rheingold SR. Targeting the PI3K/mTOR pathway in pediatric hematologic malignancies. Front Oncol. 2014;4:108.
70. Biffi G, Di Antonio M, Tannahill D, Balasubramanian S. Visualization and selective chemical targeting of RNA G-quadruplex structures in the cytoplasm of human cells. Nat Chem. 2014;6(1):75–80.
71. Niemas-Teshiba R, Matsuno R, Wang LL, Tang XX, Chiu B, Zeki J, Coburn J, Ornell K, Naranjo A, Van Ryn C, London WB, Hogarty MD, Gastier-Foster JM, Look AT, Park JR, Maris JM, Cohn SL, Seeger RC, Asgharzadeh S, Ikegaki N, Shimada H. MYC-family protein overexpression and prominent nucleolar formation represent prognostic indicators and potential therapeutic targets for aggressive high-MKI neuroblastomas: a report from the Children's Oncology Group. Oncotarget. 2018;9(5):6416–32. https://doi.org/10.18632/oncotarget.23740.
72. Hein N, Hannan KM, George AJ, Sanij E, Hannan RD. The nucleolus: an emerging target for cancer therapy. Trends Mol Med. 2013;19(11):643–54. https://doi.org/10.1016/j.molmed.2013.07.005.
73. de Jonge MJ, Dumez H, Verweij J, Yarkoni S, Snyder D, Lacombe D, Marreaud S, Yamaguchi T, Punt CJ,

van Oosterom A, Group EN. Phase I and pharmacokinetic study of halofuginone, an oral quinazolinone derivative in patients with advanced solid tumours. Eur J Cancer. 2006;42(12):1768–74. https://doi.org/10.1016/j.ejca.2005.12.027.
74. Drygin D, Lin A, Bliesath J, Ho CB, O'Brien SE, Proffitt C, Omori M, Haddach M, Schwaebe MK, Siddiqui-Jain A, Streiner N, Quin JE, Sanij E, Bywater MJ, Hannan RD, Ryckman D, Anderes K, Rice WG. Targeting RNA polymerase I with an oral small molecule CX-5461 inhibits ribosomal RNA synthesis and solid tumor growth. Cancer Res. 2011;71(4):1418–30. https://doi.org/10.1158/0008-5472.CAN-10-1728.
75. Dai MS, Arnold H, Sun XX, Sears R, Lu H. Inhibition of c-Myc activity by ribosomal protein L11. EMBO J. 2007;26(14):3332–45. https://doi.org/10.1038/sj.emboj.7601776.
76. Liao JM, Zhou X, Gatignol A, Lu H. Ribosomal proteins L5 and L11 co-operatively inactivate c-Myc via RNA-induced silencing complex. Oncogene. 2014;33(41):4916–23. https://doi.org/10.1038/onc.2013.430.
77. Keller TL, Zocco D, Sundrud MS, Hendrick M, Edenius M, Yum J, Kim YJ, Lee HK, Cortese JF, Wirth DF, Dignam JD, Rao A, Yeo CY, Mazitschek R, Whitman M. Halofuginone and other febrifugine derivatives inhibit prolyl-tRNA synthetase. Nat Chem Biol. 2012;8(3):311–7. https://doi.org/10.1038/nchembio.790.
78. Sundrud MS, Koralov SB, Feuerer M, Calado DP, Kozhaya AE, Rhule-Smith A, Lefebvre RE, Unutmaz D, Mazitschek R, Waldner H, Whitman M, Keller T, Rao A. Halofuginone inhibits TH17 cell differentiation by activating the amino acid starvation response. Science. 2009;324(5932):1334–8. https://doi.org/10.1126/science.1172638.
79. Kim DG, Lee JY, Lee JH, Cho HY, Kang BS, Jang SY, Kim MH, Guo M, Han JM, Kim SJ, Kim S. Oncogenic mutation of AIMP2/p38 inhibits its tumor-suppressive interaction with Smurf2. Cancer Res. 2016;76(11):3422–36. https://doi.org/10.1158/0008-5472.CAN-15-3255.
80. Zhou W, Chung YJ, Parrilla Castellar ER, Zheng Y, Chung HJ, Bandle R, Liu J, Tessarollo L, Batchelor E, Aplan PD, Levens D. Far upstream element binding protein plays a crucial role in embryonic development, hematopoiesis, and stabilizing myc expression levels. Am J Pathol. 2016;186(3):701–15. https://doi.org/10.1016/j.ajpath.2015.10.028.
81. Wilhelm S, Carter C, Lynch M, Lowinger T, Dumas J, Smith RA, Schwartz B, Simantov R, Kelley S. Discovery and development of sorafenib: a multikinase inhibitor for treating cancer. Nat Rev Drug Discov. 2006;5(10):835–44. https://doi.org/10.1038/nrd2130.
82. Inoue H, Hwang SH, Wecksler AT, Hammock BD, Weiss RH. Sorafenib attenuates p21 in kidney cancer cells and augments cell death in combination with DNA-damaging chemotherapy. Cancer Biol Ther. 2011;12(9):827–36. https://doi.org/10.4161/cbt.12.9.17680.
83. Gupta R, Dong Y, Solomon PD, Wettersten HI, Cheng CJ, Min JN, Henson J, Dogra SK, Hwang SH, Hammock BD, Zhu LJ, Reddel RR, Saltzman WM, Weiss RH, Chang S, Green MR, Wajapeyee N. Synergistic tumor suppression by combined inhibition of telomerase and CDKN1A. Proc Natl Acad Sci U S A. 2014;111(30):E3062–71. https://doi.org/10.1073/pnas.1411370111.
84. Cheung NK, Dyer MA. Neuroblastoma: developmental biology, cancer genomics and immunotherapy. Nat Rev Cancer. 2013;13(6):397–411. https://doi.org/10.1038/nrc3526.
85. Flynn RL, Cox KE, Jeitany M, Wakimoto H, Bryll AR, Ganem NJ, Bersani F, Pineda JR, Suva ML, Benes CH, Haber DA, Boussin FD, Zou L. Alternative lengthening of telomeres renders cancer cells hypersensitive to ATR inhibitors. Science. 2015;347(6219):273–7. https://doi.org/10.1126/science.1257216.
86. Guzi TJ, Paruch K, Dwyer MP, Labroli M, Shanahan F, Davis N, Taricani L, Wiswell D, Seghezzi W, Penaflor E, Bhagwat B, Wang W, Gu D, Hsieh Y, Lee S, Liu M, Parry D. Targeting the replication checkpoint using SCH 900776, a potent and functionally selective CHK1 inhibitor identified via high content screening. Mol Cancer Ther. 2011;10(4):591–602. https://doi.org/10.1158/1535-7163.MCT-10-0928.
87. Negi SS, Brown P. rRNA synthesis inhibitor, CX-5461, activates ATM/ATR pathway in acute lymphoblastic leukemia, arrests cells in G2 phase and induces apoptosis. Oncotarget. 2015;6(20):18094–104. https://doi.org/10.18632/oncotarget.4093.
88. Ikegaki N, Shimada H, International Neuroblastoma Pathology Committee. Subgrouping of unfavorable histology neuroblastomas with immunohistochemistry toward precision prognosis and therapy stratification. JCO Precis Oncol. 2019;3:1–7. https://doi.org/10.1200/PO.18.00312.

Genetic Predisposition

3

Apexa Modi, Emily Blauel, and Sharon J. Diskin

3.1 Familial Neuroblastoma

Familial neuroblastoma was first described in the late 1960s and early 1970s when several families with multiple generations of neuroblastoma were reported [1–3]. It is now estimated that 1–2% of neuroblastoma cases are familial and follow an autosomal dominant inheritance pattern with incomplete penetrance. Clinically, these patients present at a younger age and with multiple primary tumor sites, a phenomenon seen in other cancer predisposition syndromes [4–6]. The majority of familial neuroblastoma cases harbor inherited activating mutations in the anaplastic lymphoma kinase gene (*ALK*), while another small percentage are explained by inherited inactivating mutations in the paired-like homeobox 2B gene (*PHOX2B*). Importantly, mutations are of variable penetrance, suggesting that additional genetic interactions likely determine individual phenotypes. These rare families have provided a unique opportunity to discover genetic drivers of neuroblastoma with a large effect size and have led to a deeper understanding of the pathways driving tumorigenesis, more precise risk stratification, and novel therapeutic strategies. Table 3.1 summarizes the mutations identified to date. Genetic testing for *ALK* and *PHOX2B* mutations has become the standard of care for children with a family history of the disease. Ongoing efforts

A. Modi
Genomics and Computational Biology, Biomedical Graduate Studies, Perelman School of Medicine, University of Pennsylvania, Philadelphia, PA, USA

Division of Oncology, Children's Hospital of Philadelphia, Philadelphia, PA, USA

Center for Childhood Cancer Research, Children's Hospital of Philadelphia, Philadelphia, PA, USA

E. Blauel
Division of Oncology, Children's Hospital of Philadelphia, Philadelphia, PA, USA

Center for Childhood Cancer Research, Children's Hospital of Philadelphia, Philadelphia, PA, USA

Department of Pediatrics, Perelman School of Medicine, University of Pennsylvania, Philadelphia, PA, USA

S. J. Diskin (✉)
Genomics and Computational Biology, Biomedical Graduate Studies, Perelman School of Medicine, University of Pennsylvania, Philadelphia, PA, USA

Division of Oncology, Children's Hospital of Philadelphia, Philadelphia, PA, USA

Center for Childhood Cancer Research, Children's Hospital of Philadelphia, Philadelphia, PA, USA

Department of Pediatrics, Perelman School of Medicine, University of Pennsylvania, Philadelphia, PA, USA

Abramson Family Cancer Research Institute, Perelman School of Medicine, University of Pennsylvania, Philadelphia, PA, USA
e-mail: diskin@chop.edu

S. Asgharzadeh, F. Westermann (eds.), *Neuroblastoma*, Pediatric Oncology,
https://doi.org/10.1007/978-3-031-51292-6_3

Table 3.1 Germline mutations in familial neuroblastoma predisposition genes

Gene	Mutation	Clinical characteristics	Functional consequence	References
PHOX2B	R100L	Found in families with Hirschsprung disease and neuroblastic tumors	Missense mutation in DNA binding domain. Not dominant negative	[7] [8] [9]
	R141G	Neuroblastoma patient inherited from mother, who was not affected	Missense mutation in homeodomain	[7]
	G197D	Present in a family with multiple individuals with neuroblastoma but no evidence of autonomic dysfunction or neurocristopathy	Unknown	[10]
	676delG	Found in families with Hirschsprung disease and neuroblastoma	Overexpression causes decrease in terminal differentiation markers in sympathetic ganglion cells. Dominant negative. Unable to bind HPCAL1	[11] [9] [12]
	Polyalanine repeat mutations	Associated with congenital central hypoventilation syndrome (CCHS)	Genotype 20/33 identified in a neuroblastoma/CCHS/Hirschsprung disease patient	[13]
ALK	R1060H	Unlikely to be clinically significant. Believed to be a silent/passenger mutation	Not predicted to be damaging by algorithms. Between kinase and transmembrane domains	[14]
	G1128A	Not specified	P-loop of kinase domain Transforms NIH-3T3 cells	[15]
	T1151M T1151R	T1151R found in patient with multifocal tumors	Promotes modest constitutive ALK activation. Does not transform NIH-3T3 cells β3 Strand of kinase domain	[6] [14]
	I1183T	Unlikely to be clinically significant. Thought to be a silent/passenger mutation	N-lobe of kinase domain	[14]
	R1192P	Found in patient with multifocal tumors	β4 Strand of kinase domain. Increases k_{cat} of non-phosphorylated ALK tyrosine kinase domain by 15×. Transforms NIH-3T3 cells	[15] [6] [14]
	L1204F	Unlikely to be clinically significant. Thought to be a silent/passenger mutation	C-lobe of kinase domain	[14]
	R1231Q	Unlikely to be clinically significant. Thought to be a silent/passenger mutation	Not predicted to be damaging by algorithms αE helix of kinase domain	[14]
	I1250T	Unlikely to be clinically significant. Thought to be a silent/passenger mutation	"Kinase dead" mutation that results in reduced activity via protein instability/misfolding Phe core domain	[16] [14]
	R1275Q	Crizotinib-sensitive. Found in patient with multifocal tumors	R1275 residue accounts for ~45% of overall neuroblastoma ALK mutations (somatic and germline). Activation loop of kinase domain	[15] [17] [6]

ALK anaplastic lymphoma kinase, *PHOX2B* paired-like homeobox 2B, *HPCAL1* Hippocalcin-like protein 1

are focused on discovering the genetic cause in the ~10–15% of familial cases without an identifiable mutation in *ALK* or *PHOX2B*.

3.1.1 PHOX2B

A small subset of neuroblastoma cases present in children with co-existing anomalies of neural crest derived tissues, or neurocristopothies, such as Hirschsprung disease and congenital central hypoventilation syndrome (CCHS) [18, 19]. In 2003, frameshift mutations in the paired-like homeobox 2B gene (*PHOX2B*) were described in patients with CCHS [20]. In 2004, germline PHOX2B mutations were also identified in neuroblastoma patients, making *PHOX2B* the first *bona fide* neuroblastoma predisposition gene [7, 11]. This discovery prompted further work on the effect of *PHOX2B* germline mutations and phenotypic differences of individual mutations. The *PHOX2B* gene is mapped to chromosome 4p12 and codes for a "master regulator" transcription factor that is involved in neural crest cell differentiation into noradrenergic neurons [21]. Functional studies demonstrated that germline *PHOX2B* mutations lead to a dominant negative block on terminal neural crest differentiation, thereby promoting malignant transformation [9, 22, 23]. Germline *PHOX2B* mutations account for approximately 5–10% of familial neuroblastoma and have also been detected in approximately 2% of sporadic neuroblastoma cases [24, 25].

3.1.2 ALK

The discovery of germline *ALK* mutations in neuroblastoma was first described in 2008 when a large genetic linkage study of twenty families collected through international efforts identified a signal at chromosome 2p23-24 [15]. Re-sequencing of the region revealed several mutations in the kinase domain of *ALK*. The *ALK* gene is located on chromosome 2p23 and codes for a receptor tyrosine kinase receptor that is involved in signaling pathways driving proliferation or differentiation. We now know that germline mutations in *ALK* account for approximately 75% of familial neuroblastoma cases, making *ALK* mutations the predominant familial neuroblastoma predisposition gene. In parallel to the identification of germline mutations in *ALK*, somatic mutations in sporadic neuroblastoma tumors were identified, including both point mutations and DNA copy number amplifications [26–28]. Somatic mutations in *ALK* are also seen in other malignancies, such as anaplastic large cell lymphoma and non-small cell lung carcinoma where translocation events result in activation of *ALK* fusion transcripts [29]. A later comprehensive study of 1596 sporadic primary neuroblastoma tumors revealed that *ALK* is somatically mutated in 8% of cases [14].

These important discoveries prompted further work on the role of *ALK* in neuroblastoma and phenotypic differences of individual mutations. Functional studies demonstrated that recurrent point mutations in the kinase domain of *ALK* result in constitutive activation of the ALK receptor (via phosphorylation) with unregulated downstream signaling in a "gain-of-function" process [30]. Similar to *PHOX2B, ALK* mutations exhibit a strong association between genotype and phenotype; mutations that more strongly activate *ALK* are also more highly penetrant. For example, the germline F1174V mutation is known to potently activate ALK and is also associated clinically with neonatal onset and multifocal disease [14, 31]. Across all neuroblastoma-predisposing *ALK* mutations in the aggregate, penetrance is estimated to be approximately 50% [14, 31]. Additional genetic modifiers influencing to the observed incomplete penetrance remain to be identified. Collectively, these studies identified ALK as an attractive therapeutic target for both small molecule inhibition and immunotherapy, with both modalities currently under study in neuroblastoma [32, 33]. Essential studies of therapy resistance are also being evaluated [34–36].

3.2 Sporadic Neuroblastoma

The vast majority of neuroblastoma cases are considered "sporadic" (non-familial), and we now know that common genetic polymorphisms contribute substantially to disease initiation and phenotypic presentation of this subset. The advent of high density single nucleotide polymorphism (SNP) genotyping using microarrays in 1998 [37] led to a breakthrough in understanding the underlying genetic basis of complex diseases. This technology was utilized to perform genome-wide association studies (GWAS), an approach that involves discovering significant differences in allele frequencies in case-control studies [38]. The first pediatric cancer GWAS was published in 2008 and utilized neuroblastoma samples collected through the Children's Oncology Group [39]. This seminal work provided the first evidence that sporadic neuroblastoma was indeed a genetic disease. Over the next decade, GWAS efforts revealed substantial insights into the genetic basis of sporadic neuroblastoma predisposition (Table 3.2; Fig. 3.1), with certain variants enriched for, or associating with, a specific phenotype. In addition, functional studies of candidate genes at GWAS loci have revealed how germline variants and/or target genes also contribute to maintenance of the malignant phenotype and/or progression of the disease. More recently, large sequencing studies have begun to reveal rare variants in known cancer predisposition genes, predicted to have larger effect size, that may contribute to neuroblastoma pathogenesis. This section reviews our current knowledge of the genetic basis of sporadic neuroblastoma. Ongoing GWAS and sequencing studies will undoubtedly uncover additional genetic determinants of this heterogeneous malignancy and efforts aimed at understanding how common and rare variants interact to drive tumor formation are underway.

Table 3.2 Common variants associated with neuroblastoma

Genomic location	Variant	Candidate gene(s)	*P*-value	Odds ratio (95% CI)	Ref/Alt Allele[a]	MAF[b] European cases/controls	Enriched clinical or biological subset	Populations studied[c]					References
								EA	UK	IT	AA	SC	
Genome-wide association study (most significant SNP from the original study is shown)													
1q21.1	(hg18) chr1: 147,292,384-147,435,422	NBPF23	3.0×10^{-17}	2.49 (2.02–3.05)	143-kb deletion	0.16/0.09	None	✓					[40]
1q23.3	rs1027702	DUSP12[e]	2.1×10^{-6}	2.01 (1.47–2.79)	C/**T**	Not reported	Low-risk	✓		✓			[41]
2q34	rs1033069	SPAG16[f]	6.4×10^{-5}	Not reported	G/**A**	Not reported	High-risk	✓			✓		[42]
2q35	rs6435862	BARD1	8.7×10^{-18}	1.68 (1.49–1.90)	T/**G**	0.40/0.29	High-risk	✓	✓	✓	✓	✓	[43–49]
3p21.31	rs80059929	KIF15	6.5×10^{-12}	2.95 (2.17–4.02)	**A**/T	0.09/0.04	MYCN amp	✓					[50]
3q25	rs6441201	MLF1 RSRC1	1.2×10^{-11}	1.23 (1.16–1.31)	G/**A**	0.52/0.47	None	✓	✓	✓	✓		[51]
4p16	rs3796727	CPZ	1.3×10^{-12}	1.30 (1.21–1.40)	G/**A**	0.35/0.30	None	✓	✓	✓			[51]
5q11.2	rs2619046	DDX4[e]	2.9×10^{-6}	1.48 (1.21–1.79)	C/**T**	Not reported	Low-risk	✓		✓			[41]
5q11.2	rs10055201	IL31RA[e]	6.5×10^{-7}	1.49 (1.23–1.81)	A/**G**	Not reported	Low-risk	✓					[41]
6q16	rs4336470	HACE1	2.7×10^{-11}	1.26 (1.18–1.35)	**C**/T	0.30/0.35	None	✓		✓	✓	✓[i]	[52, 53]
6q16	rs17065417	LIN28B	1.2×10^{-8}	1.38 (1.23–1.54)	**A**/C	0.08/0.11	None	✓		✓	✓	✓[h]	[52, 54–56]
6p22	rs6939340	CASC15 NBAT1	9.3×10^{-15}	1.37 (1.27–1.49)	A/**G**	0.56/0.47	High-risk	✓	✓	✓	✓[g]	✓	[39, 57–60]
11p11.2	rs11037575	HSD17B12[e]	4.2×10^{-7}	1.67 (1.35–2.08)	**C**/T	Not reported	Low-risk	✓		✓		✓	[41, 61]
11p15.4	rs2168101[d]	LMO1	7.5×10^{-29}	0.65 (0.60–0.70)	**G**/T	0.24/0.31	High-risk	✓	✓	✓	✓[g]	✓[h]	[62–65]

(continued)

Table 3.2 (continued)

Genomic location	Variant	Candidate gene(s)	*P*-value	Odds ratio (95% CI)	Ref/Alt Allele[a]	MAF[b] European cases/controls	Enriched clinical or biological subset	Populations studied[c]					References
								EA	UK	IT	AA	SC	
11q22.2	rs10895322	MMP20	2.6×10^{-9}	2.89 (1.99–4.10)	A/**G**	0.16/0.06	11q deletion	✓					[66]
17p13.1	rs35850753	TP53	3.4×10^{-12}	2.7 (2.0–3.6)	T/**C**	0.04/0.02	None	✓		✓	✓		[67]
Candidate gene-based approaches													
8p21	rs1059111	NEFL	4.9×10^{-3}	0.86 (0.77–0.95)	T/**A**	0.12/0.13	None	✓		✓			[68]
12p13	rs34330	CDKN1B	0.002	1.15 (1.06–1.24)	C/**T**	0.26/0.23	None	✓		✓			[69]

[a] Risk allele is displayed in bold
[b] MAF=Minor Allele Frequency
[c] Association replicated unless otherwise noted. *EA* European American, *UK* United Kingdom, *IT* Italian, *AA* African American, *SC* Southern Chinese
[d] This was not the top SNP in the original study, but was demonstrated as the causal SNP in Oldridge et al. 2015
[e] Gene-based study: P-values were calculated at the gene level rather than the SNP level, and allele frequencies were not provided
[f] Case-only study (association with high-risk neuroblastoma was tested): Odds ratio and control MAF were not reported
[g] This association did not replicate
[h] A different SNP at the same locus was analyzed
[i] Association represents a combined analysis of five SNPs

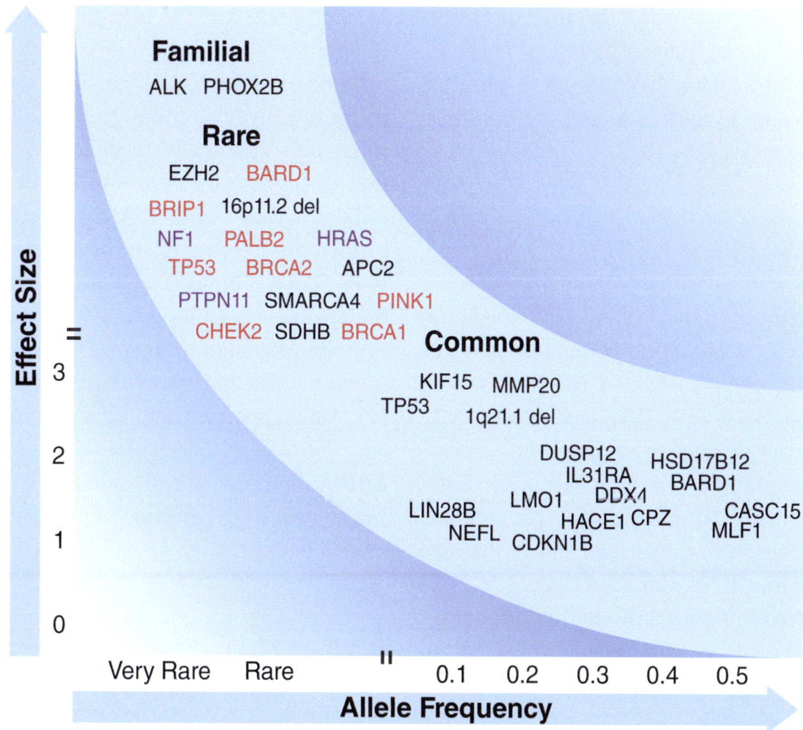

Fig. 3.1 Model of genetic basis of neuroblastoma. Variants contributing to neuroblastoma risk range from very rare variants of large effect (top left) to common variants of small effect (bottom right). Familial mutations in *ALK* and *PHOX2B* have been identified through linkage-based studies and evaluation of cases with associated conditions. Sequencing studies of sporadic neuroblastoma have identified other rare damaging germline variants in cancer-associated genes, but their true frequency and impact is unknown. Notably, several mutations affect genes involved in DNA repair (red) and Ras-MAPK signaling (purple). Common polymorphisms identified through GWAS also predispose to neuroblastoma; these common variants are plotted at the observed minor allele frequencies and odds ratios. Figure modified from Ritenour et al. [70]

3.3 Common Variants Identified by Genome-Wide Association Study (GWAS)

GWAS efforts have identified common DNA alleles associated with neuroblastoma at over a dozen loci (Table 3.2). These genetic associations have implicated an array of candidate genes including cancer susceptibility candidate 15 (*CASC15*), neuroblastoma associated transcript 1 (*NBAT1*), BRCA1 associated RING domain 1 (*BARD1*), LIM domain only 1 (*LMO1*), dual specificity phosphatase 12 (*DUSP12*), DEAD (Asp-Glu-Ala-Asp) box polypeptide 4 (*DDX4*), interleukin 31 receptor A (*IL31RA*), hydroxysteroid (17B) dehydrogenase 12 (*HSD17B12*), HECT domain and ankyrin repeat containing E3 ubiquitin protein ligase 1 (*HACE1*) , lin-28 homolog B (*LIN28B*), tumor protein P53 (*TP53*), arginine/serine-rich coiled-coil 1 (*RSRC1*), myeloid leukemia factor 1 (*MLF1*), carboxypeptidase Z (*CPZ*), matrix metalloproteinase 20 (*MMP20*), kinesin family member 15 (*KIF15*), and the neuroblastoma breakpoint family 23 gene (*NBPF23*) [39–41, 43, 50–52, 62, 66, 67]. Through GWAS efforts, it quickly became apparent that neuroblastoma-associated risk alleles were enriched in distinct disease subsets, suggesting that an inherited genetic basis may partially explain the observed clinical heterogeneity. Moreover, in addition to identifying genes influencing tumor initiation, these studies revealed oncogenes critical for tumor maintenance and progression that may ultimately be exploitable through novel therapies. Here, we highlight several major GWAS-related contributions to our current understanding of neuroblastoma tumorigenesis.

3.3.1 CASC15 and NBAT1

In the first neuroblastoma GWAS, SNP allele frequencies were statistically compared between 1032 neuroblastoma cases and 2034 controls of European ancestry [39]. Variants at the 6p22 locus were found to be associated with neuroblastoma and significantly enriched in the high-risk subset with poor outcome. As genome annotation improved, it was later shown that two long non-coding RNA (lncRNA) genes at 6p22 play a key role in neuroblastoma tumorigenesis. *NBAT1* (previously known as cancer susceptibility candidate 14 gene, *CASC14*) was shown to be differentially expressed between low- and high-risk neuroblastomas, with CpG methylation as its promoter associated with decreased expression in high risk patients [57]. In parallel, Russell et al. showed that the antisense lncRNA, *CASC15* is also down-regulated in high-risk patients, with a short isoform of the gene (*CASC15-S*) being the most abundantly expressed transcript at the 6p22 locus. Silencing of *CASC15-S* increased cell proliferation and migration in vitro [58], while recent studies by Mondal et. al showed that both *CASC15-S* and *NBAT1* bind USP36 to regulate expression of the developmental transcription factor SOX9 [59]. However, a causal variant at the 6p22 locus remains to be identified.

3.3.2 BARD1

The discovery of genetic variants enriched in aggressive disease prompted a second GWAS focused on the high-risk subset of neuroblastoma and identified a strong association within the *BARD1* gene at chromosome 2q25 [43–45]. BARD1 typically forms a heterodimer with BRCA1, increasing its stability, and allowing for tumor suppression via DNA-damage repair [71]. In neuroblastoma, the identified risk alleles correlated with an oncogenic isoform of *BARD1*, referred to as *BARD1β* [46]. *BARD1β* was shown to have growth promoting effects in neuroblastoma cells potentially mediated by its stabilization of the Aurora family of kinases (AURKA) [46]. A causal variant driving splicing has yet to be identified. However, the association of BARD1 with AURKA kinases may provide an avenue for therapeutic targeting given available therapeutics. Recent studies suggest full-length *BARD1* functions as a tumor suppressor in neuroblastoma [47, 48], supporting dual roles for *BARD1* in cancer. Further evidence for the importance of *BARD1* in tumorigenesis is indicated by the identification of rare germline mutations [72], as discussed below.

3.3.3 LMO1

A subsequent GWAS compared 1627 neuroblastoma cases to 3254 controls of European ancestry and identified an association at 11p15.4 mapping to the *LMO1* gene [62]. *LMO1* is part of the LMO family of transcriptional co-regulators (LMO1–4) that have each been implicated as oncogenes in various cancers [73, 74]. Initial studies in patient tumors and cell lines with risk alleles for *LMO1* and/or DNA amplification encompassing the gene, showed increased *LMO1* expression [62]. In vitro knockdown and overexpression studies demonstrated an oncogenic role for LMO1 in neuroblastoma. A later study utilizing genotype imputation in a larger patient cohort identified a causal variant at 11p15.4; this SNP mapped to a region of open chromatin and altered a canonical GATA transcription factor binding site [63]. The protective allele for this non-coding variant, rs2168101, disrupted binding of the GATA3 transcription factor in a neuroblastoma-specific super enhancer region within *LMO1* leading to decreased expression [63]. In contrast, the risk allele promoted GATA3 binding and increased *LMO1* expression. Synergy between LMO1 and MYCN expression was recently described in zebrafish models of neuroblastoma, where co-expression increased penetrance of neuroblastoma to 80% from the 20–30% observed with increased MYCN expression alone [64].

3.3.4 HACE1 and LIN28B

As the number of cases genotyped increased, two new neuroblastoma-associated loci mapping to 6q16-q21 were discovered in 2012 implicating the *HACE1* and *LIN28B* genes [52]. *HACE1* is an E3 ubiquitin ligase thought to be a tumor suppressor in multiple cancers based on its ability to inhibit anchorage-independent growth [75]. The exact role of *HACE1* and underlying genetic variation in neuroblastoma remains to be determined, though decreased *HACE1* expression correlates with reduced survival. *LIN28B* is an RNA-binding protein most widely known for its role in suppressing the let-7 family of miRNAs [76]. The risk alleles at the *LIN28B* locus correlated with increased *LIN28B* expression. Silencing of LIN28B in neuroblastoma cells resulted in decreased cell growth, suggesting an oncogenic role [52]. In parallel to the GWAS identifying a role for *LIN28B* in neuroblastoma, it was shown that LIN28B expression leads to elevated MYCN expression, blocked differentiation of normal neuroblast cells, and induced neuroblastoma in mouse models [54]. More recently, Schnepp et al. showed that LIN28B targets the oncogene RAN, promoting its expression and subsequent phosphorylation of Aurora kinase A, (AURKA) [55]. Altogether, given that LIN28B was independently shown to increase MYCN expression and impact AURKA, a regulatory axis involving LIN28B-RAN-AURKA-MYCN was proposed. Since AURKA has been targeted with small molecule inhibitors [77, 78], a combinatorial therapeutic approach may be possible for this signaling network.

3.3.5 TP53

In an analysis of 10,290 individuals across three independent case-control cohorts identified two SNPs, rs78378222 and rs35850753, very strongly associated with neuroblastoma predisposition [67]. This SNP maps to the 3′ untranslated region of *TP53* and disrupts its polyadenylation signal, destabilizing the *TP53* transcript and resulting in p53 haploinsufficiency [67, 79]. The rs35850753 SNP maps to the 5′ UTR of the Δ133 isoform, a truncated p53 variant that acts uniquely as an oncogene via dominant-negative inhibition of full-length p53 [80]. Thus, this SNP may predispose to neuroblastoma by causing disproportionate transcription or aberrant mRNA stabilization of the oncogenic Δ133p53 variant.

3.3.6 MLF1, RSRC1, and CPZ

Through the use of genome-wide genotype imputation, two new neuroblastoma-susceptibility loci were discovered at chromosome 3q35 in 2017. The first signal mapped to the *RSCR1* and *MLF1* genes and the second at chromosome 4p16 near the *CPZ* gene [51]. CPZ influences Wnt signaling in chick embryos, suggesting a role in development [81]. *RSRC1* has been shown to be involved in brain development and schizophrenia [82], while *MLF1* is overexpressed in AML and lung cancer [83] and shows evidence as an oncogene in neuroblastoma cells [51]. Further study of *CPZ*, *MLF1*, and *RSCR1* are needed to identify causal SNPs and the potential role of these genes in neuroblastoma.

3.3.7 Additional Neuroblastoma-Associated Loci and Genes

Several other studies of neuroblastoma cases genotyped for GWAS purposes have revealed genetic variants driving either overall disease or specific subsets. A gene-based study restricted to low-risk neuroblastoma patients revealed *DUSP12*, *IL31RA*, and *HSD17B12* as putative neuroblastoma predisposition genes enriched in this more benign form of the disease [41]. Besides risk group, neuroblastomas can be stratified based on common chromosomal abnormalities that independently predict poor outcome, including *MYCN* amplification at 2p24 which often correlates with 17q gain and 1p deletion and inversely associates with chr11q deletion. In a comparison of neuroblastoma cases with and without 11q deleted tumors, common variants in *MMP20* were associated with 11q deleted tumors and decreased *MMP20* expression [66]. Similarly, a GWAS study of *MYCN* amplified vs. non-amplified cases identified an association signal at 3p21.31 within *KIF15* [50], further highlighting how stratification based on somatic events can be used to find neuroblastoma subset-specific variants influencing predisposition. SNPs are not the only genetic aberration to be associated with neuroblastoma susceptibility and predisposition, common copy number variation (CNV) has been as well, particularly involving a 140-kb deletion at 1q21.1 [40]. Within the deleted region a novel transcript, *NBPF23*, was discovered with homology to the NBPF family of genes and thought to have tumor suppressive properties [84]. Further study of these genes and the study of CNVs in larger patient cohorts could reveal novel neuroblastoma susceptibility loci. Finally, given the high multiple testing burden of traditional GWAS, to identify genetic variants with moderate effect, a candidate gene analysis was performed with eight a-priori selected genes [68]. A minor allele at 8p21 was found to increase neurofilament light (NEFL) expression, which correlated with increased survival. A more recent study identified a second candidate loci with the risk allele lowering expression of cyclin dependent kinase inhibitor 1B (*CDKN1B*), a cell cycle gene that is known to regulate proliferation and differentiation in neuroblastoma cells [69].

3.3.8 Genetic Susceptibility in Non-European Populations

GWAS discovery efforts to date have focused on cases of European ancestry, due to issues related to statistical power (the majority of neuroblastoma cases collected through the COG are of European descent). However, a retrospective analysis of COG clinical data from 3539 cases revealed that African American and Native American neuroblastoma patients have a significantly higher prevalence of aggressive disease and lower survival rates than those of European, Hispanics, and Asian ancestry [85]. This finding suggested a potential underlying genetic predisposition and a trans-population analysis later confirmed that common genetic variation influences neuroblastoma phenotype and contributes to the observed ethnic disparities in survival [42]. As shown in Table 3.2, many GWAS-identified loci have been studied and replicated in various combinations of cohorts including cases from the United Kingdom, Italy, African Americans, and Southern Chinese. Ongoing GWAS are focused on discovering variants that associate with neuroblastoma in non-European populations. These important studies of under-represented populations have been enabled by years of sample collection and data generation.

3.4 Rare Germline Structural Variants

Large constitutional chromosomal rearrangements have been observed in some neuroblastoma patients, often co-occurring with congenital abnormalities and/or intellectual disability. These structural events include deletions overlapping chromosome bands 1p36 [86, 87] and 11q14–23 [88–90], and duplications of a critical region on chromosome 2p24 [91]. These recurrently observed events correspond to established genomic syndromes, notably monosomy 1p36, partial trisomy 2p, and 11q interstitial deletion syndrome. Isolated reports involving other genomic loci have been observed, but are of uncertain significance [92–96]. Notably, neuroblastoma is overrepresented in Turner syndrome (monosomy X), but underrepresented in triple X syndrome, Klinefelter syndrome (XXY), and Down syndrome, suggesting genes or variants exist on chromosomes X and 21 that may be protective against developing neuroblastoma [97–100]. A recent study of 5,585 neuroblastoma cases and 23,505 cancer-free children as controls identified a 550-Kb deletion at 16p11.2 significantly enriched in neuroblastoma [101]. This deletion corresponds to a known microdeletion syndrome that affects approximately one in 3,000 children and confers risk for diverse developmental phenotypes including autism spectrum disorder and other neurodevelopmental disorders [102–108].

3.5 Rare Variants

Rare germline variants (<1% in the population) are predicted to have a larger effect size and contribute more significantly to neuroblastoma susceptibility than common polymorphisms identified by GWAS [109]. Early reports of genes harboring rare germline variants possibly contributing to neuroblastoma predisposition were reported in the context of genetic syndromes; these include *TP53* in Li Fraumeni syndrome [110], *NF1* in neurofibromatosis type 1 [111], *PTPN11* in Noonan syndrome [112, 113], *HRAS* in Costello syndrome *HRAS* [113], *SDHB* in familial paraganglioma/pheochromocytoma [114], and *EZH2* in Weaver syndrome [115]. In 2013, Pugh et al. published the results of a sequencing study of 240 high-risk neuroblastoma tumors and matched normal samples. In addition to confirming the *TP53* association previously observed, this study showed enrichment of rare germline variants in *CHEK2*, *PINK1*, and *BARD1* [72]. The identification of rare variants in *BARD1* was particularly noteworthy given the established association of common variants at the *BARD1* locus and neuroblastoma [43]. Subsequent studies revealed additional potentially pathogenic germline variants in *BARD1* [116]. Recently, large next-generation germline sequencing efforts have been undertaken to identify rare variants diverse childhood cancers, including neuroblastoma [72, 117–120]. These studies reported rare germline variants in *ALK*, *APC*, *BARD1*, *BRCA1*, *BRCA2*, *PALB2*, *SDHB*, and *SMARCA4,* among other known cancer predisposition genes. Notably, several of the rare variants identified are in genes critical for DNA repair and maintenance of genomic integrity, including *BARD1*, *BRCA1*, *BRCA2*, and *PALB2*. Collectively, these variants suggest that defects in DNA repair may contribute to neuroblastoma pathogenesis. However, with the exception of pathogenic *ALK* mutations, whether these rare variants contribute directly to neuroblastoma or predispose to cancer later in life has yet to be determined.

3.6 Future Directions

Substantial advances have been made to define the genetic basis of neuroblastoma predisposition; however, gaps in our knowledge exist and additional genetic determinants remain to be identified. Figure 3.1 depicts our current understanding of neuroblastoma genetic susceptibility. Variants range from highly penetrant mutations in familial neuroblastoma (top left) to common variants with modest effect size in sporadic cases (bottom right). We can expect additional germline variants, both common and rare, to be identified in the coming years; however, several key questions remain. For example, the "causal" variant(s) at most GWAS loci remain elusive and the interaction of common and rare variants in tumor initiation is unknown. Moreover, we have only a nascent understanding of the clinical and functional relevance of many rare germline mutations in neuroblastoma patients. Heritability of rare mutations has not been studied due to lack of parental DNA, an obstacle being addressed in recent sequencing efforts, such as those supported by the Gabriella Miller Kids First (GMKF) program. Here, germline DNA from hundreds of patient-parent trios will be sequenced, allowing the first assessment of heritability of rare mutations in sporadic neuroblastoma. The coming years will continue to build on the many important discoveries of the past decade with respect to neuroblastoma genetic predisposition.

References

1. Chatten J, Voorhess ML. Familial neuroblastoma. Report of a kindred with multiple disorders, including neuroblastomas in four siblings. N Engl J Med. 1967;277(23):1230–6. https://doi.org/10.1056/NEJM196712072772304.
2. Wong KY, Hanenson IB, Lampkin BC. Familial neuroblastoma. Am J Dis Child. 1971;121(5):415–6.
3. Hardy PC, Nesbit ME Jr. Familial neuroblastoma: report of a kindred with a high incidence of infantile tumors. J Pediatr. 1972;80(1):74–7.

4. Kushner BH, Gilbert F, Helson L. Familial neuroblastoma. Case reports, literature review, and etiologic considerations. Cancer. 1986;57(9):1887–93.
5. Brodeur GM. Neuroblastoma: biological insights into a clinical enigma. Nat Rev Cancer. 2003;3(3):203–16. https://doi.org/10.1038/nrc1014.
6. Bourdeaut F, Ferrand S, Brugieres L, Hilbert M, Ribeiro A, Lacroix L, Benard J, Combaret V, Michon J, Valteau-Couanet D, Isidor B, Rialland X, Poiree M, Defachelles AS, Peuchmaur M, Schleiermacher G, Pierron G, Gauthier-Villars M, Janoueix-Lerosey I, Delattre O, Comite Neuroblastome of the Societe Francaise de C. ALK germline mutations in patients with neuroblastoma: a rare and weakly penetrant syndrome. Eur J Hum Genet. 2012;20(3):291–7. https://doi.org/10.1038/ejhg.2011.195.
7. Trochet D, Bourdeaut F, Janoueix-Lerosey I, Deville A, de Pontual L, Schleiermacher G, Coze C, Philip N, Frebourg T, Munnich A, Lyonnet S, Delattre O, Amiel J. Germline mutations of the paired-like homeobox 2B (PHOX2B) gene in neuroblastoma. Am J Hum Genet. 2004;74(4):761–4. https://doi.org/10.1086/383253.
8. Bourdeaut F, Trochet D, Janoueix-Lerosey I, Ribeiro A, Deville A, Coz C, Michiels JF, Lyonnet S, Amiel J, Delattre O. Germline mutations of the paired-like homeobox 2B (PHOX2B) gene in neuroblastoma. Cancer Lett. 2005;228(1-2):51–8. https://doi.org/10.1016/j.canlet.2005.01.055.
9. Pei D, Luther W, Wang W, Paw BH, Stewart RA, George RE. Distinct neuroblastoma-associated alterations of PHOX2B impair sympathetic neuronal differentiation in zebrafish models. PLoS Genet. 2013;9(6):e1003533. https://doi.org/10.1371/journal.pgen.1003533.
10. McConville C, Reid S, Baskcomb L, Douglas J, Rahman N. PHOX2B analysis in non-syndromic neuroblastoma cases shows novel mutations and genotype-phenotype associations. Am J Med Genet A. 2006;140(12):1297–301. https://doi.org/10.1002/ajmg.a.31278.
11. Mosse YP, Laudenslager M, Khazi D, Carlisle AJ, Winter CL, Rappaport E, Maris JM. Germline PHOX2B mutation in hereditary neuroblastoma. Am J Hum Genet. 2004;75(4):727–30. https://doi.org/10.1086/424530.
12. Wang W, Zhong Q, Teng L, Bhatnagar N, Sharma B, Zhang X, Luther W, Haynes LP, Burgoyne RD, Vidal M, Volchenboum S, Hill DE, George RE. Mutations that disrupt PHOXB interaction with the neuronal calcium sensor HPCAL1 impede cellular differentiation in neuroblastoma. Oncogene. 2014;33(25):3316–24. https://doi.org/10.1038/onc.2013.290.
13. Armstrong AE, Weese-Mayer DE, Mian A, Maris JM, Batra V, Gosiengfiao Y, Reichek J, Madonna MB, Bush JW, Shore RM, Walterhouse DO. Treatment of neuroblastoma in congenital central hypoventilation syndrome with a PHOX2B polyalanine repeat expansion mutation: new twist on a neurocristopathy syndrome. Pediatr Blood Cancer. 2015;62(11):2007–10. https://doi.org/10.1002/pbc.25572.
14. Bresler SC, Weiser DA, Huwe PJ, Park JH, Krytska K, Ryles H, Laudenslager M, Rappaport EF, Wood AC, McGrady PW, Hogarty MD, London WB, Radhakrishnan R, Lemmon MA, Mosse YP. ALK mutations confer differential oncogenic activation and sensitivity to ALK inhibition therapy in neuroblastoma. Cancer Cell. 2014;26(5):682–94. https://doi.org/10.1016/j.ccell.2014.09.019.
15. Mosse YP, Laudenslager M, Longo L, Cole KA, Wood A, Attiyeh EF, Laquaglia MJ, Sennett R, Lynch JE, Perri P, Laureys G, Speleman F, Kim C, Hou C, Hakonarson H, Torkamani A, Schork NJ, Brodeur GM, Tonini GP, Rappaport E, Devoto M, Maris JM. Identification of ALK as a major familial neuroblastoma predisposition gene. Nature. 2008;455(7215):930–5. https://doi.org/10.1038/nature07261.
16. Schonherr C, Ruuth K, Eriksson T, Yamazaki Y, Ottmann C, Combaret V, Vigny M, Kamaraj S, Palmer RH, Hallberg B. The neuroblastoma ALK(I1250T) mutation is a kinase-dead RTK in vitro and in vivo. Transl Oncol. 2011;4(4):258–65.
17. Bresler SC, Wood AC, Haglund EA, Courtright J, Belcastro LT, Plegaria JS, Cole K, Toporovskaya Y, Zhao H, Carpenter EL, Christensen JG, Maris JM, Lemmon MA, Mosse YP. Differential inhibitor sensitivity of anaplastic lymphoma kinase variants found in neuroblastoma. Sci Transl Med. 2011;3(108):108–14. https://doi.org/10.1126/scitranslmed.3002950.
18. Michna BA, McWilliams NB, Krummel TM, Hartenberg MA, Salzberg AM. Multifocal ganglioneuroblastoma coexistent with total colonic aganglionosis. J Pediatr Surg. 1988;23(1):57–9.
19. Stovroff M, Dykes F, Teague WG. The complete spectrum of neurocristopathy in an infant with congenital hypoventilation, Hirschsprung's disease, and neuroblastoma. J Pediatr Surg. 1995;30(8):1218–21.
20. Amiel J, Laudier B, Attie-Bitach T, Trang H, de Pontual L, Gener B, Trochet D, Etchevers H, Ray P, Simonneau M, Vekemans M, Munnich A, Gaultier C, Lyonnet S. Polyalanine expansion and frameshift mutations of the paired-like homeobox gene PHOX2B in congenital central hypoventilation syndrome. Nat Genet. 2003;33(4):459–61. https://doi.org/10.1038/ng1130.
21. Pattyn A, Morin X, Cremer H, Goridis C, Brunet JF. The homeobox gene Phox2b is essential for the development of autonomic neural crest derivatives. Nature. 1999;399(6734):366–70. https://doi.org/10.1038/20700.
22. Raabe EH, Laudenslager M, Winter C, Wasserman N, Cole K, LaQuaglia M, Maris DJ, Mosse YP, Maris JM. Prevalence and functional consequence of PHOX2B mutations in neuroblastoma. Oncogene. 2008;27(4):469–76. https://doi.org/10.1038/sj.onc.1210659.

23. Nagashimada M, Ohta H, Li C, Nakao K, Uesaka T, Brunet JF, Amiel J, Trochet D, Wakayama T, Enomoto H. Autonomic neurocristopathy-associated mutations in PHOX2B dysregulate Sox10 expression. J Clin Invest. 2012;122(9):3145–58. https://doi.org/10.1172/JCI63401.
24. Van Limpt V, Schramm A, van Lakeman A, Sluis P, Chan A, van Noesel M, Baas F, Caron H, Eggert A, Versteeg R. The Phox2B homeobox gene is mutated in sporadic neuroblastomas. Oncogene. 2004;23(57):9280–8. https://doi.org/10.1038/sj.onc.1208157.
25. Serra A, Haberle B, Konig IR, Kappler R, Suttorp M, Schackert HK, Roesner D, Fitze G. Rare occurrence of PHOX2b mutations in sporadic neuroblastomas. J Pediatr Hematol Oncol. 2008;30(10):728–32. https://doi.org/10.1097/MPH.0b013e3181772141.
26. Janoueix-Lerosey I, Lequin D, Brugieres L, Ribeiro A, de Pontual L, Combaret V, Raynal V, Puisieux A, Schleiermacher G, Pierron G, Valteau-Couanet D, Frebourg T, Michon J, Lyonnet S, Amiel J, Delattre O. Somatic and germline activating mutations of the ALK kinase receptor in neuroblastoma. Nature. 2008;455(7215):967–70. https://doi.org/10.1038/nature07398.
27. Chen Y, Takita J, Choi YL, Kato M, Ohira M, Sanada M, Wang L, Soda M, Kikuchi A, Igarashi T, Nakagawara A, Hayashi Y, Mano H, Ogawa S. Oncogenic mutations of ALK kinase in neuroblastoma. Nature. 2008;455(7215):971–4. https://doi.org/10.1038/nature07399.
28. George RE, Sanda T, Hanna M, Frohling S, Luther W 2nd, Zhang J, Ahn Y, Zhou W, London WB, McGrady P, Xue L, Zozulya S, Gregor VE, Webb TR, Gray NS, Gilliland DG, Diller L, Greulich H, Morris SW, Meyerson M, Look AT. Activating mutations in ALK provide a therapeutic target in neuroblastoma. Nature. 2008;455(7215):975–8. https://doi.org/10.1038/nature07397.
29. Morris SW, Kirstein MN, Valentine MB, Dittmer KG, Shapiro DN, Saltman DL, Look AT. Fusion of a kinase gene, ALK, to a nucleolar protein gene, NPM, in non-Hodgkin's lymphoma. Science. 1994;263(5151):1281–4.
30. Mosse YP. Anaplastic lymphoma kinase as a cancer target in pediatric malignancies. Clin Cancer Res. 2016;22(3):546–52. https://doi.org/10.1158/1078-0432.CCR-14-1100.
31. Devoto M, Specchia C, Laudenslager M, Longo L, Hakonarson H, Maris J, Mosse Y. Genome-wide linkage analysis to identify genetic modifiers of ALK mutation penetrance in familial neuroblastoma. Hum Hered. 2011;71(2):135–9. https://doi.org/10.1159/000324843.
32. Schonherr C, Ruuth K, Yamazaki Y, Eriksson T, Christensen J, Palmer RH, Hallberg B. Activating ALK mutations found in neuroblastoma are inhibited by Crizotinib and NVP-TAE684. Biochem J. 2011;440(3):405–13. https://doi.org/10.1042/BJ20101796.
33. Mosse YP, Lim MS, Voss SD, Wilner K, Ruffner K, Laliberte J, Rolland D, Balis FM, Maris JM, Weigel BJ, Ingle AM, Ahern C, Adamson PC, Blaney SM. Safety and activity of crizotinib for paediatric patients with refractory solid tumours or anaplastic large-cell lymphoma: a Children's Oncology Group phase 1 consortium study. Lancet Oncol. 2013;14(6):472–80. https://doi.org/10.1016/S1470-2045(13)70095-0.
34. Carpenter EL, Haglund EA, Mace EM, Deng D, Martinez D, Wood AC, Chow AK, Weiser DA, Belcastro LT, Winter C, Bresler SC, Vigny M, Mazot P, Asgharzadeh S, Seeger RC, Zhao H, Guo R, Christensen JG, Orange JS, Pawel BR, Lemmon MA, Mosse YP. Antibody targeting of anaplastic lymphoma kinase induces cytotoxicity of human neuroblastoma. Oncogene. 2012;31(46):4859–67. https://doi.org/10.1038/onc.2011.647.
35. Wang Y, Wang L, Guan S, Cao W, Wang H, Chen Z, Zhao Y, Yu Y, Zhang H, Pang JC, Huang SL, Akiyama Y, Yang Y, Sun W, Xu X, Shi Y, Zhang H, Kim ES, Muscal JA, Lu F, Yang J. Novel ALK inhibitor AZD3463 inhibits neuroblastoma growth by overcoming crizotinib resistance and inducing apoptosis. Sci Rep. 2016;6:19423. https://doi.org/10.1038/srep19423.
36. Lu J, Guan S, Zhao Y, Yu Y, Woodfield SE, Zhang H, Yang KL, Bieerkehazhi S, Qi L, Li X, Gu J, Xu X, Jin J, Muscal JA, Yang T, Xu GT, Yang J. The second-generation ALK inhibitor alectinib effectively induces apoptosis in human neuroblastoma cells and inhibits tumor growth in a TH-MYCN transgenic neuroblastoma mouse model. Cancer Lett. 2017;400:61–8. https://doi.org/10.1016/j.canlet.2017.04.022.
37. Wang DG, Fan J-B, Siao C-J, Berno A, Young P, Sapolsky R, Ghandour G, Perkins N, Winchester E, Spencer J, Kruglyak L, Stein L, Hsie L, Topaloglou T, Hubbell E, Robinson E, Mittmann M, Morris MS, Shen N, Kilburn D, Rioux J, Nusbaum C, Rozen S, Hudson TJ, Lipshutz R, Chee M, Lander ES. Large-scale identification, mapping, and genotyping of single-nucleotide polymorphisms in the human genome. Science. 1998;280(5366):1077.
38. Hirschhorn JN, Daly MJ. Genome-wide association studies for common diseases and complex traits. Nat Rev Genet. 2005;6(2):95–108. https://doi.org/10.1038/nrg1521.
39. Maris JM, Mosse YP, Bradfield JP, Hou C, Monni S, Scott RH, Asgharzadeh S, Attiyeh EF, Diskin SJ, Laudenslager M, Winter C, Cole KA, Glessner JT, Kim C, Frackelton EC, Casalunovo T, Eckert AW, Capasso M, Rappaport EF, McConville C, London WB, Seeger RC, Rahman N, Devoto M, Grant SF, Li H, Hakonarson H. Chromosome 6p22 locus associated with clinically aggressive neuroblastoma. N Engl J Med. 2008;358(24):2585–93. https://doi.org/10.1056/NEJMoa0708698.
40. Diskin SJ, Hou C, Glessner JT, Attiyeh EF, Laudenslager M, Bosse K, Cole K, Mossé YP, Wood

A, Lynch JE, Pecor K, Diamond M, Winter C, Wang K, Kim C, Geiger EA, McGrady PW, Blakemore AIF, London WB, Shaikh TH, Bradfield J, Grant S, Li H, Devoto M, Rappaport ER, Hakonarson H, Maris JM. Copy number variation at 1q21.1 associated with neuroblastoma. Nature. 2009;459(7249):987–91. https://doi.org/10.1038/nature08035.
41. Nguyen LB, Diskin SJ, Capasso M, Wang K, Diamond MA, Glessner J, Kim C, Attiyeh EF, Mosse YP, Cole K, Iolascon A, Devoto M, Hakonarson H, Li HK, Maris JM, Schork NJ. Phenotype restricted genome-wide association study using a gene-centric approach identifies three low-risk neuroblastoma susceptibility loci. PLoS Genet. 2011;7(3):1002026. https://doi.org/10.1371/journal.pgen.1002026.
42. Gamazon ER, Pinto N, Konkashbaev A, Im HK, Diskin SJ, London WB, Maris JM, Dolan ME, Cox NJ, Cohn SL. Trans-population analysis of genetic mechanisms of ethnic disparities in neuroblastoma survival. J Natl Cancer Inst. 2013;105(4):503. https://doi.org/10.1093/jnci/djs503.
43. Capasso M, Devoto M, Hou C, Asgharzadeh S, Glessner JT, Attiyeh EF, Mosse YP, Kim C, Diskin SJ, Cole KA, Bosse K, Diamond M, Laudenslager M, Winter C, Bradfield JP, Scott RH, Jagannathan J, Garris M, McConville C, London WB, Seeger RC, Grant SF, Li H, Rahman N, Rappaport E, Hakonarson H, Maris JM. Common variations in BARD1 influence susceptibility to high-risk neuroblastoma. Nat Genet. 2009;41(6):718–23. https://doi.org/10.1038/ng.374.
44. Capasso M, Diskin SJ, Totaro F, Longo L, de Mariano M, Russo R, Cimmino F, Hakonarson H, Tonini GP, Devoto M, Maris JM, Iolascon A. Replication of GWAS-identified neuroblastoma risk loci strengthens the role of BARD1 and affirms the cumulative effect of genetic variations on disease susceptibility. Carcinogenesis. 2013;34(3):605–11. https://doi.org/10.1093/carcin/bgs380.
45. Latorre V, Diskin SJ, Diamond MA, Zhang H, Hakonarson H, Maris JM, Devoto M. Replication of neuroblastoma SNP association at the BARD1 locus in African-Americans. Cancer Epidemiol Biomark Prev. 2012;21(4):658–63. https://doi.org/10.1158/1055-9965.EPI-11-0830.
46. Bosse KR, Diskin SJ, Cole KA, Wood AC, Schnepp RW, Norris G, Nguyen LB, Jagannathan J, Laquaglia M, Winter C, Diamond M, Hou C, Attiyeh EF, Mosse YP, Pineros V, Dizin E, Zhang Y, Asgharzadeh S, Seeger RC, Capasso M, Pawel BR, Devoto M, Hakonarson H, Rappaport EF, Irminger-Finger I, Maris JM. Common variation at BARD1 results in the expression of an oncogenic isoform that influences neuroblastoma susceptibility and oncogenicity. Cancer Res. 2012;72(8):2068–78. https://doi.org/10.1158/0008-5472.CAN-11-3703.
47. Cimmino F, Avitabile M, Diskin SJ, Vaksman Z, Pignataro P, Formicola D, Cardinale A, Testori A, Koster J, de Torres C, Devoto M, Maris JM, Iolascon A, Capasso M. Fine mapping of 2q35 high-risk neuroblastoma locus reveals independent functional risk variants and suggests full-length BARD1 as tumor-suppressor. Int J Cancer. 2018;143(11):2828–37. https://doi.org/10.1002/ijc.31822.
48. Cimmino F, Avitabile M, Lasorsa VA, Pezone L, Cardinale A, Montella A, Cantalupo S, Iolascon A, Capasso M. Functional characterization of full-length BARD1 strengthens its role as a tumor suppressor in neuroblastoma. J Cancer. 2020;11(6):1495–504. https://doi.org/10.7150/jca.36164.
49. Zhang R, Zou Y, Zhu J, Zeng X, Yang T, Wang F, He J, Xia H. The association between GWAS-identified BARD1 gene SNPs and neuroblastoma susceptibility in a Southern Chinese population. Int J Med Sci. 2016;13(2):133–8. https://doi.org/10.7150/ijms.13426.
50. Hungate EA, Applebaum MA, Skol AD, Vaksman Z, Diamond M, McDaniel L, Volchenboum SL, Stranger BE, Maris JM, Diskin SJ, Onel K, Cohn SL. Evaluation of genetic predisposition for MYCN-amplified neuroblastoma. J Natl Cancer Inst. 2017;109(10):1–4. https://doi.org/10.1093/jnci/djx093.
51. McDaniel LD, Conkrite KL, Chang X, Capasso M, Vaksman Z, Oldridge DA, Zachariou A, Horn M, Diamond M, Huo C, Iolascon A, Hakonarson H, Rahman N, Devoto M, Diskin SJ. Common variants upstream of MLF1 at 3q25 and within CPZ at 4p16 associated with neuroblastoma. PLoS Genet. 2017;13(5):1006787. https://doi.org/10.1371/journal.pgen.1006787.
52. Diskin SJ, Capasso M, Schnepp RW, Cole KA, Attiyeh EF, Hou C, Diamond M, Carpenter EL, Winter C, Lee H, Jagannathan J, Latorre V, Iolascon A, Hakonarson H, Devoto M, Maris JM. Common variation at 6q16 within HACE1 and LIN28B influences susceptibility to neuroblastoma. Nat Genet. 2012;44(10):1126–30. https://doi.org/10.1038/ng.2387.
53. Zhang Z, Zhang R, Zhu J, Wang F, Yang T, Zou Y, He J, Xia H. Common variations within HACE1 gene and neuroblastoma susceptibility in a Southern Chinese population. Onco Targets Ther. 2017;10:703–9. https://doi.org/10.2147/OTT.S129042.
54. Molenaar JJ, Domingo-Fernández R, Ebus ME, Lindner S, Koster J, Drabek K, Mestdagh P, van Sluis P, Valentijn LJ, van Nes J, Broekmans M, Haneveld F, Volckmann R, Bray I, Heukamp L, Sprüssel A, Thor T, Kieckbusch K, Klein-Hitpass L, Fischer M, Vandesompele J, Schramm A, van Noesel MM, Varesio L, Speleman F, Eggert A, Stallings RL, Caron HN, Versteeg R, Schulte JH. LIN28B induces neuroblastoma and enhances MYCN levels via let-7 suppression. Nat Genet. 2012;44(11):1199–206. https://doi.org/10.1038/ng.2436.
55. Schnepp RW, Khurana P, Attiyeh EF, Raman P, Chodosh SE, Oldridge DA, Gagliardi ME, Conkrite KL, Asgharzadeh S, Seeger RC, Madison BB, Rustgi AK, Maris JM, Diskin SJ. A LIN28B-RAN-AURKA signaling network promotes neuroblastoma

tumorigenesis. Cancer Cell. 2015;28(5):599–609. https://doi.org/10.1016/j.ccell.2015.09.012.
56. He J, Yang T, Zhang R, Zhu J, Wang F, Zou Y, Xia H. Potentially functional polymorphisms in the LIN28B gene contribute to neuroblastoma susceptibility in Chinese children. J Cell Mol Med. 2016;20(8):1534–41. https://doi.org/10.1111/jcmm.12846.
57. Pandey GK, Mitra S, Subhash S, Hertwig F, Kanduri M, Mishra K, Fransson S, Ganeshram A, Mondal T, Bandaru S, Östensson M, Akyürek LM, Abrahamsson J, Pfeifer S, Larsson E, Shi L, Peng Z, Fischer M, Martinsson T, Hedborg F, Kogner P, Kanduri C. The risk-associated long noncoding RNA NBAT-1 controls neuroblastoma progression by regulating cell proliferation and neuronal differentiation. Cancer Cell. 2014;26(5):722–37. https://doi.org/10.1016/j.ccell.2014.09.014.
58. Russell MR, Penikis A, Oldridge DA, Alvarez-Dominguez JR, McDaniel L, Diamond M, Padovan O, Raman P, Li Y, Wei JS, Zhang S, Gnanchandran J, Seeger R, Asgharzadeh S, Khan J, Diskin SJ, Maris JM, Cole KA. CASC15-S is a tumor suppressor lncRNA at the 6p22 neuroblastoma susceptibility locus. Cancer Res. 2015;75(15):3155–66. https://doi.org/10.1158/0008-5472.CAN-14-3613.
59. Mondal T, Juvvuna PK, Kirkeby A, Mitra S, Kosalai ST, Traxler L, Hertwig F, Wernig-Zorc S, Miranda C, Deland L, Volland R, Bartenhagen C, Bartsch D, Bandaru S, Engesser A, Subhash S, Martinsson T, Caren H, Akyurek LM, Kurian L, Kanduri M, Huarte M, Kogner P, Fischer M, Kanduri C. Sense-antisense lncrna pair encoded by locus 6p22.3 determines neuroblastoma susceptibility via the USP36-CHD7-SOX9 regulatory axis. Cancer Cell. 2018;33(3):417–34. https://doi.org/10.1016/j.ccell.2018.01.020.
60. He J, Zhang R, Zou Y, Zhu J, Yang T, Wang F, Xia H. Evaluation of GWAS-identified SNPs at 6p22 with neuroblastoma susceptibility in a Chinese population. Tumour Biol. 2016;37(2):1635–9. https://doi.org/10.1007/s13277-015-3936-7.
61. Zhang Z, Zou Y, Zhu J, Zhang R, Yang T, Wang F, Xia H, He J, Feng Z. HSD17B12 gene rs11037575 C>T polymorphism confers neuroblastoma susceptibility in a Southern Chinese population. Onco Targets Ther. 2017;10:1969–75. https://doi.org/10.2147/OTT.S136006.
62. Wang K, Diskin SJ, Zhang H, Attiyeh EF, Winter C, Hou C, Schnepp RW, Diamond M, Bosse K, Mayes PA, Glessner J, Kim C, Frackelton E, Garris M, Wang Q, Glaberson W, Chiavacci R, Le N, Jagannathan J, Saeki N, Sasaki H, Grant SFA, Iolascon A, Mosse YP, Cole KA, Li H, Devoto M, McGrady PW, London WB, Capasso M, Rahman N, Hakonarson H, Maris JM. Integrative genomics identifies LMO1 as a neuroblastoma oncogene. Nature. 2011;469(7329):216–20. https://doi.org/10.1038/nature09609.
63. Oldridge DA, Wood AC, Weichert-Leahey N, Crimmins I, Sussman R, Winter C, McDaniel LD, Diamond M, Hart LS, Zhu S, Durbin AD, Abraham BJ, Anders L, Tian L, Zhang S, Wei JS, Khan J, Bramlett K, Rahman N, Capasso M, Iolascon A, Gerhard DS, Guidry Auvil JM, Young RA, Hakonarson H, Diskin SJ, Thomas Look A, Maris JM. Genetic predisposition to neuroblastoma mediated by a LMO1 super-enhancer polymorphism. Nature. 2015;528(7582):418–21. https://doi.org/10.1038/nature15540.
64. Zhu S, Zhang X, Weichert-Leahey N, Dong Z, Zhang C, Lopez G, Tao T, He S, Wood AC, Oldridge D, Ung CY, van Ree JH, Khan A, Salazar BM, Lummertz da Rocha E, Zimmerman MW, Guo F, Cao H, Hou X, Weroha SJ, Perez-Atayde AR, Neuberg DS, Meves A, McNiven MA, van Deursen JM, Li H, Maris JM, Look AT. LMO1 synergizes with MYCN to promote neuroblastoma initiation and metastasis. Cancer Cell. 2017;2017:1–14. https://doi.org/10.1016/j.ccell.2017.08.002.
65. He J, Zhong W, Zeng J, Zhu J, Zhang R, Wang F, Yang T, Zou Y, Xia H. LMO1 gene polymorphisms contribute to decreased neuroblastoma susceptibility in a Southern Chinese population. Oncotarget. 2016;7(16):22770–8. https://doi.org/10.18632/oncotarget.8178.
66. Chang X, Zhao Y, Hou C, Glessner J, McDaniel L, Diamond MA, Thomas K, Li J, Wei Z, Liu Y, Guo Y, Mentch FD, Qiu H, Kim C, Evans P, Vaksman Z, Diskin SJ, Attiyeh EF, Sleiman P, Maris JM, Hakonarson H. Common variants in MMP20 at 11q22.2 predispose to 11q deletion and neuroblastoma risk. Nat Commun. 2017;8(1):569. https://doi.org/10.1038/s41467-017-00408-8.
67. Diskin SJ, Capasso M, Diamond M, Oldridge DA, Conkrite K, Bosse KR, Russell MR, Iolascon A, Hakonarson H, Devoto M, Maris JM. Rare variants in TP53 and susceptibility to neuroblastoma. J Natl Cancer Inst. 2014;106(4):47. https://doi.org/10.1093/jnci/dju047.
68. Capasso M, Diskin S, Cimmino F, Acierno G, Totaro F, Petrosino G, Pezone L, Diamond M, McDaniel L, Hakonarson H, Iolascon A, Devoto M, Maris JM. Common genetic variants in NEFL influence gene expression and neuroblastoma risk. Cancer Res. 2014;74(23):6913–24. https://doi.org/10.1158/0008-5472.CAN-14-0431.
69. Capasso M, McDaniel LD, Cimmino F, Cirino A, Formicola D, Russell MR, Raman P, Cole KA, Diskin SJ. The functional variant rs34330 of CDKN1B is associated with risk of neuroblastoma. J Cell Mol Med. 2017;20(10):1–7. https://doi.org/10.1111/jcmm.13226.
70. Ritenour LE, Randall MP, Bosse KR, Diskin SJ. Genetic susceptibility to neuroblastoma: current knowledge and future directions. Cell Tissue Res. 2018;372(2):287–307. https://doi.org/10.1007/s00441-018-2820-3.
71. Wu LC, Wang ZW, Tsan JT, Spillman MA, Phung A, Xu XL, Yang M-CW, Hwang L-Y, Bowcock AM, Baer R. Identification of a RING protein that can

interact in vivo with the BRCA1 gene product. Nat Genet. 1996;14(4):430–40.
72. Pugh TJ, Morozova O, Attiyeh EF, Asgharzadeh S, Wei JS, Auclair D, Carter SL, Cibulskis K, Hanna M, Kiezun A, Kim J, Lawrence MS, Lichenstein L, McKenna A, Pedamallu CS, Ramos AH, Shefler E, Sivachenko A, Sougnez C, Stewart C, Ally A, Birol I, Chiu R, Corbett RD, Hirst M, Jackman SD, Kamoh B, Khodabakshi AH, Krzywinski M, Lo A, Moore RA, Mungall KL, Qian J, Tam A, Thiessen N, Zhao Y, Cole KA, Diamond M, Diskin SJ, Mosse YP, Wood AC, Ji L, Sposto R, Badgett T, London WB, Moyer Y, Gastier-Foster JM, Smith MA, Guidry Auvil JM, Gerhard DS, Hogarty MD, Jones SJ, Lander ES, Gabriel SB, Getz G, Seeger RC, Khan J, Marra MA, Meyerson M, Maris JM. The genetic landscape of high-risk neuroblastoma. Nat Genet. 2013;45(3):279–84. https://doi.org/10.1038/ng.2529.
73. Boehm T, Baer R, Lavenir I, Forster A, Waters JJ, Nacheva E, Rabbitts TH. The mechanism of chromosomal translocation t(11;14) involving the T-cell receptor C delta locus on human chromosome 14q11 and a transcribed region of chromosome 11p15. EMBO J. 1988;7(2):385–94.
74. Royer-Pokora B, Loos U, Ludwig WD. TTG-2, a new gene encoding a cysteine-rich protein with the LIM motif, is overexpressed in acute T-cell leukaemia with the t(11;14)(p13;q11). Oncogene. 1991;6(10):1887–93.
75. Zhang L, Anglesio MS, O'Sullivan M, Zhang F, Yang G, Sarao R. The E3 ligase HACE1 is a critical chromosome 6q21 tumor suppressor involved in multiple cancers. Nat Med. 2007;13(9):1060–9. https://doi.org/10.1038/nm1621.
76. Johnson SM, Grosshans H, Shingara J, Byrom M, Jarvis R, Cheng A, Labourier E, Reinert KL, Brown D, Slack FJ. RAS is regulated by the let-7 microRNA family. Cell. 2005;120(5):635–47. https://doi.org/10.1016/j.cell.2005.01.014.
77. Otto T, Horn S, Brockmann M, Eilers U, Schuttrumpf L, Popov N, Kenney AM, Schulte JH, Beijersbergen R, Christiansen H, Berwanger B, Eilers M. Stabilization of N-Myc is a critical function of Aurora A in human neuroblastoma. Cancer Cell. 2009;15(1):67–78. https://doi.org/10.1016/j.ccr.2008.12.005.
78. Mossé YP, Lipsitz E, Fox E, Teachey DT, Maris JM, Weigel B, Adamson PC, Ingle MA, Ahern CH, Blaney SM. Pediatric phase I trial and pharmacokinetic study of MLN8237, an investigational oral selective small-molecule inhibitor of aurora kinase A: a Children's Oncology Group Phase I Consortium Study. Clin Cancer Res. 2012;18(21):6058.
79. Stacey SN, Sulem P, Jonasdottir A, Masson G, Gudmundsson J, Gudbjartsson DF, Magnusson OT, Gudjonsson SA, Sigurgeirsson B, Thorisdottir K, Ragnarsson R, Benediktsdottir KR, Nexo BA, Tjonneland A, Overvad K, Rudnai P, Gurzau E, Koppova K, Hemminki K, Corredera C, Fuentelsaz V, Grasa P, Navarrete S, Fuertes F, Garcia-Prats MD, Sanambrosio E, Panadero A, De Juan A, Garcia A, Rivera F, Planelles D, Soriano V, Requena C, Aben KK, van Rossum MM, Cremers RG, van Oort IM, van Spronsen DJ, Schalken JA, Peters WH, Helfand BT, Donovan JL, Hamdy FC, Badescu D, Codreanu O, Jinga M, Csiki IE, Constantinescu V, Badea P, Mates IN, Dinu DE, Constantin A, Mates D, Kristjansdottir S, Agnarsson BA, Jonsson E, Barkardottir RB, Einarsson GV, Sigurdsson F, Moller PH, Stefansson T, Valdimarsson T, Johannsson OT, Sigurdsson H, Jonsson T, Jonasson JG, Tryggvadottir L, Rice T, Hansen HM, Xiao Y, Lachance DH, ON BP, Kosel ML, Decker PA, Thorleifsson G, Johannsdottir H, Helgadottir HT, Sigurdsson A, Steinthorsdottir V, Lindblom A, Sandler RS, Keku TO, Banasik K, Jorgensen T, Witte DR, Hansen T, Pedersen O, Jinga V, Neal DE, Catalona WJ, Wrensch M, Wiencke J, Jenkins RB, Nagore E, Vogel U, Kiemeney LA, Kumar R, Mayordomo JI, Olafsson JH, Kong A, Thorsteinsdottir U, Rafnar T, Stefansson K, Swedish Low-Risk Colorectal Cancer Study G. A germline variant in the TP53 polyadenylation signal confers cancer susceptibility. Nat Genet. 2011;43(11):1098–103. https://doi.org/10.1038/ng.926.
80. Fujita K, Mondal AM, Horikawa I, Nguyen GH, Kumamoto K, Sohn JJ, Bowman ED, Mathe EA, Schetter AJ, Pine SR, Ji H, Vojtesek B, Bourdon JC, Lane DP, Harris CC. p53 isoforms Delta133p53 and p53beta are endogenous regulators of replicative cellular senescence. Nat Cell Biol. 2009;11(9):1135–42. https://doi.org/10.1038/ncb1928.
81. Moeller C, Swindell EC, Kispert A, Eichele G. Carboxypeptidase Z (CPZ) modulates Wnt signaling and regulates the development of skeletal elements in the chicken. Development. 2003;130(21):5103–11. https://doi.org/10.1242/dev.00686.
82. Potkin SG, Turner JA, Fallon JA, Lakatos A, Keator DB, Guffanti G, Macciardi F, Fbirn. Gene discovery through imaging genetics: identification of two novel genes associated with schizophrenia. Mol Psychiatry. 2009;14(4):416–28. https://doi.org/10.1038/mp.2008.127.
83. Matsumoto N, Yoneda-Kato N, Iguchi T, Kishimoto Y, Kyo T, Sawada H, Tatsumi E, Fukuhara S. Elevated MLF1 expression correlates with malignant progression from myelodysplastic syndrome. Leukemia. 2000;14(10):1757–65.
84. Park RW, Kim T-M, Kasif S, Park PJ. Identification of rare germline copy number variations over-represented in five human cancer types. Mol Cancer. 2015;14:25. https://doi.org/10.1186/s12943-015-0292-6.
85. Henderson TO, Bhatia S, Pinto N, London WB, McGrady P, Crotty C, Sun CL, Cohn SL. Racial and ethnic disparities in risk and survival in children with neuroblastoma: a Children's Oncology Group Study. J Clin Oncol. 2011;29(1):76–82. https://doi.org/10.1200/JCO.2010.29.6103.

86. White PS, Thompson PM, Gotoh T, Okawa ER, Igarashi J, Kok M, Winter C, Gregory SG, Hogarty MD, Maris JM, Brodeur GM. Definition and characterization of a region of 1p36.3 consistently deleted in neuroblastoma. Oncogene. 2004;24:2684. https://doi.org/10.1038/sj.onc.1208306.
87. Isidor B, Le Cunff M, Boceno M, Boisseau P, Thomas C, Rival JM, David A, Le Caignec C. Complex constitutional subtelomeric 1p36.3 deletion/duplication in a mentally retarded child with neonatal neuroblastoma. Eur J Med Genet. 2008;51(6):679–84. https://doi.org/10.1016/j.ejmg.2008.06.004.
88. Mosse Y, Greshock J, King A, Khazi D, Weber BL, Maris JM. Identification and high-resolution mapping of a constitutional 11q deletion in an infant with multifocal neuroblastoma. Lancet Oncol. 2003;4(12):769–71. https://doi.org/10.1016/S1470-2045(03)01283-X.
89. Passariello A, De Brasi D, Defferrari R, Genesio R, Tufano M, Mazzocco K, Capasso M, Migliorati R, Martinsson T, Siani P, Nitsch L, Tonini GP. Constitutional 11q14-q22 chromosome deletion syndrome in a child with neuroblastoma MYCN single copy. Eur J Med Genet. 2013;56(11):626–34. https://doi.org/10.1016/j.ejmg.2013.08.005.
90. Shiohama T, Fujii K, Hino M, Shimizu K, Ohashi H, Kambe M, Nakatani Y, Mitsunaga T, Yoshida H, Ochiai H, Shimojo N. Coexistence of neuroblastoma and ganglioneuroma in a girl with a hemizygous deletion of chromosome 11q14.1–23.3. Am J Med Genet A. 2016;170(2):492–7. https://doi.org/10.1002/ajmg.a.37430.
91. Morgenstern DA, Soh SY, Stavropoulos DJ, Bowdin S, Baruchel S, Malkin D, Meyn MS, Irwin MS. Metachronous neuroblastoma in an infant with germline translocation resulting in partial trisomy 2p. J Pediatr Hematol. 2014;36(3):e193–6. https://doi.org/10.1097/MPH.0b013e3182a8f25d.
92. Lehalle D, Sanlaville D, Guimier A, Plouvier E, Leblanc T, Galmiche L, Radford I, Romana S, Colleaux L, de Pontual L, Lyonnet S, Amiel J. Multiple congenital anomalies-intellectual disability (MCA-ID) and neuroblastoma in a patient harboring a de novo 14q23.1q23.3 deletion. Am J Med Genet A. 2014;164(5):1310–7. https://doi.org/10.1002/ajmg.a.36452.
93. Hienonen T, Sammalkorpi H, Isohanni P, Versteeg R, Karikoski R, Aaltonen L. A 17p11.2 germline deletion in a patient with Smith-Magenis syndrome and neuroblastoma. J Med Genet. 2005;42(1):e3. https://doi.org/10.1136/jmg.2004.022814.
94. Van Roy N, Vandesompele J, Berx G, Staes K, Van Gele M, De Smet E, De Paepe A, Laureys G, Van Der Drift P, Versteeg R, Van Roy F, Speleman F. Localization of the 17q breakpoint of a constitutional 1;17 translocation in a patient with neuroblastoma within a 25-kb segment located between the ACCN1 and TLK2 genes and near the distal breakpoints of two microdeletions in neurofibromatosis type 1 patients. Genes Chromosomes Cancer. 2002;35(2):113–20. https://doi.org/10.1002/gcc.10034.
95. Vandepoele K, Andries V, Van Roy N, Staes K, Vandesompele J, Laureys G, De Smet E, Berx G, Speleman F, van Roy F. A constitutional translocation t(1;17)(p36.2;q11.2) in a neuroblastoma patient disrupts the human NBPF1 and ACCN1 genes. PLoS One. 2008;3(5):e2207. https://doi.org/10.1371/journal.pone.0002207.
96. Laureys GV, Speleman F, Opdenakker G, Benoit Y, Leroy J. Constitutional translocation t(1;17)(p36;q12-21) in a patient with neuroblastoma. Genes Chromosom Cancer. 1990;2(3):252–4. https://doi.org/10.1002/gcc.2870020315.
97. Blatt J, Olshan AF, Lee PA, Ross JL. Neuroblastoma and related tumors in Turner's syndrome. J Pediatr. 1997;131(5):666–70. https://doi.org/10.1016/s0022-3476(97)70090-8.
98. Satgé D, Sasco AJ, Carlsen NLT, Stiller CA, Rubie H, Hero B, de Bernardi B, de Kraker J, Coze C, Kogner P, Langmark F, Hakvoort-Cammel FGAJ, Beck D, von der Weid N, Parkes S, Hartmann O, Lippens RJJ, Kamps WA, Sommelet D. A Lack of neuroblastoma in down syndrome: a study from 11 European countries. Cancer Res. 1998;58(3):448.
99. Satgé D, Sasco AJ, Plantaz D, Bénard J, Vekemans MJ. Abnormal number of X chromosomes and neuroblastic tumors. J Pediatr Hematol. 2001;23(5):331–2. https://doi.org/10.1097/00043426-200106000-00022.
100. Satge D, Moore SW, Stiller CA, Niggli FK, Pritchard-Jones K, Bown N, Benard J, Plantaz D. Abnormal constitutional karyotypes in patients with neuroblastoma: a report of four new cases and review of 47 others in the literature. Cancer Genet Cytogenet. 2003;147(2):89–98. https://doi.org/10.1016/S0165-4608(03)00203-6.
101. Egolf LE, Vaksman Z, Lopez G, Rokita JL, Modi A, Basta PV, Hakonarson H, Olshan AF, Diskin SJ. Germline 16p11.2 microdeletion predisposes to neuroblastoma. Am J Hum Genet. 2019;105(3):658–68. https://doi.org/10.1016/j.ajhg.2019.07.020.
102. Weiss LA, Shen Y, Korn JM, Arking DE, Miller DT, Fossdal R, Saemundsen E, Stefansson H, Ferreira MA, Green T, Platt OS, Ruderfer DM, Walsh CA, Altshuler D, Chakravarti A, Tanzi RE, Stefansson K, Santangelo SL, Gusella JF, Sklar P, Wu BL, Daly MJ, Autism C. Association between microdeletion and microduplication at 16p11.2 and autism. N Engl J Med. 2008;358(7):667–75. https://doi.org/10.1056/NEJMoa075974.
103. Shinawi M, Liu P, Kang SH, Shen J, Belmont JW, Scott DA, Probst FJ, Craigen WJ, Graham BH, Pursley A, Clark G, Lee J, Proud M, Stocco A, Rodriguez DL, Kozel BA, Sparagana S, Roeder ER, McGrew SG, Kurczynski TW, Allison LJ, Amato S, Savage S, Patel A, Stankiewicz P, Beaudet AL, Cheung SW, Lupski JR. Recurrent reciprocal 16p11.2 rearrangements associated with global developmental delay, behavioural problems, dys-

morphism, epilepsy, and abnormal head size. J Med Genet. 2010;47(5):332–41. https://doi.org/10.1136/jmg.2009.073015.
104. Rosenfeld JA, Coppinger J, Bejjani BA, Girirajan S, Eichler EE, Shaffer LG, Ballif BC. Speech delays and behavioral problems are the predominant features in individuals with developmental delays and 16p11.2 microdeletions and microduplications. J Neurodev Disord. 2010;2(1):26–38. https://doi.org/10.1007/s11689-009-9037-4.
105. Walters RG, Jacquemont S, Valsesia A, de Smith AJ, Martinet D, Andersson J, Falchi M, Chen F, Andrieux J, Lobbens S, Delobel B, Stutzmann F, El-Sayed Moustafa JS, Chevre JC, Lecoeur C, Vatin V, Bouquillon S, Buxton JL, Boute O, Holder-Espinasse M, Cuisset JM, Lemaitre MP, Ambresin AE, Brioschi A, Gaillard M, Giusti V, Fellmann F, Ferrarini A, Hadjikhani N, Campion D, Guilmatre A, Goldenberg A, Calmels N, Mandel JL, Le Caignec C, David A, Isidor B, Cordier MP, Dupuis-Girod S, Labalme A, Sanlaville D, Beri-Dexheimer M, Jonveaux P, Leheup B, Ounap K, Bochukova EG, Henning E, Keogh J, Ellis RJ, Macdermot KD, van Haelst MM, Vincent-Delorme C, Plessis G, Touraine R, Philippe A, Malan V, Mathieu-Dramard M, Chiesa J, Blaumeiser B, Kooy RF, Caiazzo R, Pigeyre M, Balkau B, Sladek R, Bergmann S, Mooser V, Waterworth D, Reymond A, Vollenweider P, Waeber G, Kurg A, Palta P, Esko T, Metspalu A, Nelis M, Elliott P, Hartikainen AL, McCarthy MI, Peltonen L, Carlsson L, Jacobson P, Sjostrom L, Huang N, Hurles ME, O'Rahilly S, Farooqi IS, Mannik K, Jarvelin MR, Pattou F, Meyre D, Walley AJ, Coin LJ, Blakemore AI, Froguel P, Beckmann JS. A new highly penetrant form of obesity due to deletions on chromosome 16p11.2. Nature. 2010;463(7281):671–5. https://doi.org/10.1038/nature08727.
106. Jacquemont S, Reymond A, Zufferey F, Harewood L, Walters RG, Kutalik Z, Martinet D, Shen Y, Valsesia A, Beckmann ND, Thorleifsson G, Belfiore M, Bouquillon S, Campion D, de Leeuw N, de Vries BB, Esko T, Fernandez BA, Fernandez-Aranda F, Fernandez-Real JM, Gratacos M, Guilmatre A, Hoyer J, Jarvelin MR, Kooy RF, Kurg A, Le Caignec C, Mannik K, Platt OS, Sanlaville D, Van Haelst MM, Villatoro Gomez S, Walha F, Wu BL, Yu Y, Aboura A, Addor MC, Alembik Y, Antonarakis SE, Arveiler B, Barth M, Bednarek N, Bena F, Bergmann S, Beri M, Bernardini L, Blaumeiser B, Bonneau D, Bottani A, Boute O, Brunner HG, Cailley D, Callier P, Chiesa J, Chrast J, Coin L, Coutton C, Cuisset JM, Cuvellier JC, David A, de Freminville B, Delobel B, Delrue MA, Demeer B, Descamps D, Didelot G, Dieterich K, Disciglio V, Doco-Fenzy M, Drunat S, Duban-Bedu B, Dubourg C, El-Sayed Moustafa JS, Elliott P, Faas BH, Faivre L, Faudet A, Fellmann F, Ferrarini A, Fisher R, Flori E, Forer L, Gaillard D, Gerard M, Gieger C, Gimelli S, Gimelli G, Grabe HJ, Guichet A, Guillin O, Hartikainen AL, Heron D, Hippolyte L, Holder M, Homuth G, Isidor B, Jaillard S, Jaros Z, Jimenez-Murcia S, Helas GJ, Jonveaux P, Kaksonen S, Keren B, Kloss-Brandstatter A, Knoers NV, Koolen DA, Kroisel PM, Kronenberg F, Labalme A, Landais E, Lapi E, Layet V, Legallic S, Leheup B, Leube B, Lewis S, Lucas J, MacDermot KD, Magnusson P, Marshall C, Mathieu-Dramard M, McCarthy MI, Meitinger T, Mencarelli MA, Merla G, Moerman A, Mooser V, Morice-Picard F, Mucciolo M, Nauck M, Ndiaye NC, Nordgren A, Pasquier L, Petit F, Pfundt R, Plessis G, Rajcan-Separovic E, Ramelli GP, Rauch A, Ravazzolo R, Reis A, Renieri A, Richart C, Ried JS, Rieubland C, Roberts W, Roetzer KM, Rooryck C, Rossi M, Saemundsen E, Satre V, Schurmann C, Sigurdsson E, Stavropoulos DJ, Stefansson H, Tengstrom C, Thorsteinsdottir U, Tinahones FJ, Touraine R, Vallee L, van Binsbergen E, Van der Aa N, Vincent-Delorme C, Visvikis-Siest S, Vollenweider P, Volzke H, Vulto-van Silfhout AT, Waeber G, Wallgren-Pettersson C, Witwicki RM, Zwolinksi S, Andrieux J, Estivill X, Gusella JF, Gustafsson O, Metspalu A, Scherer SW, Stefansson K, Blakemore AI, Beckmann JS, Froguel P. Mirror extreme BMI phenotypes associated with gene dosage at the chromosome 16p11.2 locus. Nature. 2011;478(7367):97–102. https://doi.org/10.1038/nature10406.
107. Zufferey F, Sherr EH, Beckmann ND, Hanson E, Maillard AM, Hippolyte L, Mace A, Ferrari C, Kutalik Z, Andrieux J, Aylward E, Barker M, Bernier R, Bouquillon S, Conus P, Delobel B, Faucett WA, Goin-Kochel RP, Grant E, Harewood L, Hunter JV, Lebon S, Ledbetter DH, Martin CL, Mannik K, Martinet D, Mukherjee P, Ramocki MB, Spence SJ, Steinman KJ, Tjernagel J, Spiro JE, Reymond A, Beckmann JS, Chung WK, Jacquemont S, Simons VIPC, European C. A 600 kb deletion syndrome at 16p11.2 leads to energy imbalance and neuropsychiatric disorders. J Med Genet. 2012;49(10):660–8. https://doi.org/10.1136/jmedgenet-2012-101203.
108. Malhotra D, Sebat J. CNVs: harbingers of a rare variant revolution in psychiatric genetics. Cell. 2012;148(6):1223–41. https://doi.org/10.1016/j.cell.2012.02.039.
109. Schork NJ, Murray SS, Frazer KA, Topol EJ. Common vs. rare allele hypotheses for complex diseases. Curr Opin Genet Dev. 2009;19(3):212–9. https://doi.org/10.1016/j.gde.2009.04.010.
110. Birch JM, Alston RD, McNally RJ, Evans DG, Kelsey AM, Harris M, Eden OB, Varley JM. Relative frequency and morphology of cancers in carriers of germline TP53 mutations. Oncogene. 2001;20(34):4621–8. https://doi.org/10.1038/sj.onc.1204621.
111. Origone P, Defferrari R, Mazzocco K, Lo Cunsolo C, De Bernardi B, Tonini GP. Homozygous inactivation of NF1 gene in a patient with familial NF1 and disseminated neuroblastoma. Am J Med Genet A. 2003;118A(4):309–13. https://doi.org/10.1002/ajmg.a.10167.

112. Mutesa L, Pierquin G, Janin N, Segers K, Thomee C, Provenzi M, Bours V. Germline PTPN11 missense mutation in a case of Noonan syndrome associated with mediastinal and retroperitoneal neuroblastic tumors. Cancer Genet Cytogenet. 2008;182(1):40–2. https://doi.org/10.1016/j.cancergencyto.2007.12.005.
113. Kratz CP, Rapisuwon S, Reed H, Hasle H, Rosenberg PS. Cancer in Noonan, Costello, cardiofaciocutaneous and LEOPARD syndromes. Am J Med Genet C Semin Med Genet. 2011;157C(2):83–9. https://doi.org/10.1002/ajmg.c.30300.
114. Schimke RN, Collins DL, Stolle CA. Paraganglioma, neuroblastoma, and a SDHB mutation: resolution of a 30-year-old mystery. Am J Med Genet A. 2010;152A(6):1531–5. https://doi.org/10.1002/ajmg.a.33384.
115. Tatton-Brown K, Murray A, Hanks S, Douglas J, Armstrong R, Banka S, Bird LM, Clericuzio CL, Cormier-Daire V, Cushing T, Flinter F, Jacquemont ML, Joss S, Kinning E, Lynch SA, Magee A, McConnell V, Medeira A, Ozono K, Patton M, Rankin J, Shears D, Simon M, Splitt M, Strenger V, Stuurman K, Taylor C, Titheradge H, Van Maldergem L, Temple IK, Cole T, Seal S, Childhood Overgrowth C, Rahman N. Weaver syndrome and EZH2 mutations: clarifying the clinical phenotype. Am J Med Genet A. 2013;161A(12):2972–80. https://doi.org/10.1002/ajmg.a.36229.
116. Mody RJ, Wu YM, Lonigro RJ, Cao X, Roychowdhury S, Vats P, Frank KM, Prensner JR, Asangani I, Palanisamy N, Dillman JR, Rabah RM, Kunju LP, Everett J, Raymond VM, Ning Y, Su F, Wang R, Stoffel EM, Innis JW, Roberts JS, Robertson PL, Yanik G, Chamdin A, Connelly JA, Choi S, Harris AC, Kitko C, Rao RJ, Levine JE, Castle VP, Hutchinson RJ, Talpaz M, Robinson DR, Chinnaiyan AM. Integrative clinical sequencing in the management of refractory or relapsed cancer in youth. JAMA. 2015;314(9):913–25. https://doi.org/10.1001/jama.2015.10080.
117. Zhang J, Walsh MF, Wu G, Edmonson MN, Gruber TA, Easton J, Hedges D, Ma X, Zhou X, Yergeau DA, Wilkinson MR, Vadodaria B, Chen X, McGee RB, Hines-Dowell S, Nuccio R, Quinn E, Shurtleff SA, Rusch M, Patel A, Becksfort JB, Wang S, Weaver MS, Ding L, Mardis ER, Wilson RK, Gajjar A, Ellison DW, Pappo AS, Pui CH, Nichols KE, Downing JR. Germline mutations in predisposition genes in pediatric cancer. N Engl J Med. 2015;373(24):2336–46. https://doi.org/10.1056/NEJMoa1508054.
118. Parsons DW, Roy A, Yang Y, Wang T, Scollon S, Bergstrom K, Kerstein RA, Gutierrez S, Petersen AK, Bavle A, Lin FY, Lopez-Terrada DH, Monzon FA, Hicks MJ, Eldin KW, Quintanilla NM, Adesina AM, Mohila CA, Whitehead W, Jea A, Vasudevan SA, Nuchtern JG, Ramamurthy U, McGuire AL, Hilsenbeck SG, Reid JG, Muzny DM, Wheeler DA, Berg SL, Chintagumpala MM, Eng CM, Gibbs RA, Plon SE. Diagnostic yield of clinical tumor and germline whole-exome sequencing for children with solid tumors. JAMA Oncol. 2016;2(5):616–24. https://doi.org/10.1001/jamaoncol.2015.5699.
119. Kim J, Gianferante M, Karyadi DM, Hartley SW, Frone MN, Luo W, Robison LL, Armstrong GT, Bhatia S, Dean M, Yeager M, Zhu B, Song L, Sampson JN, Yasui Y, Leisenring WM, Brodie SA, de Andrade KC, Fortes FP, Goldstein AM, Khincha PP, Machiela MJ, McMaster ML, Nickerson ML, Oba L, Pemov A, Pinheiro M, Rotunno M, Santiago K, Wegman-Ostrosky T, Diver WR, Teras L, Freedman ND, Hicks BD, Zhu B, Wang M, Jones K, Hutchinson AA, Dagnall C, Savage SA, Tucker MA, Chanock SJ, Morton LM, Stewart DR, Mirabello L. Frequency of pathogenic germline variants in cancer-susceptibility genes in the childhood cancer survivor study. JNCI Cancer Spectr. 2021;5(2):7. https://doi.org/10.1093/jncics/pkab007.
120. Fiala EM, Jayakumaran G, Mauguen A, Kennedy JA, Bouvier N, Kemel Y, Fleischut MH, Maio A, Salo-Mullen EE, Sheehan M, Arnold AG, Latham A, Carlo MI, Cadoo K, Murkherjee S, Slotkin EK, Trippett T, Glade Bender J, Meyers PA, Wexler L, Dela Cruz FS, Cheung N-K, Basu E, Kentsis A, Ortiz M, Francis JH, Dunkel IJ, Khakoo Y, Gilheeney S, Farouk Sait S, Forlenza CJ, Sulis M, Karajannis M, Modak S, Gerstle JT, Heaton TE, Roberts S, Yang C, Jairam S, Vijai J, Topka S, Friedman DN, Stadler ZK, Robson M, Berger MF, Schultz N, Ladanyi M, O'Reilly RJ, Abramson DH, Ceyhan-Birsoy O, Zhang L, Mandelker D, Shukla NN, Kung AL, Offit K, Zehir A, Walsh MF. Prospective pan-cancer germline testing using MSK-IMPACT informs clinical translation in 751 patients with pediatric solid tumors. Nat Can. 2021;2(3):357–65. https://doi.org/10.1038/s43018-021-00172-1.

Somatic Genomic Alterations in Neuroblastoma

4

Pauline Depuydt, Gudrun Schleiermacher, and Katleen De Preter

4.1 Recurrent Somatic Mutations

Next generation sequencing approaches have indicated that most neuroblastoma tumors harbor only few mutations, with an average of 10–20 predicted nonsynonymous variations in coding regions per genome, indicating an exonic mutation frequency of 0.2–0.4 per Mb [1–5]. The frequency of somatic events strongly correlates with tumor stage, as lower stage tumors harbor a lower number of mutations [2].

The most frequent recurrent somatic mutation in neuroblastoma concerns the gene *ALK* (anaplastic lymphoma kinase), with mutations activating the tyrosine kinase domain in approximately 10% of all cases at diagnosis [6–9]. In high-risk neuroblastoma, genetic alterations of ALK (clonal mutations and amplifications) have been shown to be independent predictors of poorer survival [10]. The somatic *ALK-F1174L* mutation appears to contribute to a more aggressive phenotype [11], but unlike *ALK-R1275Q* mutations, these specific mutations are not found in familial neuroblastoma and are not tolerated in the germline [9, 11, 12]. The oncogenic role of activating *ALK* mutations in neuroblastoma has been demonstrated in vitro and in vivo in both zebrafish and mouse models, with co-activation of ALK-F1174L and MYCN producing a synergistic effect for neuroblastoma tumorigenesis in mice and zebrafish [13–15]. Small molecule inhibitors targeting the activated kinase domain of ALK are available, making this a promising target for molecular therapy, but still require more specific development [7, 16, 17].

Other recurrent mutations in neuroblastoma target distinct cellular pathways and include *PTPN11* mutations (in 3% of cases) [5], regulators of the RAC/Rho pathway involved in neuritogenesis, such as *TIAM1*, as well as genes in the RAS-MAPK pathway (mainly in relapse cases) [2, 18, 19].

Interestingly, genes involved in chromatin remodeling have been found to be targeted in a significant number of cases, either by mutations or by structural variations, including mutations in the *ARID1A*/*ARID1B* genes [3] or *SMARCA4* [20]. Somatic alterations of *ATRX* are associ-

P. Depuydt
Center for Medical Genetics, Ghent University, Ghent, Belgium

Cancer Research Institute Ghent, Ghent, Belgium

G. Schleiermacher
U830 INSERM, Recherche Translationelle en Oncologie Pédiatrique (RTOP) and Department of Pediatric Oncology, Institut Curie, Paris, France

K. De Preter (✉)
Center for Medical Genetics, Ghent University, Ghent, Belgium

Cancer Research Institute Ghent, Ghent, Belgium

Center for Medical Biotechnology, VIB-UGent, Ghent, Belgium
e-mail: katleen.depreter@ugent.be

S. Asgharzadeh, F. Westermann (eds.), *Neuroblastoma*, Pediatric Oncology,
https://doi.org/10.1007/978-3-031-51292-6_4

ated with an absence of the ATRX protein in the nucleus and with an increase in telomere length. This occurs due to activation of a telomere maintenance mechanism termed alternative lengthening of telomeres (ALT) [21], which may be associated with primary chemotherapy resistance. *ATRX* alterations appear to be more frequent in older children and occur in mutually exclusive fashion with *MYCN* amplification [4, 22]. Recurrent genomic rearrangements of the promotor region of the *telomerase reverse transcriptase* (*TERT*) gene on chromosome 5p15.33 have been described in >10% of neuroblastoma cases and result in *TERT* upregulation due to enhancer hijacking. *TERT* rearrangements occur in mutually exclusive fashion with *MYCN* amplification and *ATRX* mutations [5, 23, 24]. A recent study has shown that clinical neuroblastoma subgroups are defined by telomere maintenance and RAS and p53 pathways alterations [25].

4.2 Recurrent DNA Copy Number Alterations

In contrast to the sparse somatic mutations, DNA copy number alterations are present in almost all neuroblastoma tumors [26, 27] and may lead to deregulation of neurodevelopmental processes [28]. Based on the proportion of the chromosome involved, three types of copy number alterations can be distinguished, i.e., numerical, large segmental, and small focal alterations. In-depth analysis of these copy number variations has led to new insights into neuroblastoma biology and oncogenesis.

4.2.1 Numerical Chromosome Alterations

With respect to whole-chromosome alterations, also called numerical chromosome alterations, gains of chromosome 17 are most frequently observed in neuroblastoma tumors, followed by gain of chromosome 7 and loss of chromosomes 14, 3, and 4 [27]. These alterations probably arise from defects in mitotic cell division and lead to tumors displaying a near-triploid genome [29, 30].

4.2.2 Segmental Chromosome Alterations

The most frequently observed segmental alteration in neuroblastoma cells is chromosome arm 17q gain, however, the breakpoints on chromosome 17q occur over nearly the whole chromosome arm and are not recurrent. Other common segmental alterations are 1q and 2p gain and 1p, 3p, 4p, 11q, and 14q loss. Many studies have attempted to define the smallest region of overlap (SRO) of recurring copy number alterations, aiming to identify candidate oncogenes and tumor suppressor genes located in these regions (1p [31–43], 3p [37, 44, 45], 11q [37, 46–49], 14q [50], 17q [37, 51–55]). However, in many cases these SROs remain relatively large. Integration of copy number data with expression and/or methylation data can further assist to define the candidate onco- and tumor suppressor genes. In the SRO of chromosome 1p loss, *CHD5* was put forward as a candidate tumor suppressor, as Fujita et al. and Koyama et al. could show that the remaining allele is commonly hypermethylated [56, 57]. *BIRC5* was proposed as a candidate oncogene on 17q, given the association of high expression levels with poor survival outcome [58]. The identification of both inactivating mutations in and (focal) deletions encompassing the genes *ARID1A* (on 1p36.11) and *ARID1B* (6q25.3) has put these chromatin remodeling genes forward as new (haplo-insufficient) tumor suppressor genes in neuroblastoma [3].

4.2.3 Focal Copy Number Alterations

Focal alterations specifically target a small region containing only a few genes and can help to further pinpoint the oncogenic drivers or tumor suppressor genes located in chromosomal regions of gain or loss. Three Mb is commonly used as upper size limit for focal alterations.

A typical example of a focal aberration is amplification of the *MYCN* oncogene. Amplicons are genomic regions with 8 to thousand copies. In 1983, the observation of amplified genomic region at 2p24.1 led to the identification of the *MYCN* (proto-)oncogene in aggressive neuroblastoma tumors [59]. Amplification of the *MYCN* oncogene occurs in approximately 20–25% of all neuroblastomas and 40% of high-risk tumors. It remains one of the most important genetic alterations associated with advanced stages of disease, an aggressive phenotype and poor outcome, and is the main genetic marker to be used in clinical practice for risk stratification and adaptation of treatment intensity [60–64]. Although closely associated with poor survival in localized disease and in infants, its prognostic impact in metastatic disease of older children with an overall poor outcome is less pronounced. At a cytogenetic level, amplification of the *MYCN* oncogene occurs either as double-minute chromosomes (DM) [65] or homogeneously staining regions (HSR) integrated into various chromosomes [65–67], which contain between 10 to over 100 ectopic copies of the *MYCN* oncogene. The oncogenic role of *MYCN* has been clearly demonstrated as its ectopic expression in the neural crest, is sufficient to drive neuroblastoma tumorigenesis in zebrafish and mouse model systems [15, 68, 69], and is based on an upregulation of genes involved in cell proliferation and on the repression of genes involved in differentiation and apoptosis [70].

Other, rare amplifications encompass genes such as *ALK* (2p23.1), *ODC1* (2p25.1), *LIN28B* (6q16.3), *CDK4* (12q14.1), *PPM1D* (17q23.2), *MDM2* (12q15), and *CCND1* (11q13.3) and are most often accompanied by *MYCN* amplification [52, 71–77].

In addition to these amplifications, focal homozygous deletions of the tumor suppressor genes *CDKN2A* (9p21.3), *KIF1B* (1p36.22), and *NF1* (17q11.2) have been described [37, 78–80], as well as hemizygous focal deletions of *PTPRD* (9p23), *ARID1B* (6q25.3), *APAF1* (12q23.1), *ELAVL4* (1p33), and *RGS5* (1q23.3) [3, 81, 82].

A meta-analysis study of Kumps et al. [82] indicated that focal DNA copy number imbalances in neuroblastoma target genes that are implicated in MYCN signaling, are possibly selected to reinforce *MYCN* oncogene addiction, including *CDK4*, *TERT*, *ODC1*, *MDM2*, the miR-17-92 cluster, and *PTPRD* (Fig. 4.1) [70, 82]. Furthermore, loss of let-7 family members at 3p and 11q has been shown to lead to upregulation of *MYCN* [83]. Also the genes *CDKN2A*, *CCND1*, *CHD5*, *LIN28B*, and *ALK* present in copy number alterations are connected in the

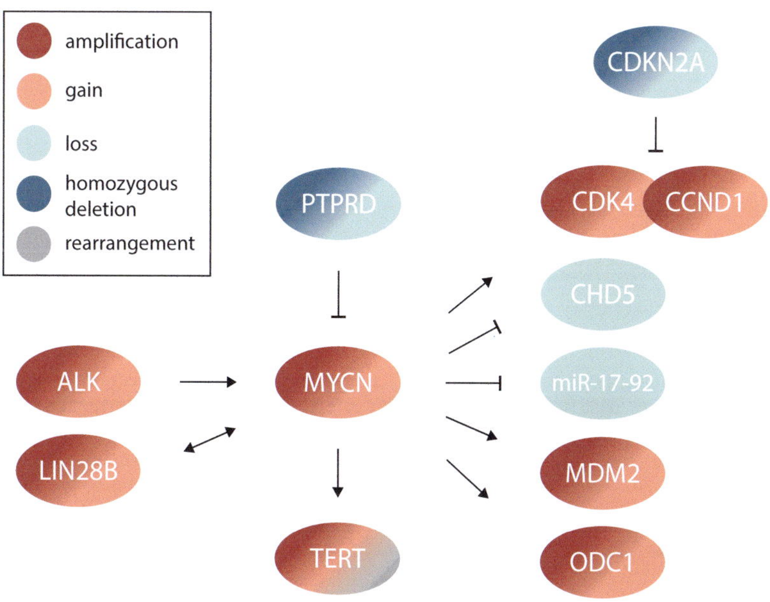

Fig. 4.1 Genes affected by somatic genomic alterations cooperate in MYCN signaling pathway. Cooperation of genes dysregulated in neuroblastoma by various genomic mechanisms and implicated in MYCN signaling. These gene likely reinforce MYCN oncogene addiction and lead to upregulation of MYCN

same signaling pathway. These findings emphasize the importance of the MYC(N) signaling pathway, even in *MYCN*-nonamplified tumors.

4.3 Molecular Subgroups Based on Somatic Genetic Alterations

Based on the co-occurrence of certain copy number alterations in neuroblastoma tumors, distinct genomic subgroups can be distinguished (Fig. 4.2).

A first group consists of tumors harboring numerical chromosome alterations (NCA) only. The remaining tumors are characterized by segmental chromosome alterations (SCA) with or without numerical alterations, often including 17q gain, and can be further divided in two groups. A second group consists of SCA tumors without *MYCN* amplification (MNA), which frequently present with 11q loss and 14q loss. Interestingly, these tumors often present with a higher number of segmental alterations and are more prevalent in older patients [84]. Finally, in a third group *MYCN* amplification (MNA) is observed, frequently associated with 1p loss and occurring at a younger age. With respect to telomere maintenance mechanisms, NCA tumors do not show telomere elongation, while SCA tumors

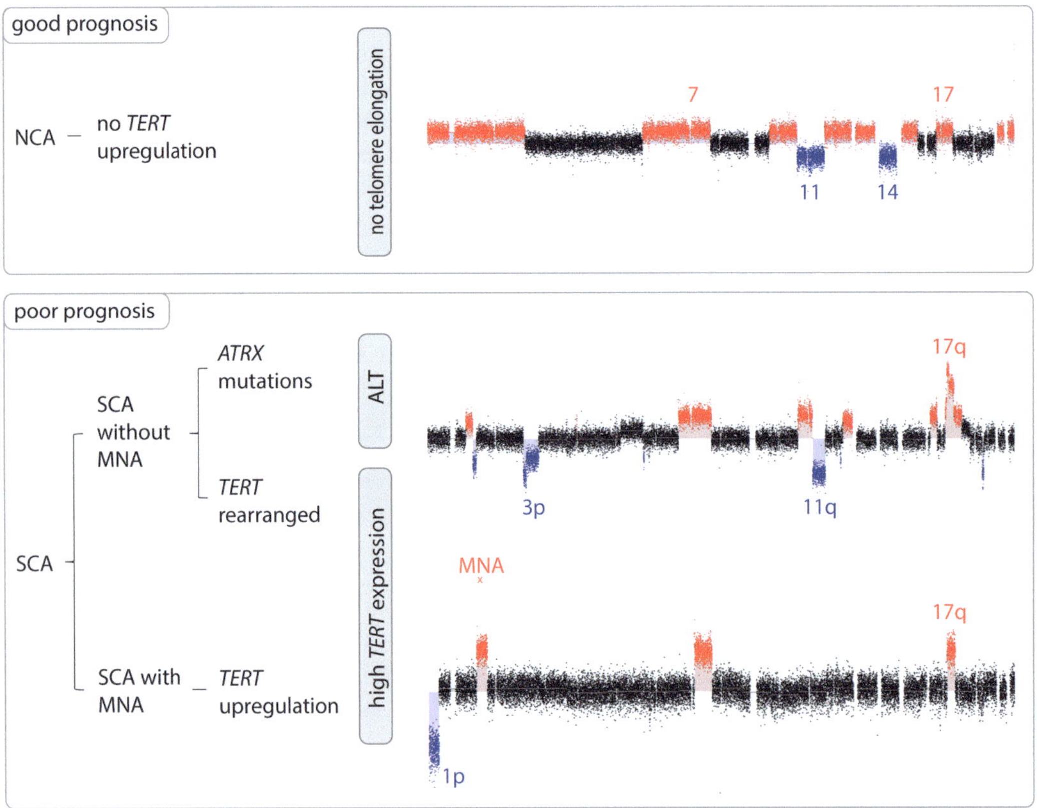

Fig. 4.2 Molecular subgroups based on copy number profile. Tumors with numerical chromosome alterations (NCA) only are characterized by absence of telomere elongation and are associated with good prognosis. Tumors with segmental chromosome alterations (SCA) typically display telomere maintenance mechanisms, either through alternative lengthening of telomeres (ALT) or through increased telomerase activity due to high TERT expression. Based on the copy number profile, a group of SCA tumors with MYCN amplification (MNA) and a group without MNA can be distinguished. MNA frequently occurs with 1p loss and 17q gain, while the group without MNA frequently presents with 17q gain and 11q loss. Both groups of tumors with SCA are associated with poor prognosis

display different maintenance mechanisms. In tumors with SCA and MNA, *TERT* is upregulated by *MYCN*, leading to telomerase activation. In tumors with SCA without MNA, two other mechanisms are observed. About half of those tumors display *TERT* rearrangements, also leading to upregulation of *TERT*, while the other half is characterized by *ATRX* mutations, which activates the ALT mechanism [23–25, 85, 86].

These three main groups were first described by Brodeur et al. [87, 88], predominantly based on karyotyping and FISH data. This observation was confirmed in later studies using hierarchical clustering of genome-wide comparative genomic hybridization (CGH) data [89] and array CGH data [76]. Another report on a large cohort of almost 500 primary neuroblastoma tumors described two additional groups, i.e., a group of cases with a mix of NCA and SCA and a group of cases with NCA with *MYCN* amplification. Using this method, 98% of patients could be unambiguously classified [27].

The main molecular subgroups are considered to be entirely distinct tumor types, that is, in general tumors with only numerical alterations are believed not to progress into the segmental type. Recently however, some observations have suggested otherwise. The existence of cases with a mixed pattern of NCA and SCA that closely resemble the pattern of NCA tumors suggests that these mixed cases progressed from tumors containing only NCA. Moreover, some patients present with SCA at relapse while only NCA were detected at diagnosis [90]. These reports indicate that progression from the favorable to unfavorable type may occur sporadically. This might be due to either an occurrence of new chromosome breakpoints during disease progression or spatial intratumor heterogeneity, with some alterations occurring either only at certain tumor sites, or at a subclonal level within the tumor [91].

4.4 Risk Stratification Based on Somatic Genetic Alterations

The presence of certain copy number alterations has been associated with patient outcome. The most well-known prognostic genetic biomarker for neuroblastoma is *MYCN* amplification status. The presence of *MYCN* amplification is associated with advanced stage of disease [60] and with decreased event-free survival [61]. This association is strongest in patients with low- and intermediate-risk disease. Within the subgroup of high-risk neuroblastoma tumors, the presence of *MYCN* amplification is associated with decreased survival time, however not with 10-year survival probability [77, 84]. Larger segmental alterations are also predictive of poor outcome. Gain of chromosome 17q is a strong prognostic factor associated with adverse outcome [92, 93], as well as loss of 1p and 11q [84, 94, 95]. In localized resectable tumors, loss and gain of a region on 1p and 1q, respectively, were associated with an increased risk of relapse [96]. A similar study including localized and stage 4S tumors identified losses of chromosome 3p and 11q as predictive for worse outcome [97]. *TERT* rearrangements on 5p15.33 define another subgroup of patients with increased risk [23, 24, 86]. A recent mechanistical classification suggests that patients whose tumors harbor telomere maintenance mechanisms in combination with RAS and/or p53 pathway mutations have the poorest outcome [25].

Furthermore, specific copy number alterations were reported to be associated with metastasis to the central nervous system, including gain of 18q22.1 and the *TERT* locus [98]. A meta-analysis study including 556 high-risk neuroblastoma copy number profiles revealed that the presence of distal 6q losses is linked with poor prognosis within high-risk neuroblastoma patients [77]. Interestingly, loss of 6q was observed more frequently in relapse tumors compared to primary tumors, indicating that these alterations play a role in more aggressive disease [19]. In the same meta-analysis study [77], the presence of amplifications in regions not encompassing *MYCN* (including the genes *ODC1*, *ALK*, *TERT*, *LIN28B*, *MYC*, *CCND1*, *CDK4*, and *MDM2*) were shown to be linked with poor prognosis within high-risk neuroblastoma patients [77], pointing to opportunities for alternative therapies for those patients.

More importantly, the overall copy number profile is associated with patient outcome and disease stage. Low-stage tumors (including the spontaneously regressing stage 4S/MS tumors) generally present with numerical alterations while segmental and focal alterations are abundant in high-stage tumors [89, 99]. Accordingly, tumors with only numerical alterations have a favorable prognosis, while the presence of segmental alterations is indicative of poor survival outcome [27, 87]. Moreover, the accumulation of segmental alterations in the genome, or in other words the number of breakpoints, is also predictive of outcome. Patients with a higher number of breakpoints show poorer survival than patients with fewer breakpoints [90], even within the subgroup of high-risk patients [77]. The prognostic power of the presence of segmental alterations is currently being confirmed in a prospective trial for low- and intermediate-risk patients (LINES), in which treatment intensity, particularly in the low-risk patient group, is adapted based on the overall genomic profile. Indeed, in the absence of SCA, an observational attitude may be proposed for patients with low-risk disease in the absence of clinical symptoms, whereas the presence of SCA will motivate a more intensive treatment regimen, with the aim to improve patient outcome with minimal treatment burden (https://clinicaltrials.gov/ct2/show/NCT01728155). For localized resectable MYCN-nonamplified neuroblastoma, age dependency of the prognostic impact of tumor genomics have been shown [100].

4.5 DNA Copy Number Profiling Technologies

Given that neuroblastoma is a copy number disease, the advances in neuroblastoma research have coincided with the development of copy number profiling techniques (Fig. 4.3). The analysis of copy number alterations in cells has revolutionized during the past decades from microscopy-based methods to array-based approaches and now also sequencing-based techniques. Karyotyping, the visualization of individual chromosomes in the metaphase of the cell cycle, has been used since the 1960s to detect chromosomal imbalances in tumor samples, which are recognized as abnormally shaped chromosomes such as double minutes, homogeneously stained regions, and 1;17 translocations [101–103]. In addition, multi-color karyotyping can be used for in-depth study of translocations [104]. Later fluorescence in situ hybridization (FISH) was introduced to detect specific genomic aberrations. This microscopy-based technique uses fluorescently labeled probes to visualize the status of a specific genomic locus. This method has been used frequently in the diagnostic setting of neuroblastoma for the detection of *MYCN* amplification, 17q gain, 1p deletion, 1;17 translocations, etc. [105–110]. To overcome the problem of limited resolution of karyotyping, comparative genomic hybridization (CGH) was developed in the 1990s. With this technique, differentially labeled tumor and reference DNA are hybridized on metaphase chromosomes. By analyzing the ratio of the signal from the tumor versus the signal from the reference DNA, the DNA copy number status of the tumor could be determined genome-wide. Application of this technique on hundreds of neuroblastoma samples further illustrated the extensive genetic heterogeneity of this type of tumors [53, 111–113]. A few years later a variant of this technique, array CGH (aCGH), was developed, in which the tumor and reference DNA are hybridized on oligonucleotide probes fixed on a glass slide [76, 81, 114–119]. In addition, genome-wide SNP arrays (SNPa) allowed to determine allelic imbalances on top of copy number status [37, 120]. This approach had the advantage of informing on copy-neutral loss of heterozygosity (LOH), however, the precise prognostic impact of the rarely occurring copy-neutral LOH in neuroblastoma remains to be determined. A more targeted method is multiplex ligation-dependent probe amplification (MLPA), which is a PCR-based method to determine the copy number of a set of genomic regions of interest. MPLA has been proven valuable to interrogate the most common chromosomal alterations in neuroblastoma [121, 122]. With the introduction of second-generation sequencing, many laboratories are using shallow whole genome sequencing (or low coverage

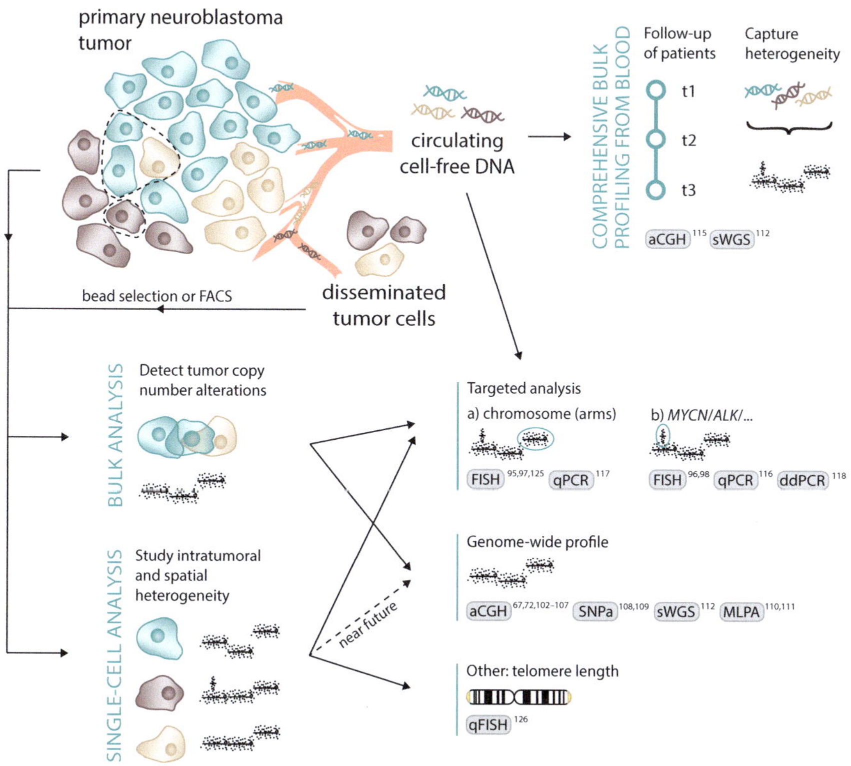

Fig. 4.3 Overview of copy number profiling techniques. Biopsies of the primary tumor or disseminated tumor cells are used to obtain a copy number profile of tumor cells. Bulk analysis can be performed to get information about copy number alterations present in the tumor, either on a targeted or genome-wide level. In contrast, single-cell analysis is valuable to study intratumoral and spatial heterogeneity. Single-cell analyses currently mainly focus on targeted analysis, while more recent genome-wide profiling allow to obtain a complete view of copy number alterations in single cells. In addition, liquid biopsies can be used to study copy number alterations in cell-free DNA originating from tumor cells (genome-wide or targeted level). This method has the advantage of capturing copy number alteration present in different cells of the tumor, which can be missed with conventional biopsies, as well as providing the opportunity to analyze copy number profiles over time during follow-up of the patients. *aCGH* array comparative genomic hybridization, *SNPa* single nucleotide polymorphism array, *sWGS* shallow whole genome sequencing, *MLPA* multiplex ligation-dependent probe amplification, *FISH* fluorescence in situ hybridization, *qFISH* quantitative FISH, *qPCR* quantitative PCR, *ddPCR* digital droplet PCR, *FACS* fluorescence-activated cell sorting

whole genome sequencing) (sWGS) for copy number profiling [123]. With this sequencing method, tumor DNA is sequenced at low coverage (approximately 0.5×). The genome is divided in windows of a certain size (e.g., 100 kb, depending on the coverage), and the number of reads in each window is then used as a measure for the copy number.

For most of above techniques DNA isolated from fresh tumor cells is used. As tumor tissue is not readily available for all patients, Vandewoestyne et al. developed a method to determine the tumor DNA copy number from disseminated tumor cells (DTCs) from the bone marrow [124]. Interestingly, the presence of specific alterations in DTCs can play an important role in understanding and preventing the occurrence of relapses [125]. More recently, several studies reported on the successful copy number profiling and mutation analysis of the tumor using circulating cell-free DNA (cfDNA) isolated from the patient's blood, applying sWGS, arrays, targeted sequencing, or qPCR [123, 126–130]. Another frequently used method to detect genomic aberrations in cfDNA is digital droplet PCR (ddPCR). This technique has been applied to check amplifications/gains and/or mutations of *MYCN* and *ALK* in the blood of high-risk neuroblastoma patients [131, 132]. These recent advancements in the field of liquid biopsies now present the opportunity to analyze the tumor copy number profile and the mutated genes over time, i.e., during therapy and follow-up of the patient [133, 134]. Moreover, these first reports provide evidence that clonal and spatial tumor heterogeneity is captured better by looking at the cfDNA. Alternatively, the introduction of single cell genomics will help us to further map the genomic heterogeneity present in tumors [135].

In neuroblastoma, intratumor heterogeneity has been first described by Squire et al. [136] for *MYCN* amplification and later by Ambros et al. [137] for both *MYCN* amplification and 1p loss, in contradiction to previous studies reporting only consistent presence of *MYCN* amplification in several samples of the same patient [138]. A later study performed on a large cohort confirmed that heterogeneity of *MYCN* amplification is rare, occurring in only 20 out of 1341 patients [139]. Recently, Berbegall et al. confirmed these findings and, in addition, reported also intratumor heterogeneity for 1p and 11q loss and 2p and 17q gain associated with heterogeneous *MYCN* amplification [140]. In another study, intratumoral diversity of multiple numerical (as well as segmental) alterations could be demonstrated [141]. A study on telomere length in single cells highlighted the association of intratumor diversity of telomere length with disease progression [142]. Furthermore, single-cell targeted sequencing of DTCs revealed that *ALK* mutations can be reliably detected at single-cell level [143].

In summary, molecular genetic characterization and in particular analysis of copy number alterations are an integral part of diagnostic procedures for neuroblastoma patients and are required to predict survival outcome and inform therapy stratification. At diagnosis, *MYCN* amplification is evaluated most frequently using FISH [144], while an overall copy number profile is nowadays generally obtained using sWGS. Panel and/or whole exome or whole genome sequencing add additional information.

References

1. Brady SW, Liu Y, Ma X, Gout AM, Hagiwara K, Zhou X, Wang J, Macias M, Chen X, Easton J, Mulder HL, Rusch M, Wang L, Nakitandwe J, Lei S, Davis EM, Naranjo A, Cheng C, Maris JM, Downing JR, Cheung NV, Hogarty MD, Dyer MA, Zhang J. Pan-neuroblastoma analysis reveals age- and signature-associated driver alterations. Nat Commun. 2020;11(1):5183. https://doi.org/10.1038/s41467-020-18987-4.
2. Molenaar JJ, Koster J, Zwijnenburg DA, van Sluis P, Valentijn LJ, van der Ploeg I, Hamdi M, van Nes J, Westerman BA, van Arkel J, Ebus ME, Haneveld F, Lakeman A, Schild L, Molenaar P, Stroeken P, van Noesel MM, Ora I, Santo EE, Caron HN, Westerhout EM, Versteeg R. Sequencing of neuroblastoma identifies chromothripsis and defects in neuritogenesis genes. Nature. 2012;483(7391):589–93. https://doi.org/10.1038/nature10910.
3. Sausen M, Leary RJ, Jones S, Wu J, Reynolds CP, Liu X, Blackford A, Parmigiani G, Diaz LA Jr, Papadopoulos N, Vogelstein B, Kinzler KW, Velculescu VE, Hogarty MD. Integrated genomic analyses identify ARID1A and ARID1B alterations in the childhood cancer neuroblastoma. Nat Genet. 2013;45(1):12–7. https://doi.org/10.1038/ng.2493.
4. Cheung NKV, Zhang JH, Lu C, Parker M, Bahrami A, Tickoo SK, Heguy A, Pappo AS, Federico S, Dalton J, Cheung IY, Ding L, Fulton R, Wang JW, Chen X, Becksfort J, Wu JR, Billups CA, Ellison D, Mardis ER, Wilson RK, Downing JR, Dyer MA, Washin SJ. Association of age at diagnosis and genetic mutations in patients with neuroblastoma. JAMA. 2012;307(10):1062–71. https://doi.org/10.1001/jama.2012.228.
5. Pugh TJ, Morozova O, Attiyeh EF, Asgharzadeh S, Wei JS, Auclair D, Carter SL, Cibulskis K, Hanna M, Kiezun A, Kim J, Lawrence MS, Lichenstein L, McKenna A, Pedamallu CS, Ramos AH, Shefler E, Sivachenko A, Sougnez C, Stewart C, Ally A, Birol I, Chiu R, Corbett RD, Hirst M, Jackman SD, Kamoh B, Khodabakshi AH, Krzywinski M, Lo A, Moore RA, Mungall KL, Qian J, Tam A, Thiessen N, Zhao Y, Cole KA, Diamond M, Diskin SJ, Mosse YP, Wood AC, Ji L, Sposto R, Badgett T, London WB, Moyer Y, Gastier-Foster JM, Smith MA, Guidry Auvil JM, Gerhard DS, Hogarty MD, Jones SJ, Lander ES, Gabriel SB, Getz G, Seeger RC, Khan J, Marra MA, Meyerson M, Maris JM. The genetic landscape of high-risk neuroblastoma. Nat Genet. 2013;45(3):279–84. https://doi.org/10.1038/ng.2529.
6. Chen Y, Takita J, Choi YL, Kato M, Ohira M, Sanada M, Wang L, Soda M, Kikuchi A, Igarashi T, Nakagawara A, Hayashi Y, Mano H, Ogawa S. Oncogenic mutations of ALK kinase in neuroblastoma. Nature. 2008;455(7215):971–4. https://doi.org/10.1038/nature07399.

7. George RE, Sanda T, Hanna M, Frohling S, Luther W 2nd, Zhang J, Ahn Y, Zhou W, London WB, McGrady P, Xue L, Zozulya S, Gregor VE, Webb TR, Gray NS, Gilliland DG, Diller L, Greulich H, Morris SW, Meyerson M, Look AT. Activating mutations in ALK provide a therapeutic target in neuroblastoma. Nature. 2008;455(7215):975–8. https://doi.org/10.1038/nature07397.
8. Janoueix-Lerosey I, Lequin D, Brugieres L, Ribeiro A, de Pontual L, Combaret V, Raynal V, Puisieux A, Schleiermacher G, Pierron G, Valteau-Couanet D, Frebourg T, Michon J, Lyonnet S, Amiel J, Delattre O. Somatic and germline activating mutations of the ALK kinase receptor in neuroblastoma. Nature. 2008;455(7215):967–70. https://doi.org/10.1038/nature07398.
9. Mosse YP, Laudenslager M, Longo L, Cole KA, Wood A, Attiyeh EF, Laquaglia MJ, Sennett R, Lynch JE, Perri P, Laureys G, Speleman F, Kim C, Hou C, Hakonarson H, Torkamani A, Schork NJ, Brodeur GM, Tonini GP, Rappaport E, Devoto M, Maris JM. Identification of ALK as a major familial neuroblastoma predisposition gene. Nature. 2008;455(7215):930–5. https://doi.org/10.1038/nature07261.
10. Bellini A, Potschger U, Bernard V, Lapouble E, Baulande S, Ambros PF, Auger N, Beiske K, Bernkopf M, Betts DR, Bhalshankar J, Bown N, de Preter K, Clement N, Combaret V, Font de Mora J, George SL, Jimenez I, Jeison M, Marques B, Martinsson T, Mazzocco K, Morini M, Muhlethaler-Mottet A, Noguera R, Pierron G, Rossing M, Taschner-Mandl S, Van Roy N, Vicha A, Chesler L, Balwierz W, Castel V, Elliott M, Kogner P, Laureys G, Luksch R, Malis J, Popovic-Beck M, Ash S, Delattre O, Valteau-Couanet D, Tweddle DA, Ladenstein R, Schleiermacher G. Frequency and prognostic impact of ALK amplifications and mutations in the European Neuroblastoma Study Group (SIOPEN) high-risk neuroblastoma trial (HR-NBL1). J Clin Oncol. 2021;39(30):3377–90. https://doi.org/10.1200/JCO.21.00086.
11. De Brouwer S, De Preter K, Kumps C, Zabrocki P, Porcu M, Westerhout EM, Lakeman A, Vandesompele J, Hoebeeck J, Van Maerken T, De Paepe A, Laureys G, Schulte JH, Schramm A, Van Den Broecke C, Vermeulen J, Van Roy N, Beiske K, Renard M, Noguera R, Delattre O, Janoueix-Lerosey I, Kogner P, Martinsson T, Nakagawara A, Ohira M, Caron H, Eggert A, Cools J, Versteeg R, Speleman F. Meta-analysis of neuroblastomas reveals a skewed ALK mutation spectrum in tumors with MYCN amplification. Clin Cancer Res. 2010;16(17):4353–62. https://doi.org/10.1158/1078-0432.CCR-09-2660.
12. Janoueix-Lerosey I, Schleiermacher G, Delattre O. Molecular pathogenesis of peripheral neuroblastic tumors. Oncogene. 2010;29(11):1566–79. https://doi.org/10.1038/onc.2009.518.
13. Heukamp LC, Thor T, Schramm A, De Preter K, Kumps C, De Wilde B, Odersky A, Peifer M, Lindner S, Spruessel A, Pattyn F, Mestdagh P, Menten B, Kuhfittig-Kulle S, Kunkele A, Konig K, Meder L, Chatterjee S, Ullrich RT, Schulte S, Vandesompele J, Speleman F, Buttner R, Eggert A, Schulte JH. Targeted expression of mutated ALK induces neuroblastoma in transgenic mice. Sci Transl Med. 2012;4(141):141–91. https://doi.org/10.1126/scitranslmed.3003967.
14. Berry T, Luther W, Bhatnagar N, Jamin Y, Poon E, Sanda T, Pei D, Sharma B, Vetharoy WR, Hallsworth A, Ahmad Z, Barker K, Moreau L, Webber H, Wang W, Liu Q, Perez-Atayde A, Rodig S, Cheung NK, Raynaud F, Hallberg B, Robinson SP, Gray NS, Pearson AD, Eccles SA, Chesler L, George RE. The ALK(F1174L) mutation potentiates the oncogenic activity of MYCN in neuroblastoma. Cancer Cell. 2012;22(1):117–30. https://doi.org/10.1016/j.ccr.2012.06.001.
15. Zhu S, Lee JS, Guo F, Shin J, Perez-Atayde AR, Kutok JL, Rodig SJ, Neuberg DS, Helman D, Feng H, Stewart RA, Wang W, George RE, Kanki JP, Look AT. Activated ALK collaborates with MYCN in neuroblastoma pathogenesis. Cancer Cell. 2012;21(3):362–73. https://doi.org/10.1016/j.ccr.2012.02.010.
16. Schulte JH, Eggert A. ALK inhibitors in neuroblastoma: a sprint from bench to bedside. Clin Cancer Res. 2021;27(13):3507–9. https://doi.org/10.1158/1078-0432.CCR-21-0627.
17. Mosse YP, Lim MS, Voss SD, Wilner K, Ruffner K, Laliberte J, Rolland D, Balis FM, Maris JM, Weigel BJ, Ingle AM, Ahern C, Adamson PC, Blaney SM. Safety and activity of crizotinib for paediatric patients with refractory solid tumours or anaplastic large-cell lymphoma: a Children's Oncology Group phase 1 consortium study. Lancet Oncol. 2013;14(6):472–80. https://doi.org/10.1016/S1470-2045(13)70095-0.
18. Fransson S, Martinez-Monleon A, Johansson M, Sjoberg RM, Bjorklund C, Ljungman G, Ek T, Kogner P, Martinsson T. Whole-genome sequencing of recurrent neuroblastoma reveals somatic mutations that affect key players in cancer progression and telomere maintenance. Sci Rep. 2020;10(1):22432. https://doi.org/10.1038/s41598-020-78370-7.
19. Eleveld TF, Oldridge DA, Bernard V, Koster J, Colmet Daage L, Diskin SJ, Schild L, Bentahar NB, Bellini A, Chicard M, Lapouble E, Combaret V, Legoix-Ne P, Michon J, Pugh TJ, Hart LS, Rader J, Attiyeh EF, Wei JS, Zhang S, Naranjo A, Gastier-Foster JM, Hogarty MD, Asgharzadeh S, Smith MA, Guidry Auvil JM, Watkins TB, Zwijnenburg DA, Ebus ME, van Sluis P, Hakkert A, van Wezel E, van der Schoot CE, Westerhout EM, Schulte JH, Tytgat GA, Dolman ME, Janoueix-Lerosey I, Gerhard DS, Caron HN, Delattre O, Khan J, Versteeg R, Schleiermacher G, Molenaar JJ, Maris JM. Relapsed neuroblastomas show frequent RAS-MAPK pathway mutations. Nat Genet. 2015;47(8):864–71. https://doi.org/10.1038/ng.3333.

20. Bellini A, Bessoltane-Bentahar N, Bhalshankar J, Clement N, Raynal V, Baulande S, Bernard V, Danzon A, Chicard M, Colmet-Daage L, Pierron G, Le Roux L, Planchon JM, Combaret V, Lapouble E, Corradini N, Thebaud E, Gambart M, Valteau-Couanet D, Michon J, Louis-Brennetot C, Janoueix-Lerosey I, Defachelles AS, Bourdeaut F, Delattre O, Schleiermacher G. Study of chromatin remodeling genes implicates SMARCA4 as a putative player in oncogenesis in neuroblastoma. Int J Cancer. 2019;145(10):2781–91. https://doi.org/10.1002/ijc.32361.
21. Hartlieb SA, Sieverling L, Nadler-Holly M, Ziehm M, Toprak UH, Herrmann C, Ishaque N, Okonechnikov K, Gartlgruber M, Park YG, Wecht EM, Savelyeva L, Henrich KO, Rosswog C, Fischer M, Hero B, Jones DTW, Pfaff E, Witt O, Pfister SM, Volckmann R, Koster J, Kiesel K, Rippe K, Taschner-Mandl S, Ambros P, Brors B, Selbach M, Feuerbach L, Westermann F. Alternative lengthening of telomeres in childhood neuroblastoma from genome to proteome. Nat Commun. 2021;12(1):1269. https://doi.org/10.1038/s41467-021-21247-8.
22. Zeineldin M, Federico S, Chen X, Fan Y, Xu B, Stewart E, Zhou X, Jeon J, Griffiths L, Nguyen R, Norrie J, Easton J, Mulder H, Yergeau D, Liu Y, Wu J, Van Ryn C, Naranjo A, Hogarty MD, Kaminski MM, Valentine M, Pruett-Miller SM, Pappo A, Zhang J, Clay MR, Bahrami A, Vogel P, Lee S, Shelat A, Sarthy JF, Meers MP, George RE, Mardis ER, Wilson RK, Henikoff S, Downing JR, Dyer MA. MYCN amplification and ATRX mutations are incompatible in neuroblastoma. Nat Commun. 2020;11(1):913. https://doi.org/10.1038/s41467-020-14682-6.
23. Peifer M, Hertwig F, Roels F, Dreidax D, Gartlgruber M, Menon R, Kramer A, Roncaioli JL, Sand F, Heuckmann JM, Ikram F, Schmidt R, Ackermann S, Engesser A, Kahlert Y, Vogel W, Altmuller J, Nurnberg P, Thierry-Mieg J, Thierry-Mieg D, Mariappan A, Heynck S, Mariotti E, Henrich KO, Gloeckner C, Bosco G, Leuschner I, Schweiger MR, Savelyeva L, Watkins SC, Shao C, Bell E, Hofer T, Achter V, Lang U, Theissen J, Volland R, Saadati M, Eggert A, de Wilde B, Berthold F, Peng Z, Zhao C, Shi L, Ortmann M, Buttner R, Perner S, Hero B, Schramm A, Schulte JH, Herrmann C, O'Sullivan RJ, Westermann F, Thomas RK, Fischer M. Telomerase activation by genomic rearrangements in high-risk neuroblastoma. Nature. 2015;526(7575):700–4. https://doi.org/10.1038/nature14980.
24. Valentijn LJ, Koster J, Zwijnenburg DA, Hasselt NE, van Sluis P, Volckmann R, van Noesel MM, George RE, Tytgat GA, Molenaar JJ, Versteeg R. TERT rearrangements are frequent in neuroblastoma and identify aggressive tumors. Nat Genet. 2015;47(12):1411–4. https://doi.org/10.1038/ng.3438.
25. Ackermann S, Cartolano M, Hero B, Welte A, Kahlert Y, Roderwieser A, Bartenhagen C, Walter E, Gecht J, Kerschke L, Volland R, Menon R, Heuckmann JM, Gartlgruber M, Hartlieb S, Henrich KO, Okonechnikov K, Altmuller J, Nurnberg P, Lefever S, de Wilde B, Sand F, Ikram F, Rosswog C, Fischer J, Theissen J, Hertwig F, Singhi AD, Simon T, Vogel W, Perner S, Krug B, Schmidt M, Rahmann S, Achter V, Lang U, Vokuhl C, Ortmann M, Buttner R, Eggert A, Speleman F, O'Sullivan RJ, Thomas RK, Berthold F, Vandesompele J, Schramm A, Westermann F, Schulte JH, Peifer M, Fischer M. A mechanistic classification of clinical phenotypes in neuroblastoma. Science. 2018;362(6419):1165–70. https://doi.org/10.1126/science.aat6768.
26. Schleiermacher G, Mosseri V, London WB, Maris JM, Brodeur GM, Attiyeh E, Haber M, Khan J, Nakagawara A, Speleman F, Noguera R, Tonini GP, Fischer M, Ambros I, Monclair T, Matthay KK, Ambros P, Cohn SL, Pearson ADJ. Segmental chromosomal alterations have prognostic impact in neuroblastoma: a report from the INRG project. Br J Cancer. 2012;107(8):1418–22. https://doi.org/10.1038/bjc.2012.375.
27. Janoueix-Lerosey I, Schleiermacher G, Michels E, Mosseri V, Ribeiro A, Lequin D, Vermeulen J, Couturier J, Peuchmaur M, Valent A, Plantaz D, Rubie H, Valteau-Couanet D, Thomas C, Combaret V, Rousseau R, Eggert A, Michon J, Speleman F, Delattre O. Overall genomic pattern is a predictor of outcome in neuroblastoma. J Clin Oncol. 2009;27(7):1026–33. https://doi.org/10.1200/Jco.2008.16.0630.
28. Lopez G, Conkrite KL, Doepner M, Rathi KS, Modi A, Vaksman Z, Farra LM, Hyson E, Noureddine M, Wei JS, Smith MA, Asgharzadeh S, Seeger RC, Khan J, Auvil JG, Gerhard DS, Maris JM, Diskin SJ. Somatic structural variation targets neurodevelopmental genes and identifies SHANK2 as a tumor suppressor in neuroblastoma. Genome Res. 2020;30(9):1228–42. https://doi.org/10.1101/gr.252106.119.
29. Thompson SL, Compton DA. Examining the link between chromosomal instability and aneuploidy in human cells. J Cell Biol. 2008;180(4):665–72. https://doi.org/10.1083/jcb.200712029.
30. Thompson SL, Compton DA. Chromosomes and cancer cells. Chromosom Res. 2011;19(3):433–44. https://doi.org/10.1007/s10577-010-9179-y.
31. White PS, Thompson PM, Seifried BA, Sulman EP, Jensen SJ, Guo C, Maris JM, Hogarty MD, Allen C, Biegel JA, Matise TC, Gregory SG, Reynolds CP, Brodeur GM. Detailed molecular analysis of 1p36 in neuroblastoma. Med Pediatr Oncol. 2001;36(1):37–41. https://doi.org/10.1002/1096-911X(20010101)36:1<37::AID-MPO1010>3.0.CO;2-L.
32. Bauer A, Savelyeva L, Claas A, Praml C, Berthold F, Schwab M. Smallest region of overlapping deletion in 1p36 in human neuroblastoma: a 1 Mbp cosmid and PAC contig. Genes Chromosomes

Cancer. 2001;31(3):228–39. https://doi.org/10.1002/gcc.1139.
33. White PS, Maris JM, Sulman EP, Jensen SJ, Kyemba SM, Beltinger CP, Allen C, Kramer DL, Biegel JA, Brodeur GM. Molecular analysis of the region of distal 1p commonly deleted in neuroblastoma. Eur J Cancer. 1997;33(12):1957–61. https://doi.org/10.1016/s0959-8049(97)00311-0.
34. Hogarty MD, Liu XY, Guo C, Thompson PM, Weiss MJ, White PS, Sulman EP, Brodeur GM, Maris JM. Identification of a 1-megabase consensus region of deletion at 1p36.3 in primary neuroblastomas. Med Pediatr Oncol. 2000;35(6):512–5. https://doi.org/10.1002/1096-911x(20001201)35:6<512::Aid-Mpo2>3.0.Co;2-D.
35. Caron H, Spieker N, Godfried M, Veenstra M, van Sluis P, de Kraker J, Voûte P, Versteeg R. Chromosome bands 1p35-36 contain two distinct neuroblastoma tumor suppressor loci, one of which is imprinted. Genes Chromosomes Cancer. 2001;30(2):168–74. https://doi.org/10.1002/1098-2264(200102)30:2<168::Aid-gcc1072>3.0.Co;2-e.
36. White PS, Thompson PM, Gotoh T, Okawa ER, Igarashi J, Kok M, Winter C, Gregory SG, Hogarty MD, Maris JM, Brodeur GM. Definition and characterization of a region of 1p36.3 consistently deleted in neuroblastoma. Oncogene. 2005;24(16):2684–94. https://doi.org/10.1038/sj.onc.1208306.
37. Caren H, Erichsen J, Olsson L, Enerback C, Sjoberg RM, Abrahamsson J, Kogner P, Martinsson T. High-resolution array copy number analyses for detection of deletion, gain, amplification and copy-neutral LOH in primary neuroblastoma tumors: four cases of homozygous deletions of the CDKN2A gene. BMC Genomics. 2008;9:353. https://doi.org/10.1186/1471-2164-9-353.
38. Martinsson T, Sjoberg RM, Hedborg F, Kogner P. Deletion of chromosome 1p loci and microsatellite instability in neuroblastomas analyzed with short-tandem repeat polymorphisms. Cancer Res. 1995;55(23):5681–6.
39. Maris JM, Guo C, Blake D, White PS, Hogarty MD, Thompson PM, Rajalingam V, Gerbing R, Stram DO, Matthay KK, Seeger RC, Brodeur GM. Comprehensive analysis of chromosome 1p deletions in neuroblastoma. Med Pediatr Oncol. 2001;36(1):32–6. https://doi.org/10.1002/1096-911X(20010101)36:1<32::AID-MPO1009>3.0.CO;2-0.
40. Ohira M, Kageyama H, Mihara M, Furuta S, Machida T, Shishikura T, Takayasu H, Islam A, Nakamura Y, Takahashi M, Tomioka N, Sakiyama S, Kaneko Y, Toyoda A, Hattori M, Sakaki Y, Ohki M, Horii A, Soeda E, Inazawa J, Seki N, Kuma H, Nozawa I, Nakagawara A. Identification and characterization of a 500-kb homozygously deleted region at 1p36.2-p36.3 in a neuroblastoma cell line. Oncogene. 2000;19(37):4302–7. https://doi.org/10.1038/sj.onc.1203786.
41. Chen YZ, Soeda E, Yang HW, Takita J, Chai L, Horii A, Inazawa J, Ohki M, Hayashi Y. Homozygous deletion in a neuroblastoma cell line defined by a high-density STS map spanning human chromosome band 1p36. Genes Chromosomes Cancer. 2001;31(4):326–32. https://doi.org/10.1002/gcc.1151.
42. Martinsson T, Sjoberg RM, Hallstensson K, Nordling M, Hedborg F, Kogner P. Delimitation of a critical tumour suppressor region at distal 1p in neuroblastoma tumours. Eur J Cancer. 1997;33(12):1997–2001. https://doi.org/10.1016/S0959-8049(97)00278-5.
43. Ejeskar K, Sjoberg RM, Abel F, Kogner P, Ambros PF, Martinsson T. Fine mapping of a tumour suppressor candidate gene region in 1p36.2-3, commonly deleted in neuroblastomas and germ cell tumours. Med Pediatr Oncol. 2001;36(1):61–6. https://doi.org/10.1002/1096-911X(20010101)36:1<61::AID-MPO1016>3.0.CO;2-0.
44. Hoebeeck J, Michels E, Menten B, Van Roy N, Eggert A, Schramm A, De Preter K, Yigit N, De Smet E, De Paepe A, Laureys G, Vandesompele J, Speleman F. High resolution tiling-path BAC array deletion mapping suggests commonly involved 3p21-p22 tumor suppressor genes in neuroblastoma and more frequent tumors. Int J Cancer. 2007;120(3):533–8. https://doi.org/10.1002/ijc.22326.
45. Ejeskar K, Aburatani H, Abrahamsson J, Kogner P, Martinsson T. Loss of heterozygosity of 3p markers in neuroblastoma tumours implicate a tumour-suppressor locus distal to the FHIT gene. Br J Cancer. 1998;77(11):1787–91. https://doi.org/10.1038/bjc.1998.297.
46. Guo C, White PS, Weiss MJ, Hogarty MD, Thompson PM, Stram DO, Gerbing R, Matthay KK, Seeger RC, Brodeur GM, Maris JM. Allelic deletion at 11q23 is common in MYCN single copy neuroblastomas. Oncogene. 1999;18(35):4948–57. https://doi.org/10.1038/sj.onc.1202887.
47. Mlakar V, Jurkovic Mlakar S, Lopez G, Maris JM, Ansari M, Gumy-Pause F. 11q deletion in neuroblastoma: a review of biological and clinical implications. Mol Cancer. 2017;16(1):114. https://doi.org/10.1186/s12943-017-0686-8.
48. Maris JM, Guo C, White PS, Hogarty MD, Thompson PM, Stram DO, Gerbing R, Matthay KK, Seeger RC, Brodeur GM. Allelic deletion at chromosome bands 11q14-23 is common in neuroblastoma. Med Pediatr Oncol. 2001;36(1):24–7. https://doi.org/10.1002/1096-911x(20010101)36:1<24::Aid-Mpo1007>3.0.Co;2-7.
49. Schleiermacher G, Michon J, Huon I, d'Enghien CD, Klijanienko J, Brisse H, Ribeiro A, Mosseri V, Rubie H, Munzer C, Thomas C, Valteau-Couanet D, Auvrignon A, Plantaz D, Delattre O, Couturier J. Chromosomal CGH identifies patients with a higher risk of relapse in neuroblastoma without MYCN amplification. Br J Cancer. 2007;97(2):238–46. https://doi.org/10.1038/sj.bjc.6603820.

50. Thompson PM, Seifried BA, Kyemba SK, Jensen SJ, Guo C, Maris JM, Brodeur GM, Stram DO, Seeger RC, Gerbing R, Matthay KK, Matise TC, White PS. Loss of heterozygosity for chromosome 14q in neuroblastoma. Med Pediatr Oncol. 2001;36(1):28–31. https://doi.org/10.1002/1096-911X(20010101)36:1<28::AID-MPO1008>3.0.CO;2-0.
51. Vandesompele J, Michels E, De Preter K, Menten B, Schramm A, Eggert A, Ambros PF, Combaret V, Francotte N, Antonacci F, De Paepe A, Laureys G, Speleman F, Van Roy N. Identification of 2 putative critical segments of 17q gain in neuroblastoma through integrative genomics. Int J Cancer. 2008;122(5):1177–82. https://doi.org/10.1002/ijc.23156.
52. Saito-Ohara F, Imoto I, Inoue J, Hosoi H, Nakagawara A, Sugimoto T, Inazawa J. PPM1D is a potential target for 17q gain in neuroblastoma. Cancer Res. 2003;63(8):1876–83.
53. Plantaz D, Mohapatra G, Matthay KK, Pellarin M, Seeger RC, Feuerstein BG. Gain of chromosome 17 is the most frequent abnormality detected in neuroblastoma by comparative genomic hybridization. Am J Pathol. 1997;150(1):81–9.
54. Meddeb M, Danglot G, Chudoba I, Venuat AM, Benard J, Avet-Loiseau H, Vasseur B, Le Paslier D, Terrier-Lacombe MJ, Hartmann O, Bernheim A. Additional copies of a 25 Mb chromosomal region originating from 17q23.1-17qter are present in 90% of high-grade neuroblastomas. Genes Chromosomes Cancer. 1996;17(3):156–65.
55. Lastowska M, Cotterill S, Bown N, Cullinane C, Variend S, Lunec J, Strachan T, Pearson AD, Jackson MS. Breakpoint position on 17q identifies the most aggressive neuroblastoma tumors. Genes Chromosomes Cancer. 2002;34(4):428–36. https://doi.org/10.1002/gcc.10089.
56. Fujita T, Igarashi J, Okawa ER, Gotoh T, Manne J, Kolla V, Kim J, Zhao H, Pawel BR, London WB, Maris JM, White PS, Brodeur GM. CHD5, a tumor suppressor gene deleted from 1p36.31 in neuroblastomas. J Natl Cancer Inst. 2008;100(13):940–9. https://doi.org/10.1093/jnci/djn176.
57. Koyama H, Zhuang T, Light JE, Kolla V, Higashi M, McGrady PW, London WB, Brodeur GM. Mechanisms of CHD5 inactivation in neuroblastomas. Clin Cancer Res. 2012;18(6):1588–97. https://doi.org/10.1158/1078-0432.CCR-11-2644.
58. Islam A, Kageyama H, Takada N, Kawamoto T, Takayasu H, Isogai E, Ohira M, Hashizume K, Kobayashi H, Kaneko Y, Nakagawara A. High expression of survivin, mapped to 17q25, is significantly associated with poor prognostic factors and promotes cell survival in human neuroblastoma. Oncogene. 2000;19(5):617–23. https://doi.org/10.1038/sj.onc.1203358.
59. Schwab M, Alitalo K, Klempnauer KH, Varmus HE, Bishop JM, Gilbert F, Brodeur G, Goldstein M, Trent J. Amplified DNA with limited homology to myc cellular oncogene is shared by human neuroblastoma cell lines and a neuroblastoma tumour. Nature. 1983;305(5931):245–8. https://doi.org/10.1038/305245a0.
60. Brodeur GM, Seeger RC, Schwab M, Varmus HE, Bishop JM. Amplification of N-myc in untreated human neuroblastomas correlates with advanced disease stage. Science. 1984;224(4653):1121–4. https://doi.org/10.1126/science.6719137.
61. Seeger RC, Brodeur GM, Sather H, Dalton A, Siegel SE, Wong KY, Hammond D. Association of multiple copies of the N-myc oncogene with rapid progression of neuroblastomas. N Engl J Med. 1985;313(18):1111–6. https://doi.org/10.1056/NEJM198510313131802.
62. Thompson D, Vo KT, London WB, Fischer M, Ambros PF, Nakagawara A, Brodeur GM, Matthay KK, DuBois SG. Identification of patient subgroups with markedly disparate rates of MYCN amplification in neuroblastoma: a report from the International Neuroblastoma Risk Group project. Cancer. 2016;122(6):935–45. https://doi.org/10.1002/cncr.29848.
63. Campbell K, Gastier-Foster JM, Mann M, Naranjo AH, Van Ryn C, Bagatell R, Matthay KK, London WB, Irwin MS, Shimada H, Granger MM, Hogarty MD, Park JR, DuBois SG. Association of MYCN copy number with clinical features, tumor biology, and outcomes in neuroblastoma: a report from the Children's Oncology Group. Cancer. 2017;123(21):4224–35. https://doi.org/10.1002/cncr.30873.
64. Pinto NR, Applebaum MA, Volchenboum SL, Matthay KK, London WB, Ambros PF, Nakagawara A, Berthold F, Schleiermacher G, Park JR, Valteau-Couanet D, Pearson AD, Cohn SL. Advances in risk classification and treatment strategies for neuroblastoma. J Clin Oncol. 2015;33(27):3008–17. https://doi.org/10.1200/JCO.2014.59.4648.
65. Schwab M, Varmus HE, Bishop JM, Grzeschik KH, Naylor SL, Sakaguchi AY, Brodeur G, Trent J. Chromosome localization in normal human cells and neuroblastomas of a gene related to c-myc. Nature. 1984;308(5956):288–91. https://doi.org/10.1038/308288a0.
66. Kanda N, Schreck R, Alt F, Bruns G, Baltimore D, Latt S. Isolation of amplified DNA sequences from IMR-32 human neuroblastoma cells: facilitation by fluorescence-activated flow sorting of metaphase chromosomes. Proc Natl Acad Sci U S A. 1983;80(13):4069–73. https://doi.org/10.1073/pnas.80.13.4069.
67. Emanuel BS, Balaban G, Boyd JP, Grossman A, Negishi M, Parmiter A, Glick MC. N-myc amplification in multiple homogeneously staining regions in two human neuroblastomas. Proc Natl Acad Sci U S A. 1985;82(11):3736–40. https://doi.org/10.1073/pnas.82.11.3736.
68. Weiss WA, Aldape K, Mohapatra G, Feuerstein BG, Bishop JM. Targeted expression of MYCN

causes neuroblastoma in transgenic mice. EMBO J. 1997;16(11):2985–95. https://doi.org/10.1093/emboj/16.11.2985.

69. Althoff K, Beckers A, Bell E, Nortmeyer M, Thor T, Sprussel A, Lindner S, De Preter K, Florin A, Heukamp LC, Klein-Hitpass L, Astrahantseff K, Kumps C, Speleman F, Eggert A, Westermann F, Schramm A, Schulte JH. A Cre-conditional MYCN-driven neuroblastoma mouse model as an improved tool for preclinical studies. Oncogene. 2015;34(26):3357–68. https://doi.org/10.1038/onc.2014.269.
70. Bell E, Chen LD, Liu T, Marshall GM, Lunec J, Tweddle DA. MYCN oncoprotein targets and their therapeutic potential. Cancer Lett. 2010;293(2):144–57. https://doi.org/10.1016/j.canlet.2010.01.015.
71. Caren H, Abel F, Kogner P, Martinsson T. High incidence of DNA mutations and gene amplifications of the ALK gene in advanced sporadic neuroblastoma tumours. Biochem J. 2008;416(2):153–9. https://doi.org/10.1042/bj20081834.
72. Molenaar JJ, Domingo-Fernandez R, Ebus ME, Lindner S, Koster J, Drabek K, Mestdagh P, van Sluis P, Valentijn LJ, van Nes J, Broekmans M, Haneveld F, Volckmann R, Bray I, Heukamp L, Sprussel A, Thor T, Kieckbusch K, Klein-Hitpass L, Fischer M, Vandesompele J, Schramm A, van Noesel MM, Varesio L, Speleman F, Eggert A, Stallings RL, Caron HN, Versteeg R, Schulte JH. LIN28B induces neuroblastoma and enhances MYCN levels via let-7 suppression. Nat Genet. 2012;44(11):1199–206. https://doi.org/10.1038/ng.2436.
73. Hogarty MD, Norris MD, Davis K, Liu XY, Evageliou NF, Hayes CS, Pawel B, Guo R, Zhao HQ, Sekyere E, Keating J, Thomas W, Cheng NC, Murray J, Smith J, Sutton R, Venn N, London WB, Buxton A, Gilmour SK, Marshall GM, Haber M. ODC1 is a critical determinant of MYCN oncogenesis and a therapeutic target in neuroblastoma. Cancer Res. 2008;68(23):9735–45. https://doi.org/10.1158/0008-5472.Can-07-6866.
74. Rader J, Russell MR, Hart LS, Nakazawa MS, Belcastro LT, Martinez D, Li Y, Carpenter EL, Attiyeh EF, Diskin SJ, Kim S, Parasuraman S, Caponigro G, Schnepp RW, Wood AC, Pawel B, Cole KA, Maris JM. Dual CDK4/CDK6 inhibition induces cell-cycle arrest and senescence in neuroblastoma. Clin Cancer Res. 2013;19(22):6173–82. https://doi.org/10.1158/1078-0432.CCR-13-1675.
75. Corvi R, Savelyeva L, Breit S, Wenzel A, Handgretinger R, Barak J, Oren M, Amler L, Schwab M. Non-syntenic amplification of MDM2 and MYCN in human neuroblastoma. Oncogene. 1995;10(6):1081–6.
76. Michels E, Vandesompele J, De Preter K, Hoebeeck J, Vermeulen J, Schramm A, Molenaar JJ, Menten B, Marques B, Stallings RL, Combaret V, Devalck C, De Paepe A, Versteeg R, Eggert A, Laureys G, Van Roy N, Speleman F. ArrayCGH-based classification of neuroblastoma into genomic subgroups. Genes Chromosomes Cancer. 2007;46(12):1098–108. https://doi.org/10.1002/gcc.20496.
77. Depuydt P, Boeva V, Hocking TD, Cannoodt R, Ambros IM, Ambros PF, Asgharzadeh S, Attiyeh EF, Combaret V, Defferrari R, Fischer M, Hero B, Hogarty MD, Irwin MS, Koster J, Kreissman S, Ladenstein R, Lapouble E, Laureys G, London WB, Mazzocco K, Nakagawara A, Noguera R, Ohira M, Park JR, Potschger U, Theissen J, Tonini GP, Valteau-Couanet D, Varesio L, Versteeg R, Speleman F, Maris JM, Schleiermacher G, De Preter K. Genomic amplifications and distal 6q loss: novel markers for poor survival in high-risk neuroblastoma patients. J Natl Cancer Inst. 2018;110(10):1084–93. https://doi.org/10.1093/jnci/djy022.
78. Yang HW, Chen YZ, Takita J, Soeda E, Piao HY, Hayashi Y. Genomic structure and mutational analysis of the human KIF1B gene which is homozygously deleted in neuroblastoma at chromosome 1p36.2. Oncogene. 2001;20(36):5075–83. https://doi.org/10.1038/sj.onc.1204456.
79. The I, Murthy AE, Hannigan GE, Jacoby LB, Menon AG, Gusella JF, Bernards A. Neurofibromatosis type 1 gene mutations in neuroblastoma. Nat Genet. 1993;3(1):62–6. https://doi.org/10.1038/ng0193-62.
80. Martinsson T, Sjoberg RM, Hedborg F, Kogner P. Homozygous deletion of the neurofibromatosis-1 gene in the tumor of a patient with neuroblastoma. Cancer Genet Cytogenet. 1997;95(2):183–9. https://doi.org/10.1016/s0165-4608(96)00259-2.
81. Stallings RL, Nair P, Maris JM, Catchpoole D, McDermott M, O'Meara A, Breatnach F. High-resolution analysis of chromosomal breakpoints and genomic instability identifies PTPRD as a candidate tumor suppressor gene in neuroblastoma. Cancer Res. 2006;66(7):3673–80. https://doi.org/10.1158/0008-5472.Can-05-4154.
82. Kumps C, Fieuw A, Mestdagh P, Menten B, Lefever S, Pattyn F, De Brouwer S, Sante T, Schulte JH, Schramm A, Van Roy N, Van Maerken T, Noguera R, Combaret V, Devalck C, Westermann F, Laureys G, Eggert A, Vandesompele J, De Preter K, Speleman F. Focal DNA copy number changes in neuroblastoma target MYCN regulated genes. PLoS One. 2013;8(1):e52321. https://doi.org/10.1371/journal.pone.0052321.
83. Powers JT, Tsanov KM, Pearson DS, Roels F, Spina CS, Ebright R, Seligson M, de Soysa Y, Cahan P, Theissen J, Tu HC, Han A, Kurek KC, LaPier GS, Osborne JK, Ross SJ, Cesana M, Collins JJ, Berthold F, Daley GQ. Multiple mechanisms disrupt the let-7 microRNA family in neuroblastoma. Nature. 2016;535(7611):246–51. https://doi.org/10.1038/nature18632.
84. Caren H, Kryh H, Nethander M, Sjoberg RM, Trager C, Nilsson S, Abrahamsson J, Kogner P, Martinsson T. High-risk neuroblastoma tumors with 11q-deletion display a poor prognostic, chromosome instability phenotype with later onset. Proc

Natl Acad Sci U S A. 2010;107(9):4323–8. https://doi.org/10.1073/pnas.0910684107.

85. Hertwig F, Peifer M, Fischer M. Telomere maintenance is pivotal for high-risk neuroblastoma. Cell Cycle. 2016;15(3):311–2. https://doi.org/10.1080/15384101.2015.1125243.
86. Koneru B, Lopez G, Farooqi A, Conkrite KL, Nguyen TH, Macha SJ, Modi A, Rokita JL, Urias E, Hindle A, Davidson H, McCoy K, Nance J, Yazdani V, Irwin MS, Yang S, Wheeler DA, Maris JM, Diskin SJ, Reynolds CP. Telomere maintenance mechanisms define clinical outcome in high-risk neuroblastoma. Cancer Res. 2020;80(12):2663–75. https://doi.org/10.1158/0008-5472.CAN-19-3068.
87. Brodeur GM, Maris JM, Yamashiro DJ, Hogarty MD, White PS. Biology and genetics of human neuroblastomas. J Pediatr Hematol Oncol. 1997;19(2):93–101. https://doi.org/10.1097/00043426-199703000-00001.
88. Brodeur GM. Neuroblastoma: biological insights into a clinical enigma. Nat Rev Cancer. 2003;3(3):203–16. https://doi.org/10.1038/nrc1014.
89. Vandesompele J, Baudis M, De Preter K, Van Roy N, Ambros P, Bown N, Brinkschmidt C, Christiansen H, Combaret V, Lastowska M, Nicholson J, O'Meara A, Plantaz D, Stallings R, Brichard B, Van den Broecke C, De Bie S, De Paepe A, Laureys G, Speleman F. Unequivocal delineation of clinicogenetic subgroups and development of a new model for improved outcome prediction in neuroblastoma. J Clin Oncol. 2005;23(10):2280–99. https://doi.org/10.1200/JCO.2005.06.104.
90. Schleiermacher G, Janoueix-Lerosey I, Ribeiro A, Klijanienko J, Couturier J, Pierron G, Mosseri V, Valent A, Auger N, Plantaz D, Rubie H, Valteau-Couanet D, Bourdeaut F, Combaret V, Bergeron C, Michon J, Delattre O. Accumulation of segmental alterations determines progression in neuroblastoma. J Clin Oncol. 2010;28(19):3122–30. https://doi.org/10.1200/JCO.2009.26.7955.
91. Andersson N, Bakker B, Karlsson J, Valind A, Holmquist Mengelbier L, Spierings DCJ, Foijer F, Gisselsson D. Extensive clonal branching shapes the evolutionary history of high-risk pediatric cancers. Cancer Res. 2020;80(7):1512–23. https://doi.org/10.1158/0008-5472.CAN-19-3468.
92. Lastowska M, Cotterill S, Pearson AD, Roberts P, McGuckin A, Lewis I, Bown N. Gain of chromosome arm 17q predicts unfavourable outcome in neuroblastoma patients. U.K. Children's Cancer Study Group and the U.K. Cancer Cytogenetics Group. Eur J Cancer. 1997;33(10):1627–33. https://doi.org/10.1016/s0959-8049(97)00282-7.
93. Bown N, Cotterill S, Lastowska M, O'Neill S, Pearson AD, Plantaz D, Meddeb M, Danglot G, Brinkschmidt C, Christiansen H, Laureys G, Speleman F, Nicholson J, Bernheim A, Betts DR, Vandesompele J, Van Roy N. Gain of chromosome arm 17q and adverse outcome in patients with neuroblastoma. N Engl J Med. 1999;340(25):1954–61. https://doi.org/10.1056/NEJM199906243402504.
94. Attiyeh EF, London WB, Mosse YP, Wang Q, Winter C, Khazi D, McGrady PW, Seeger RC, Look AT, Shimada H, Brodeur GM, Cohn SL, Matthay KK, Maris JM, Children's Oncology G. Chromosome 1p and 11q deletions and outcome in neuroblastoma. N Engl J Med. 2005;353(21):2243–53. https://doi.org/10.1056/NEJMoa052399.
95. Luttikhuis ME, Powell JE, Rees SA, Genus T, Chughtai S, Ramani P, Mann JR, McConville CM. Neuroblastomas with chromosome 11q loss and single copy MYCN comprise a biologically distinct group of tumours with adverse prognosis. Br J Cancer. 2001;85(4):531–7. https://doi.org/10.1054/bjoc.2001.1960.
96. Parodi F, Passoni L, Massimo L, Luksch R, Gambini C, Rossi E, Zuffardi O, Pistoia V, Pezzolo A. Identification of novel prognostic markers in relapsing localized resectable neuroblastoma. OMICS. 2011;15(3):113–21. https://doi.org/10.1089/omi.2010.0085.
97. Spitz R, Hero B, Ernestus K, Berthold F. Deletions in chromosome arms 3p and 11q are new prognostic markers in localized and 4s neuroblastoma. Clin Cancer Res. 2003;9(1):52–8.
98. Cobrinik D, Ostrovnaya I, Hassimi M, Tickoo SK, Cheung IY, Cheung NK. Recurrent pre-existing and acquired DNA copy number alterations, including focal TERT gains, in neuroblastoma central nervous system metastases. Genes Chromosomes Cancer. 2013;52(12):1150–66. https://doi.org/10.1002/gcc.22110.
99. Lavarino C, Cheung NK, Garcia I, Domenech G, de Torres C, Alaminos M, Rios J, Gerald WL, Kushner B, LaQuaglia M, Mora J. Specific gene expression profiles and chromosomal abnormalities are associated with infant disseminated neuroblastoma. BMC Cancer. 2009;9:44. https://doi.org/10.1186/1471-2407-9-44.
100. Ambros IM, Tonini GP, Potschger U, Gross N, Mosseri V, Beiske K, Berbegall AP, Benard J, Bown N, Caron H, Combaret V, Couturier J, Defferrari R, Delattre O, Jeison M, Kogner P, Lunec J, Marques B, Martinsson T, Mazzocco K, Noguera R, Schleiermacher G, Valent A, Van Roy N, Villamon E, Janousek D, Pribill I, Glogova E, Attiyeh EF, Hogarty MD, Monclair TF, Holmes K, Valteau-Couanet D, Castel V, Tweddle DA, Park JR, Cohn S, Ladenstein R, Beck-Popovic M, De Bernardi B, Michon J, Pearson ADJ, Ambros PF. Age dependency of the prognostic impact of tumor genomics in localized resectable MYCN-nonamplified neuroblastomas. J Clin Oncol. 2020;38(31):3685–97. https://doi.org/10.1200/JCO.18.02132.
101. Gilbert F, Feder M, Balaban G, Brangman D, Lurie DK, Podolsky R, Rinaldt V, Vinikoor N, Weisband J. Human neuroblastomas and abnormalities of chromosomes 1 and 17. Cancer Res. 1984;44(11):5444–9.

102. Brodeur GM, Green AA, Hayes FA, Williams KJ, Williams DL, Tsiatis AA. Cytogenetic features of human neuroblastomas and cell lines. Cancer Res. 1981;41(11 Pt 1):4678–86.
103. Kaneko Y, Kanda N, Maseki N, Sakurai M, Tsuchida Y, Takeda T, Okabe I, Sakurai M. Different karyotypic patterns in early and advanced stage neuroblastomas. Cancer Res. 1987;47(1):311–8.
104. Schleiermacher G, Janoueix-Lerosey I, Combaret V, Derre J, Couturier J, Aurias A, Delattre O. Combined 24-color karyotyping and comparative genomic hybridization analysis indicates predominant rearrangements of early replicating chromosome regions in neuroblastoma. Cancer Genet Cytogenet. 2003;141(1):32–42. https://doi.org/10.1016/s0165-4608(02)00644-1.
105. Van Roy N, Laureys G, Cheng NC, Willem P, Opdenakker G, Versteeg R, Speleman F. 1;17 translocations and other chromosome 17 rearrangements in human primary neuroblastoma tumors and cell lines. Genes Chromosomes Cancer. 1994;10(2):103–14. https://doi.org/10.1002/gcc.2870100205.
106. Lastowska M, Roberts P, Pearson AD, Lewis I, Wolstenholme J, Bown N. Promiscuous translocations of chromosome arm 17q in human neuroblastomas. Genes Chromosomes Cancer. 1997;19(3):143–9.
107. Van Roy N, Van Limbergen H, Vandesompele J, Van Gele M, Poppe B, Salwen H, Laureys G, Manoel N, De Paepe A, Speleman F. Combined M-FISH and CGH analysis allows comprehensive description of genetic alterations in neuroblastoma cell lines. Genes Chromosomes Cancer. 2001;32(2):126–35. https://doi.org/10.1002/gcc.1174.
108. Mathew P, Valentine MB, Bowman LC, Rowe ST, Nash MB, Valentine VA, Cohn SL, Castleberry RP, Brodeur GM, Look AT. Detection of MYCN gene amplification in neuroblastoma by fluorescence in situ hybridization: a pediatric oncology group study. Neoplasia. 2001;3(2):105–9. https://doi.org/10.1038/sj.neo.7900146.
109. Spitz R, Hero B, Ernestus K, Berthold F. FISH analyses for alterations in chromosomes 1, 2, 3, and 11 define high-risk groups in neuroblastoma. Med Pediatr Oncol. 2003;41(1):30–5. https://doi.org/10.1002/mpo.10313.
110. Shapiro DN, Valentine MB, Rowe ST, Sinclair AE, Sublett JE, Roberts WM, Look AT. Detection of N-myc gene amplification by fluorescence in situ hybridization. Diagnostic utility for neuroblastoma. Am J Pathol. 1993;142(5):1339–46.
111. Vandesompele J, Van Roy N, Van Gele M, Laureys G, Ambros P, Heimann P, Devalck C, Schuuring E, Brock P, Otten J, Gyselinck J, De Paepe A, Speleman F. Genetic heterogeneity of neuroblastoma studied by comparative genomic hybridization. Genes Chromosomes Cancer. 1998;23(2):141–52. https://doi.org/10.1002/(sici)1098-2264(199810)23:2<141::aid-gcc7>3.0.co;2-2.
112. Van Roy N, Jauch A, Van Gele M, Laureys G, Versteeg R, De Paepe A, Cremer T, Speleman F. Comparative genomic hybridization analysis of human neuroblastomas: detection of distal 1p deletions and further molecular genetic characterization of neuroblastoma cell lines. Cancer Genet Cytogenet. 1997;97(2):135–42. https://doi.org/10.1016/s0165-4608(96)00362-7.
113. Brinkschmidt C, Christiansen H, Terpe HJ, Simon R, Boecker W, Lampert F, Stoerkel S. Comparative genomic hybridization (Cgh) analysis of neuroblastomas—an important methodological approach in paediatric tumour pathology. J Pathol. 1997;181(4):394–400. https://doi.org/10.1002/(sici)1096-9896(199704)181:4<394::Aid-path800>3.0.Co;2-1.
114. Spitz R, Oberthuer A, Zapatka M, Brors B, Hero B, Ernestus K, Oestreich J, Fischer M, Simon T, Berthold F. Oligonucleotide array-based comparative genomic hybridization (aCGH) of 90 neuroblastomas reveals aberration patterns closely associated with relapse pattern and outcome. Genes Chromosomes Cancer. 2006;45(12):1130–42. https://doi.org/10.1002/gcc.20376.
115. Michels E, De Preter K, Van Roy N, Speleman F. Detection of DNA copy number alterations in cancer by array comparative genomic hybridization. Genet Med. 2007;9(9):574–84. https://doi.org/10.1097/gim.0b013e318145b25b.
116. Squire JA, Pei J, Marrano P, Beheshti B, Bayani J, Lim G, Moldovan L, Zielenska M. High-resolution mapping of amplifications and deletions in pediatric osteosarcoma by use of CGH analysis of cDNA microarrays. Genes Chromosomes Cancer. 2003;38(3):215–25. https://doi.org/10.1002/gcc.10273.
117. Selzer RR, Richmond TA, Pofahl NJ, Green RD, Eis PS, Nair P, Brothman AR, Stallings RL. Analysis of chromosome breakpoints in neuroblastoma at sub-kilobase resolution using fine-tiling oligonucleotide array CGH. Genes Chromosomes Cancer. 2005;44(3):305–19. https://doi.org/10.1002/gcc.20243.
118. Chen QR, Bilke S, Wei JS, Whiteford CC, Cenacchi N, Krasnoselsky AL, Greer BT, Son CG, Westermann F, Berthold F, Schwab M, Catchpoole D, Khan J. cDNA array-CGH profiling identifies genomic alterations specific to stage and MYCN-amplification in neuroblastoma. BMC Genomics. 2004;5(70):70. https://doi.org/10.1186/1471-2164-5-70.
119. Beheshti B, Braude I, Marrano P, Thorner P, Zielenska M, Squire JA. Chromosomal localization of DNA amplifications in neuroblastoma tumors using cDNA microarray comparative genomic hybridization. Neoplasia. 2003;5(1):53–62. https://doi.org/10.1016/S1476-5586(03)80017-9.
120. George RE, Attiyeh EF, Li S, Moreau LA, Neuberg D, Li C, Fox EA, Meyerson M, Diller L, Fortina P, Look AT, Maris JM. Genome-wide analysis of neuroblastomas using high-density single nucleotide

polymorphism arrays. PLoS One. 2007;2(2):e255. https://doi.org/10.1371/journal.pone.0000255.
121. Combaret V, Iacono I, Brejon S, Schleiermacher G, Pierron G, Couturier J, Bergeron C, Blay JY. Analysis of genomic alterations in neuroblastoma by multiplex ligation-dependent probe amplification and array comparative genomic hybridization: a comparison of results. Cancer Genet. 2012;205(12):657–64. https://doi.org/10.1016/j.cancergen.2012.11.002.
122. Costa RA, Seuanez HN. Investigation of major genetic alterations in neuroblastoma. Mol Biol Rep. 2018;45(3):287–95. https://doi.org/10.1007/s11033-018-4161-4.
123. Van Roy N, Van Der Linden M, Menten B, Dheedene A, Vandeputte C, Van Dorpe J, Laureys G, Renard M, Sante T, Lammens T, De Wilde B, Speleman F, De Preter K. Shallow whole genome sequencing on circulating cell-free DNA allows reliable noninvasive copy-number profiling in neuroblastoma patients. Clin Cancer Res. 2017;23(20):6305–14. https://doi.org/10.1158/1078-0432.CCR-17-0675.
124. Vandewoestyne M, Kumps C, Swerts K, Menten B, Lammens T, Philippe J, De Preter K, Laureys G, Van Roy N, Speleman F, Deforce D. Isolation of disseminated neuroblastoma cells from bone marrow aspirates for pretreatment risk assessment by array comparative genomic hybridization. Int J Cancer. 2012;130(5):1098–108. https://doi.org/10.1002/ijc.26133.
125. Abbasi MR, Rifatbegovic F, Brunner C, Mann G, Ziegler A, Potschger U, Crazzolara R, Ussowicz M, Benesch M, Ebetsberger-Dachs G, Chan GCF, Jones N, Ladenstein R, Ambros IM, Ambros PF. Impact of disseminated neuroblastoma cells on the identification of the relapse-seeding clone. Clin Cancer Res. 2017;23(15):4224–32. https://doi.org/10.1158/1078-0432.CCR-16-2082.
126. Chicard M, Boyault S, Colmet Daage L, Richer W, Gentien D, Pierron G, Lapouble E, Bellini A, Clement N, Iacono I, Brejon S, Carrere M, Reyes C, Hocking T, Bernard V, Peuchmaur M, Corradini N, Faure-Conter C, Coze C, Plantaz D, Defachelles AS, Thebaud E, Gambart M, Millot F, Valteau-Couanet D, Michon J, Puisieux A, Delattre O, Combaret V, Schleiermacher G. Genomic copy number profiling using circulating free tumor DNA highlights heterogeneity in neuroblastoma. Clin Cancer Res. 2016;22(22):5564–73. https://doi.org/10.1158/1078-0432.CCR-16-0500.
127. Combaret V, Audoynaud C, Iacono I, Favrot MC, Schell M, Bergeron C, Puisieux A. Circulating MYCN DNA as a tumor-specific marker in neuroblastoma patients. Cancer Res. 2002;62(13):3646–8.
128. Combaret V, Brejon S, Iacono I, Schleiermacher G, Pierron G, Ribeiro A, Bergeron C, Marabelle A, Puisieux A. Determination of 17q gain in patients with neuroblastoma by analysis of circulating DNA. Pediatr Blood Cancer. 2011;56(5):757–61. https://doi.org/10.1002/pbc.22816.
129. Peneder P, Stutz AM, Surdez D, Krumbholz M, Semper S, Chicard M, Sheffield NC, Pierron G, Lapouble E, Totzl M, Erguner B, Barreca D, Rendeiro AF, Agaimy A, Boztug H, Engstler G, Dworzak M, Bernkopf M, Taschner-Mandl S, Ambros IM, Myklebost O, Marec-Berard P, Burchill SA, Brennan B, Strauss SJ, Whelan J, Schleiermacher G, Schaefer C, Dirksen U, Hutter C, Boye K, Ambros PF, Delattre O, Metzler M, Bock C, Tomazou EM. Multimodal analysis of cell-free DNA whole-genome sequencing for pediatric cancers with low mutational burden. Nat Commun. 2021;12(1):3230. https://doi.org/10.1038/s41467-021-23445-w.
130. Cimmino F, Lasorsa VA, Vetrella S, Iolascon A, Capasso M. A targeted gene panel for circulating tumor DNA sequencing in neuroblastoma. Front Oncol. 2020;10:596191. https://doi.org/10.3389/fonc.2020.596191.
131. Lodrini M, Sprussel A, Astrahantseff K, Tiburtius D, Konschak R, Lode HN, Fischer M, Keilholz U, Eggert A, Deubzer HE. Using droplet digital PCR to analyze MYCN and ALK copy number in plasma from patients with neuroblastoma. Oncotarget. 2017;8(49):85234–51. https://doi.org/10.18632/oncotarget.19076.
132. Peitz C, Sprussel A, Linke RB, Astrahantseff K, Grimaldi M, Schmelz K, Toedling J, Schulte JH, Fischer M, Messerschmidt C, Beule D, Keilholz U, Eggert A, Deubzer HE, Lodrini M. Multiplexed quantification of four neuroblastoma DNA targets in a single droplet digital PCR reaction. J Mol Diagn. 2020. https://doi.org/10.1016/j.jmoldx.2020.07.006.
133. Chicard M, Colmet-Daage L, Clement N, Danzon A, Bohec M, Bernard V, Baulande S, Bellini A, Deveau P, Pierron G, Lapouble E, Janoueix-Lerosey I, Peuchmaur M, Corradini N, Defachelles AS, Valteau-Couanet D, Michon J, Combaret V, Delattre O, Schleiermacher G. Whole-exome sequencing of cell-free DNA reveals temporo-spatial heterogeneity and identifies treatment-resistant clones in neuroblastoma. Clin Cancer Res. 2018;24(4):939–49. https://doi.org/10.1158/1078-0432.CCR-17-1586.
134. Berko ER, Witek GM, Matkar S, Petrova ZO, Wu MA, Smith CM, Daniels A, Kalna J, Kennedy A, Gostuski I, Casey C, Krytska K, Gerelus M, Pavlick D, Ghazarian S, Park JR, Marachelian A, Maris JM, Goldsmith KC, Radhakrishnan R, Lemmon MA, Mossé YP. Nat Commun. 2023;14(1):2601. https://doi.org/10.1038/s41467-023-38195-0. PMID: 37147298.
135. Linnarsson S, Teichmann SA. Single-cell genomics: coming of age. Genome Biol. 2016;17(97):97. https://doi.org/10.1186/s13059-016-0960-x.
136. Squire JA, Thorner P, Marrano P, Parkinson D, Ng YK, Gerrie B, Chilton-Macneill S, Zielenska M. Identification of MYCN copy number heterogeneity by direct FISH analysis of neuroblastoma preparations. Mol Diagn. 1996;1(4):281–9. https://doi.org/10.1054/MODI00100281.

137. Ambros PF, Ambros IM, Kerbl R, Luegmayr A, Rumpler S, Ladenstein R, Amann G, Kovar H, Horcher E, De Bernardi B, Michon J, Gadner H. Intratumoural heterogeneity of 1p deletions and MYCN amplification in neuroblastomas. Med Pediatr Oncol. 2001;36(1):1–4. https://doi.org/10.1002/1096-911X(20010101)36:1<1::AID-MPO1002>3.0.CO;2-L.
138. Brodeur GM, Hayes FA, Green AA, Casper JT, Wasson J, Wallach S, Seeger RC. Consistent N-myc copy number in simultaneous or consecutive neuroblastoma samples from sixty individual patients. Cancer Res. 1987;47(16):4248–53.
139. Theissen J, Boensch M, Spitz R, Betts D, Stegmaier S, Christiansen H, Niggli F, Schilling F, Schwab M, Simon T, Westermann F, Berthold F, Hero B. Heterogeneity of the MYCN oncogene in neuroblastoma. Clin Cancer Res. 2009;15(6):2085–90. https://doi.org/10.1158/1078-0432.CCR-08-1648.
140. Berbegall AP, Villamon E, Piqueras M, Tadeo I, Djos A, Ambros PF, Martinsson T, Ambros IM, Canete A, Castel V, Navarro S, Noguera R. Comparative genetic study of intratumoral heterogenous MYCN amplified neuroblastoma versus aggressive genetic profile neuroblastic tumors. Oncogene. 2016;35(11):1423–32. https://doi.org/10.1038/onc.2015.200.
141. Lundberg G, Jin Y, Sehic D, Ora I, Versteeg R, Gisselsson D. Intratumour diversity of chromosome copy numbers in neuroblastoma mediated by on-going chromosome loss from a polyploid state. PLoS One. 2013;8(3):e59268. https://doi.org/10.1371/journal.pone.0059268.
142. Pezzolo A, Pistorio A, Gambini C, Haupt R, Ferraro M, Erminio G, De Bernardi B, Garaventa A, Pistoia V. Intratumoral diversity of telomere length in individual neuroblastoma tumors. Oncotarget. 2015;6(10):7493–503. https://doi.org/10.18632/oncotarget.2115.
143. Carpenter EL, Rader J, Ruden J, Rappaport EF, Hunter KN, Hallberg PL, Krytska K, O'Dwyer PJ, Mosse YP. Dielectrophoretic capture and genetic analysis of single neuroblastoma tumor cells. Front Oncol. 2014;4:201. https://doi.org/10.3389/fonc.2014.00201.
144. Ambros PF, Ambros IM, Brodeur GM, Haber M, Khan J, Nakagawara A, Schleiermacher G, Speleman F, Spitz R, London WB, Cohn SL, Pearson AD, Maris JM. International consensus for neuroblastoma molecular diagnostics: report from the International Neuroblastoma Risk Group (INRG) Biology Committee. Br J Cancer. 2009;100(9):1471–82. https://doi.org/10.1038/sj.bjc.6605014.

5 Neuroblastoma Epigenetic Landscape: Drugging Opportunities

Veronica Veschi, Kaat Durinck, Carol J. Thiele, and Frank Speleman

5.1 Introduction

A recent review by Feinberg describes "a disrupted and unstable epigenome as a central feature of cancer" and attributes such an altered epigenetic landscape as a result of the interplay between epigenetic modifiers, mediators, and modulators [1]. Modulators are environmental cues such as inflammation or photoaging and therefore can be assumed to play little or no role in pediatric cancers, although the impact of prenatal modulating factors cannot be excluded. Epigenetic modifiers are amongst the most frequently mutated genes across all cancer entities and directly impact on downstream epigenetic mediators such as pluripotency factors that contribute to a cell-state change toward stem-cell–like phenotypes [2]. In pediatric cancers, the overall mutation burden is typically low suggesting that only a few or even a single genetic event (e.g., in rhabdoid sarcomas) can disrupt the carefully controlled transition across successive permissive epigenetic developmental states during normal differentiation leading to embryonal cancer.

The epigenetic information is encoded through three distinct regulatory processes in the nucleus: DNA methylation, chromatin modification and remodeling, and higher order DNA structure. The normal control of DNA methylation during proliferation, differentiation, and homeostasis has been studied in great detail, and perturbation of DNA methylation patterns and mutations in the enzymes controlling this process in cancer cells has been extensively reported. Second, more than 200 post-translational modifications of nucleosomal histones around which the double helix is itself wound are currently known and involve acetylation, methylation, phosphorylation, ubiquitylation, and sumoylation. Third, chromatin is organized in a 3D-space enabling, amongst other promoter-enhancer contacts. Each of these three

Veronica Veschi and Kaat Durinck contributed equally with all other contributors.

V. Veschi
Cell & Molecular Biology Section, Pediatric Oncology Branch, Center for Cancer Research, National Cancer Institute, Bethesda, MD, USA

Department of Molecular Medicine, University of La Sapienza, Rome, Italy
e-mail: veronica.veschi@uniroma1.it

K. Durinck · F. Speleman
Center for Medical Genetics, Ghent University, Ghent, Belgium

Cancer Research Institute Ghent (CRIG), Ghent, Belgium
e-mail: Kaat.Durinck@ugent.be; franki.speleman@ugent.be

C. J. Thiele (✉)
Cell & Molecular Biology Section, Pediatric Oncology Branch, Center for Cancer Research, National Cancer Institute, Bethesda, MD, USA
e-mail: thielec@mail.nih.gov

S. Asgharzadeh, F. Westermann (eds.), *Neuroblastoma*, Pediatric Oncology,
https://doi.org/10.1007/978-3-031-51292-6_5

processes are essential and interact in the dynamic epigenetic control of gene activity and transcription [1] and control the homeostatic balance of chromatin, causing it to become aberrantly restrictive or permissive, the latter being referred to as epigenetic plasticity [2].

In NB, several recent reports are providing an increasing and rapidly changing view on this epigenetic landscape. Not unexpectedly, the prototypical NB oncogene *MYCN*, amplified in half of the high-risk cases, plays a central role in this story. Indeed, MYCN stimulates a gene expression program through hijacking of the epigenetic enhancer landscape, while in the remainder of the high-risk cases a similar MYCN driven oncogenic program is activated. In this review, we focus on novel insights in the context of a growing body of knowledge on how DNA-methylation, chromatin modification, and chromatin remodeling impacts on the NB epigenome and discuss how the perturbed NB epigenome can serve as target for novel drugs.

5.2 Aberrant DNA Methylation in Neuroblastoma

5.2.1 DNA Methylation in Normal and Cancer Cells

DNA methylation is an essential process in normal development supporting key cellular functions and controls amongst others genomic imprinting, X-chromosome inactivation, repression of transposable elements, and cell lineage dependent gene transcription patterns. In cancer cells, many stable epigenetic alterations contribute to the disease process through altered gene expression patterns. In normal cells, cytosines in CpG islands and other CG-rich loci are largely unmethylated, whereas cytosines in CG-poor regions tend to be highly methylated. In many cancers, CpG islands become hypermethylated, imposing a so-called CpG island methylator phenotype (CIMP), while CG-poor regions become hypomethylated. Of further notice, many studies have now confirmed that this hypermethylation is targeted and that these de novo events are predominantly specific for CpG islands occupied by the PRC2 complex. Cancer genomes are also marked by global hypomethylation, mainly in regions associated with the nuclear envelope lamina [1, 3, 4, 5].

5.2.2 The Neuroblastoma Methylome

In NB, much of the earlier work on the epigenetic landscape was based on the study of DNA methylation. This has been recently reviewed and here we give a short summary and focus on more recent findings [6–8]. As in many other cancer types, NB DNA methylation patterns were studied by our lab and others allowing to establish prognostic methylation signatures, while also a CpG island hypermethylator phenotype (CIMP) has been reported [9–11]. A recent large scale integrated genome wide methylation study in 105 NBs was reported by Henrich et al. [9], describing the epigenetic mechanisms of transcriptional deregulation in tumors with unfavorable prognosis. Using hierarchical clustering, two major clusters were identified with all *MYCN* amplified and high-risk tumors with high MYCN activity being part of cluster 1. Integration of methylation patterns with gene expression confirmed the established role of promoter/transcription start site-associated DNA methylation in transcriptional repression and association of gene body methylation with active transcription. This study also showed that methylated intragenic CpGs that were associated with lower gene expression, were significantly enriched with enhancer elements, suggesting that methylation of intragenic enhancer elements may regulate expression of genes relevant for high-risk NB tumor development. Further, hypermethylated and transcriptionally downregulated genes were enriched for established NB tumor suppressors including *CAMTA1*, *CHD5*, and *KIF1B* and genes previously found to be impaired in NB by genetic events, together with a significant enrichment of embryonic stem cell PRC2 targets and genes involved in neuronal differentiation.

Using methyl-CpG-binding domain (MBD) sequencing data of an initial cohort of 87 primary NBs [12], further re-analysis was done to focus on stage 4S NB methylomes in search for possible stage 4S promoter methylation portraits. This allowed the identification of 393 hypermethylated and 1150 hypomethylated promoters that clearly separated stage 4S from the low stage 1/2 and high stage tumors. Further data mining revealed interesting insights that could shed light on the enigmatic biology of the spontaneously regressing and differentiating stage 4S tumors. First, motif analysis in stage 4S differentially methylated promoters revealed enrichment for binding sites for transcription factors implicated in controlling cell cycle, apoptosis, neural crest development, and neural differentiation. Amongst these genes, the E2F1 target gene encoding for the minichromosome maintenance 2 (MCM2) is potentially interesting. MCM2 is a dual function protein acting as a component of the replicative helicase and binding H3–H4 in complex with the anti-silencing function 1 (ASF1) histone chaperone. The histone-binding property of MCM2 gives the MCM2–7 helicase the ability to orchestrate histone dynamics. MCM2, together with histone co-chaperones ASF1 and FACT (crucial complexes of proteins that mediate of the MYCN signal) has an unusual mode of H3–H4 binding allowing MCM2 to dock onto a large variety of modified and variant histones H3 and H4 through hijacking of histone sites interacting with nucleosomal DNA. Also, enrichment for motifs in methylated promoters of genes implicated in neural crest development and (sympathetic) neural differentiation was found for transcription factors MSX1, EVI1, EGR3, AHR, MEF2A, YY1, PPARA, POU2F1, and GFI142, consistent with the prevailing view that it is a developmental and differentiation defect in premigratory neural crest cells that causes stage 4S tumor formation [13].

A second major observation emerging from this stage 4S neuroblastoma methylation study was the finding of an enrichment of genes with hypermethylated promoters in subtelomeric regions. Interestingly, subtelomeric DNA methylation has been shown to suppress telomere elongation in several cancer types [14, 15], but so far this has not been explored in NB. This novel finding could implicate subtelomeric DNA methylation as a possible mechanism by which telomere length and spontaneous tumor regression are controlled in NB. Finally, this study also indicated that methylation of the *hTERT* promoter could impact on telomere length in stage 4S NBs. In this context, it is of interest that a model for NB pathogenesis has been recently proposed based on recurrent genomic alterations affecting telomere length either by telomerase activation through MYCN amplification [16] or TERT rearrangements or alternative lengthening of telomeres (ALT) in a subset of high-risk NB tumors [17].

5.3 Altered Chromatin Modifications in Neuroblastoma

5.3.1 The Histone Code and Transcriptional Regulation

As mentioned above, a plethora of histone modifications determines the epigenetic state of a given cell, including acetylation and methylation, both of which have been extensively studied. Acetylated histones are more accessible to the transcriptional machinery while methylated histones may be either restrictive or permissive. The combination of modifications on each histone and/or nucleosome establishes a code that relates to the transcriptional properties of the nearby genes and has been referred to as the "histone code" [18]. Histone modifications occur at specific residues creating the basis for different patterns of higher-order combinations associated with distinct biological readouts controlling activation and suppression of gene transcription in concertation with pioneering and transcription factors. The primary protein families and principal proteins (Fig. 5.1) in this process are (1) "writers," proteins that covalently attach chemical moieties, (2) "readers" that bind to post-

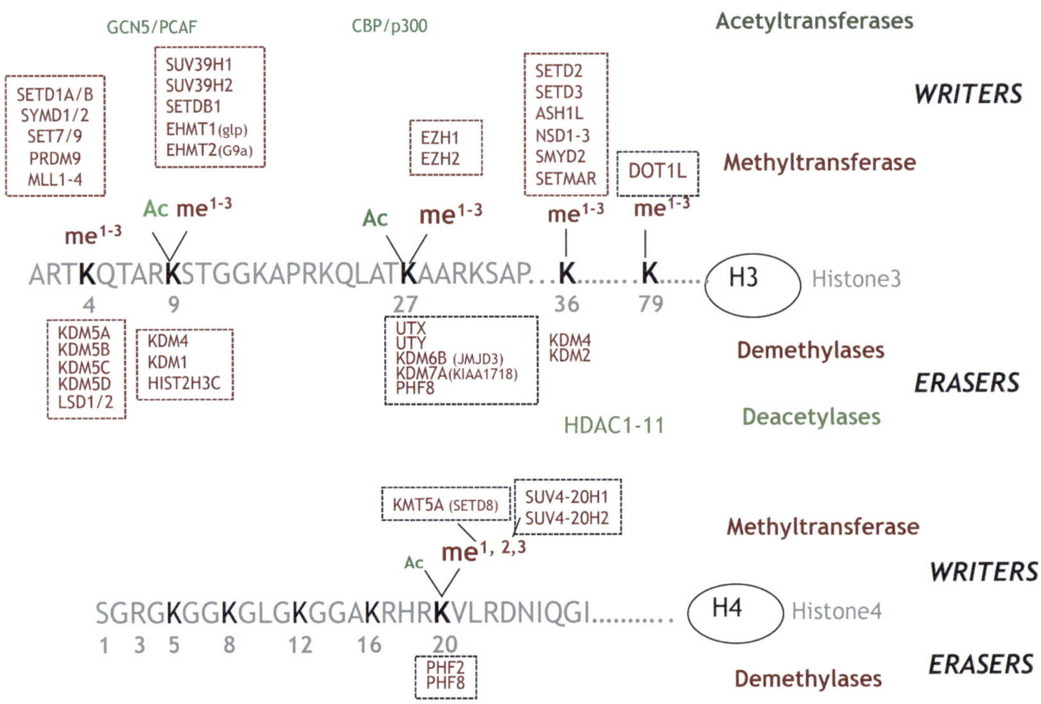

Fig. 5.1 The amino acid(AA) "tails" of histone 3(H3) and histone 4(H4) are depicted(grey). Genes encoding proteins that function to post-translationally modify specific AA residues are termed "Writers" and are depicted in boxes above the AA residues they have been shown to modify. Acetyltransferases(green) transfer acetyl(AC) groups to indicated AA residues on H3 and H4 while Methyltransferases(Red) mono-di- or tri-methylate indicated residues. Genes encoding proteins that function to remove post-translational modifications on specific residues are termed "Erasers" and are depicted in boxes below the specific AA residues. Deacetylases(green) remove Acetyl(Ac) groups while demethylases remove mono-, di-or tri-methyl(me) from indicated AA residues

translational modifications, and (3) "erasers" that enzymatically remove post-translational modifications [19]. Thus, the histone code imparts an additional level of control beyond the DNA sequence and these are linked by chromatin interacting transcription factors [20]. Through their transactivation domains, DNA binding transcription factors recruit multi-protein complexes that typically act as co-activators through recruiting various histone acetyltransferases or co-repressors. Insights into the regulation of gene transcription is evolving with our understanding of the complexities of chromatin with at least five regulated steps: (1) initiation, (2) promoter pausing, (3) mRNA capping, (4) promoter escape, and (5) transcript elongation. The chromatin architecture and RNAPolII (PolII) transcriptional activities are dynamically intertwined. PolII placed at promoters can occlude nucleosomes and promote histone H3 lysine 4 trimethylation (H3K4me3), thereby maintaining promoter accessibility to transcription factors and favoring the euchromatic state [21]. In addition, PolII promoter occupancy correlates with a hypomethylated DNA and excludes remethylation of CpG island promoters after drug-induced demethylation, thereby preventing gene silencing [22, 23]. Chromatin remodeling complexes and histone modifying enzymes are able to modulate the chromatin structure in order to either facilitate or hinder the recruitment of transcription factors and the basal transcriptional machinery to promoter regions, to ultimately promote or restrict gene transcription (see Sect. 4).

Epigenetic regulation is key to control the selection of gene programs necessary for lineage specification and cell differentiation during embryonic development. The finding that NB tumors with a good prognosis have a more differentiated histology and transcriptomes enriched in differentiation genes while those with a poor prognosis are more undifferentiated indicate that genetic alterations associated with NB affect differentiation. Thus, it is not surprising that alterations in the epigenetic machinery are being implicated in NB tumorigenesis.

5.3.2 Histone Modifications in Neuroblastoma

During development, lineage restricted gene programs are poised to be activated or repressed depending on signals received from the microenvironment. These gene programs are said to be "poised" or "bivalent" being marked by both active (H3K4me3/H3K27Ac) and suppressive (H3K27me3) histone marks at promoters and enhancers. Lineage specifying signals from the environment stimulate the activation of specific gene programs while silencing self-renewal and alternate lineage gene programs. Key players in this process are the Polycomb repressive complexes (PRC1 and PRC2) which catalyze trimethylation of histone 3 lysine 27 (H3K27me3) [20]. BMI1, a key component of PRC1, has oncogenic activity in many cancers. BMI1 expression is high in primary NB [24] and *BMI1* is a direct transcriptional target of MYCN [25] and its expression favors NB stem cell renewal [26]. Studies in TH-MYCN mice reveal that BMI1 decreases p53 stability thus enabling neuroblast (the presumed NB progenitor cell) persistence through bypass of the MYCN induced stress response [27, 28]. High expression of the PRC2 catalytic subunit EZH2 was first noted in undifferentiated, high-risk NB tumors compared to more differentiated low-risk ganglioneuroblastomas and ganglioneuromas [29]. Multiple chromosomal alterations may contribute to dysregulation of EZH2 including gains of chromosome 7 or 7q which occur in 50% of NB [30], the induction of EZH2 by MYCN and the decreased expression of miR-124, the latter being a negative regulator of EZH2 and encoded on the frequently deleted chromosome 1p36 region. Gene set enrichment analysis revealed enrichment of MYC target gene sets in upregulated genes while PRC2 target genes sets were enriched in down regulated genes in neuroblasts in the medulla of embryonic adrenal glands in the TH-MYCN mice. Further, loss of EZH2 expression or targeted inhibition of the EZH2 methylase was shown to be sufficient to suppress NB sphere formation highlighting an important role for EZH2 in the murine model of *N-myc*-driven NB tumorigenesis [31]. An unbiased genome-wide CRISPR screen identified *MYCN*-amplified human NB tumors to be particularly dependent on members of the PRC2 complex in part due to MYCN-induced increases in expression of key PRC2 components, EZH2, EED, and SUZ12 [32]. Functionally, EZH2 via H3K27me3 suppresses the 1p36 tumor suppressor CASZ1 as well as a number of other genes with tumor suppressing or differentiating activity in NB [29, 32]. EZH2 may also interact with MYCN to form complexes that suppress transcription of select genes such as the CLU tumor suppressor [33]. It is generally agreed that genetic ablation of EZH2 expression inhibits NB cell growth [29, 32, 34], while small molecule inhibitors of the EZH2 SET domain methylase inhibit but do not block growth [32]. Suppression of EZH2 activity leads to expression of a more differentiated transcriptome [29, 32], including re-expression of NGFR and TrkA [35] which enhances cell responsiveness to NGF [32, 35]. These studies support a model in which the altered expression of MYCN during sympathoadrenal differentiation leads to increased or persistent EZH2 expression which suppresses NB differentiation programs, potentially making cells less sensitive to environmental differentiation cues such as NGF.

An interrogation of the NB epigenetic landscape, utilizing an unbiased siRNA chromatin screen which comprised over 50% of the histone methylases and various chromatin modifiers, led to the identification of 53 chromatin regulators that significantly inhibited NB tumor growth in both *MYCN*-amplified and non-amplified NB cell lines [36]. Among the top hits, high expression levels of *EZH2*, *SETD8*, *BRD4*, and *TAF6L* were associated with a poor prognosis in primary NB tumors while others such as KDM4B (JMJD2B), BRD2, PRDM2 are also critical for the differentiation block. Interestingly, PRMT1, KAT5 (MYST1) and KAT8 (HTATIP) EHMT2, SUV420h1, and chromatin remodelers such as SMARCA4 were also among the top hits, suggesting epigenetic regulators critically impact on NB tumorigenesis. SETD8 was significantly associated with poor prognosis in *MYCN* non-amplified high-risk stage 4 NB patients which may result from overexpression due to gains or focal amplifications encompassing the *SETD8* (*KMT5A*) locus at chromosome 12q24 MYCN non-amplified (22%) and MYCN amplified (6%) high risk NB tumors [37, 38]. SETD8 specifically monomethylates histone H4 Lysine 20 (H4K20me1) regulating a variety of biological processes, such as gene transcription, replication origins, genome integrity, and cell-cycle progression and development [39–43].

Unlike many cancers, mutations in the tumor suppressor p53 are rare (2%) in primary NB, and while mechanisms that attenuate the activity of p53 are well known in *MYCN*-amplified high risk NB few have been described that are relevant in *MYCN*-wild type high risk NBs. Of interest, in NB, SETD8 was found to monomethylate p53 on lysine 382 (p53K382me1), decrease protein stability, and attenuate p53 pro-apoptotic and growth arrest functions [36, 44]. The identification of a small molecule inhibitor of SETD8 that reactivated the canonical p53 pathway in NB by decreasing p53K382me1 and inhibited in vivo outgrowth of NB xenograft tumors identifies SETD8 as a novel druggable target in NB.

The lysine-specific histone demethylases KDM1A (LSD1) and KDM4B (JMJD2B) have been found overexpressed in poorly differentiated NBs [25, 29, 36, 45, 46]. In embryonic stem cells, LSD1 preferentially demethylates H3K4me3, thus favoring PcG-associated H3K27me3 silencing at bivalent loci which may contribute to maintenance of stemness and the unfavorable prognosis that is associated with LSD1-overexpressing NB compared with more differentiated forms of the tumor [45]. The histone demethylase KDM4B (JMJD2B) is highly expressed in NBs and is associated with unfavorable prognosis. It physically interacts with MYCN and in the presence of MYCN localizes to a subset of gene loci important in regulating self-renewal and cell cycle progression [46]. Genetic inhibition of KDM4B function was also found to inhibit proliferation and induce differentiation [36, 46].

Ever since the first histone deacetylase inhibitors were identified, the impact of global changes in histone acetylation and deacetylation on NB proliferation and differentiation has been intensely studied [47–50]. Comprehensive genetic silencing of each of the 11 classical histone deacetylases (HDACs) indicated a complex regulatory network with HDAC8 implicated in differentiation [51], HDAC10 involved in autophagy survival [52], HDAC2 regulating a miRNA network involved in MYCN signaling [53], HDAC3 inhibiting the GRHL1 tumor suppressor [54], and HDAC5 affecting metastatic properties of NB cells [55]. High-level expression of TAF6L, a member of PCAF histone acetylases complex, was significantly associated with poor prognosis in *MYCN* non-amplified high-risk NB and its silencing induced NB cell differentiation [36]. However, an integrated understanding of the recruitment of different HATs and HDACs to distinct chromatin regions remains to be developed in the context of genome wide studies.

The bromodomain and extraterminal domain (BET) family of proteins includes BRD2, BRD3, BRD4, BRDT, which are “readers” that recognize and bind acetylated lysines on histones. BRD4 interacts with P-TEFß to facilitate RNApolII transcription, and recent studies indicate that MYC-driven transcriptional programs may be selectively affected by BET domain inhibitors (see Sect. 5.8.5).

5.4 A Role for Altered Chromatin Remodeling in Neuroblastoma

5.4.1 Chromatin Remodeling Protein Complexes and Cancer

In addition to histone modifications, ATP-dependent chromatin remodeling is a second important process involving histones implicated in epigenetic control of gene regulation. This active process controls the compaction and decompaction of DNA in the nucleus implicated in normal DNA replication, gene expression, DNA repair, and recombination. To control this broad range of essential activities, five major subfamilies of chromatin remodelers emerged during evolution: SWI/SNF, ISWI, INO80 or SWR1, CHD, and α-thalassemia mental retardation syndrome X-linked (ATRX) [56]. Perturbations in the processes controlled by these proteins are tightly linked to cancer development as further supported by the high incidence of mutations affecting components of chromatin remodeling complexes [57] with up to 20% of human cancers bearing mutations in subunits of the SWI/SNF (BAF)-related complexes [58]. The prototypical example and also first tumor in which involvement of SWI/SNF was reported is the malignant rhabdoid tumor (MRT), a very aggressive solid tumor of early childhood. The highly polymorphic (BAF) complexes are composed of a single central ATPase (BRG/SMARCA4 or BRM/SMARCA2), and several BRG/BRM-Associated Factors (BAF subunits). The latter are non-catalytic subunits contributing to targeting loci through their bromodomains, chromodomains, PHD fingers, zinc fingers, and other DNA-binding domains. Two subfamilies of BAF (Brg/Brm-associated factor) chromatin remodelers are distinguished: BAF and PBAF. Both have ATP-dependent chromatin remodeling ability to coordinate nucleosome mobilization and chromatin accessibility and recruit other proteins and the transcriptional machinery. They consist of up to 15 components, each characterized by a distinct ATPase, BRG1 (SMARCA4) and BRM (SMARCA2), respectively. PBAF differ from BAF complexes by the presence of BAF200 (ARID2) and BAF180 (PBRM1) and the lack of the BAF specific BAF250A/B (ARID1A/B). The compositions of BAF and PBAF are further complicated by the existence of multiple subunit paralogues. A total number of 29 genes encode for components for the various SWI/SNF core complexes, including four distinct neuron-specific subunits in higher vertebrates, resulting from hundreds of different combinatorial assemblies that allow highly specialized functions in a lineage restricted manner in concert with dedicated transcription factors. The functional importance of these paralogues has nicely been illustrated by several studies showing differential BAF subunit paralogue assembly through different steps in differentiation. While initial studies suggested that SWI/SNF complexes merely implicated dynamic regulation of nucleosomes to achieve open chromatin, later investigations questioned these findings. Recently, using a faithful and elegant cellular system to study subunit specific functions, it was shown that BAF complexes rapidly (in minutes) oppose both PRC1 and PRC2 without need for replication, PolII occupancy, or transcription. During this process, chromatin accessibility rapidly follows the loss of H3K27me3 and H2Aub1 and opens possible binding sites for sequence-specific or lineage-specific transcription factors in well-defined and context specific biological processes.

In this review, we will focus on the emerging role of SWI/SNF controlled remodeling, CHD5, and ATRX in the biology of NB.

5.4.2 The SWI/SNF (BAF) Chromatin Remodeling Complex in Neuroblastoma

Jubierre et al. [59] observed consistent SMARCA4/BRG1 upregulation in advanced stages of NB, with high BRG1 levels being indicative of poor outcome. As was reported for several other cancer entities, loss-of-function experiments *in vitro* and *in vivo* attributed an essential role for BRG1 in proliferation. Whole-genome transcriptome analysis further revealed that BRG1 controls the expression of key elements of oncogenic pathways such as PI3K/AKT and BCL2, providing therapeutic options (see further). Bellini et al. detected variants of potential functional importance in the SMARCA4 ATPase domain in several NB cases [60]. Using a time series of transcriptome analysis for different developmental stages of normal sympathetic ganglia and TH-MYCN-driven tumors in mice, we also observed dramatic upregulation of BRG1/SMARCA4, while in contrast BRM/SMARCA2 expression levels showed an opposite pattern [61]. These observations are in line with the normal role of BRG1/SMARCA4 in cell cycle control, and differentiation of embryonic and neuronal stem cells. The SWI/SNF-BRG1 chromatin remodeling protein plays critical roles in self-renewal, pluripotency, cell-cycle control and differentiation in embryonic stem cells, neural stem cells, and progenitor cells [62] through modulating the acetylation levels of H3K27 at the enhancers of lineage-specific genes [63].

Sequencing efforts in NB showed that like other embryonal tumors the mutational landscape is relatively silent with an average of about 5–10 mutations [64]. However, copy number alterations are very prominent in NB. As has been shown for other tumor entities, combining both mutation and copy number data can provide a more robust view on genetic alterations affecting particular genes. Notably, *ARID1A* and *ARID1B* are encoded on 1p36.11 and 6q25.3, respectively, both chromosomal regions affected in high risk NB. The study of Sausen et al. [65] reported on chromosomal and sequence alterations in ARID1A and ARID1B in 4% and 7% of investigated cases, respectively. In keeping with the more prominent involvement of structural rearrangements versus mutations in NB, mostly intragenic loss-of-function gene deletions or deletions encompassing the entire gene locus were observed. As indicated above, both ARID1 family genes are integral components of the SWI/SNF neural progenitor specific chromatin-remodeling BAF complex (npBAF), essential for the self-renewal of multipotent neural stem cells [66]. Of further notice, this study also reported nonsense mutations in the histone acetyltransferase (HAT) genes *EP300* and *CREBBP*, missense mutations in the SWI2/SNF2 family member *TTF2* gene, the histone demethylase gene *KDM5A*, and the chromatin-remodeling zinc finger gene *IKZF1*. Sausen and co-workers also found that high expression of members unique to the neural progenitor BAF complex correlated with a high-risk NB phenotype, whereas high expression of components of the neuron-specific BAF complex or downstream neuritogenesis target genes correlated with lower risk NB, suggesting that disrupted BAF complex signaling could preserve an undifferentiated sympathetic neuroblast progenitor state [67]. Further functional analysis in NB cells by Li et al. suggested that ARID1A loss could promote migration and invasion [67]. In a further study, hTERT expression was shown to be suppressed by ARID1A through co-occupancy of the hTERT promoter with the SIN3 transcription regulator family member A (SIN3A) repressor complex allowing NB differentiation to proceed [68]. Using genome editing of the syntenic 1p36 locus in primary mouse neural crest cells (NCCs), MYCN-driven tumorigenesis was shown to select for NCCs with Arid1a deletions from a pool of NCCs with randomly sized 1p36 deletions, establishing Arid1a as the MYCN-associated tumor suppressor [69]. This was further supported by disruption of ARID1A homologs in a zebrafish model which accelerated the onset and increases the penetrance of MYCN-driven neuroblastoma by increasing cell proliferation in the sympathoadrenal lineage [70].

The 6q25.3 deleted region harboring the *ARID1B* locus and affected in ultra-high risk NB also encompasses the locus of the PHF10 (BAF45A) gene encoding a SWI/SNF PBAF component [71]. Krasteva et al. discovered that proliferating neural stem and progenitor cells express complexes in which PHF10 (BAF45a), a Krüppel/PHD domain protein, is quantitatively associated with the SWI/SNF-like ATPases BRG and BRM, while a subunit switch with replacement of PHF10 is essential to allow transition from neural stem/progenitors to post-mitotic neurons. Whether and how PHF10 could contribute to NB aggressiveness in these ultra-high risk cases remains to be investigated. As for other SWI/SNF components such as ARID1A and BRG1, the mechanistic basis is intriguing as both loss-of-function and dependency characteristics can be attributed. In line with this, PHF10 was found to be essential for adult hematopoietic stem cell maintenance and myeloid lineage development [72], required for cell proliferation in normal and SV40-immortalized human fibroblast cells and embryonic lethal in mouse [73].

5.4.3 The CHD5 Chromatin Remodeler and 1p36 Tumor Suppressor

Chromodomain containing proteins were first identified as readers of methylated lysines although increasing evidence indicates that PHD and WD40 domains as well as ankyrin repeats can also recognize these regions. Chromodomain Helicase DNA Binding Protein 5 (CHD5) is a member of the chromodomain helicase DNA-binding protein, mostly expressed in neurons and forms a nucleosome remodeling and deacetylation–type (NurD) chromatin remodeling complex, similar to CHD3 and CHD4. CHD5 shares high sequence homology to these CHD3 and CHD4 family members and could have unique protein associations conferring functional specificity. In normal neuronal cells, CHD5 binds via its tandem chromodomains to H3K27me3 as well as unmethylated H4K4 and is required for terminal differentiation of neural progenitor [74]. CHD5 was shown to act as a tumor suppressor through mouse chromosomal engineering experiments and has been implicated in several tumor entities including gliomas and cancers of the colon, breast, lung, ovary, prostate, stomach, larynx, and gall bladder (and references therein) [75]. CHD5 is also located in the most frequently deleted region in MYCN amplified neuroblastoma, 1p36.31. Structurally, CHD5 is characterized by paired PHD domains and two tandem chromodomains at the N-terminal region, an SNF2-like helicase/ATPase domain in the central region, and a conserved, coiled-coil motif in the C-terminal region. CHD5 binds the unmodified N-terminus of H3 through its PHD domains at loci marked by absence of H3K4me3 and presence of H3K27me3 histone modifications. Inactivating mutations in the PHD domains of CHD5 abrogate histone 3 binding and impact on the transcriptional control of target genes. Several mechanisms for CHD5 inactivation have been identified. Overall, damaging mutations are rare. In particular in NB, only two mutations in the coding sequence, which showed significant enrichment in the relapsed tumor, were reported [76]. CHD5 may be transcriptionally silenced by DNA methylation of the promoter, silencing the remaining allele in some cancers with 1p deletion. In NBs, strongest methylation was observed in cases with both 1p loss and MYCN amplification, suggesting a possible association between MYCN amplification and the methylation status of the distal CHD5 promoter region [77]. CHD5 is regulated by the histone demethylase JMJD2A which causes transcriptional repression of CHD5 and subsequent reduced p53 expression. MiRNAs affecting CHD5 expression include several MYCN upregulated miRNAs (miR-17, miR-93, miR-106b, and miR-20b).

5.4.4 The ATR SWI/SNF-Like Chromatin Remodeling Protein, Alternative Telomere Lengthening, and More

ATRX was first discovered through the identification of loss-of-function mutations causing the α-thalassemia, mental retardation, X-linked (ATRX) syndrome [78]. Together with DAXX, ATRX forms a histone chaperone complex that deposits histone variant H3.3 into specific genomic regions enriched for H3K9me3 via its ADD domain and HP1α, including telomeres, pericentric heterochromatin, imprinted regions, retrotransposons, a subset of G-rich intragenic regions, and 3′ exons belonging to C2H2 Zinc Finger family of transcription factors. Within the ATRX/DAXX complex, DAXX was shown as the component containing H3.3 histone chaperone activity while the chromatin remodeler ATRX binds to DAXX to incorporate H3.3 into DNA. ATRX also recruits EZH2 to deposit H3K27me3 to regulate transcription.

Recently, high-throughput genome sequencing of a variety of cancers has identified inactivating mutations in the ATRX/DAXX/H3.3 complex in tumors exhibiting the alternative telomere lengthening or ALT phenotype, including pancreatic neuroendocrine tumors, glioblastoma multiforme, oligodendrogliomas, medulloblastomas, and NBs. In the latter, ATRX was predominantly affected by intragenic or gene spanning deletions in addition to missense, nonsense, and frameshift mutations mainly occurring in NBs in adolescents and young adults [79].

How ATRX loss mediates the ALT phenotype was enigmatic but recent work from the Gibbons team has provided intriguing insights. Using U2OS ALT positive osteosarcoma cells, they provide evidence that ATRX plays a pivotal role in suppressing ALT via apparently two converging pathways. First, ATRX-mediated suppression of ALT was shown to depend on the histone H3.3 chaperone DAXX and an increase in telomeric levels of histone H3.3. This is accompanied with attenuation of replication fork stalling, possibly through the suppression of G-quadruplex (G4) structures. G4 structures occur at G-rich repeats in single stranded DNA and are highly stable non-B DNA structures that represent physical barriers to the replication machinery, forming a threat to the cell as stalled forks can collapse and lead to toxic double strands breaks. In line with this, stabilization of G4 structures potentiates ALT in the presence of ATRX. Second, the authors also showed that ATRX interacts with and sequesters the MRE11-RAD50-NBS1 (MRN) complex that, in the absence of ATRX, is redistributed to ALT-associated promyelocytic leukemia (PML) nuclear bodies where it may facilitate homologous DNA repair [80].

Interestingly, in follow-up of the finding of an ATRX deficiency associated ALT phenotype in NB cells, the Fischer team discovered yet another telomere maintenance mechanism in NB cells without MYCN amplification (known to drive hTERT expression levels) and ATRX mutations/deletions, i.e., structural rearrangements including enhancer hijacking leading to hTERT activation. This has now lead to a functional classification of three major subgroups of high risk tumors with active telomere maintenance in addition to the low risk tumors with no telomere elongation exhibiting spontaneous differentiation and regression [16, 81].

5.5 The Core-Regulatory Transcription Factor Circuitry Defined Adrenergic and Mesenchymal Neuroblastoma Cell States

A detailed description of the discovery and functional exploration of the lineage specific core-regulatory transcription factor circuits (CRC) in NB are described elsewhere (Chap. 7). In the context of this chapter, we refer to these novel insights given the potential biological and translational importance, also in view of the emerging role of lineage plasticity in drug resistance development [82]. In NB, two cell types have been defined: The vast majority of NBs exhibit an adrenergic phenotype while in a smaller subset a more primitive neural crest/mesenchymal phenotype was discerned, the latter which could also be associated with therapy resistance. Thus far, developmental studies of normal maturing sympathetic neuroblasts or single cell analysis of primary NBs has not yet resolved the exact role of the neural crest/mesenchymal cells during neuroblast formation and tumor initiation and therapy relapse. Of note, the work by the Look team revealed that ARID1A knock down in human NGP neuroblastoma cells promoted the adrenergic-to-mesenchymal transition with changes in enhancer-mediated gene expression due to alterations in the genomic occupancies of distinct SWI/SNF assemblies, BAF, and PBAF. Also, our analysis of the dynamic regulated TH-MYCN mouse NB transcriptomes identified MEIS2 as a novel CRC member and putative gene implicated in the early steps of tumor formation [61].

5.6 Noncoding RNAs and Epigenetic Regulation

Over the past decade, our view on noncoding RNA has dramatically changed from "junk" transcriptional products to functional regulatory molecules. MiRNAs emerged as important actors in controlling an additional level for regulation of gene transcript abundance or translation and a crucial role for several tumor suppressor miRNAs, and oncomirs were established in various cancers including neuroblastoma [83]. Some of these miRNAs control the expression of important epigenetic regulators as illustrated by the miR-137 tumor suppressor and its target gene KDM1A (LSD1) [84]. For details on the role of miRNAs including their impact on epigenetic regulation we refer to previous reviews.

In addition to the well-known miRNAs, more recently, additional classes of noncoding RNAs emerged including circular and long noncoding RNAs. Long non-coding RNAs (lncRNAs) have been recognized as highly versatile players in the regulation of gene expression in development and human disease, particularly cancer. LncRNAs have versatile functions and can act either in *cis* or in *trans* and mainly do this in concert with interacting proteins. *Cis* regulation of gene expression by lncRNAs can act through (1) direct regulation of the expression of neighboring genes through the ability to recruit regulatory factors to the locus and/or modulate their function, (2) the act of transcription itself and/or splicing thus conferring a gene-regulation functionality that is independent of the sequence of the RNA transcript, or (3) through dependency on DNA elements within the lncRNA promoter or gene locus and thus completely independent of the encoded RNA or its production [85]. Trans-regulating lncRNA-controlled mechanisms include (1) regulation of chromatin states and gene expression at regions distant from their transcription site, (2) control of nuclear structure and organization, and (3) interaction with and regulation of the behavior of proteins and/or other RNA molecules.

In cancer cells, hundreds of lncRNAs can become dysregulated and multiple lncRNAs have demonstrated functions as tumor-suppressors or oncogenes [86]. Furthermore, studies have demonstrated that dysregulation of lncRNAs results in alterations of the epigenome in cancer cells, potentially providing a novel mechanism for the massive epigenomic alterations observed in many tumors [87, 88] including coordination of chromatin dynamics, regulation of DNA methylation, modulation of other non-coding RNAs and mRNA stability, and control of epigenetic substrate availability through altered tumor metabolism.

Evidence is now emerging that lncRNAs are also playing important roles in neuroblastoma [89–93]. Reminiscent to previous work showing translational and posttranslational control of MYC activity through at least five lncRNAs located on 8q24 in the vicinity of the MYC locus, recent studies in NB identified two noncoding RNAs, MYCN opposite strand (MYCNOS or NCYM), a *cis*-natural antisense transcript and lncUSMycN, both located within a 130-kb genomic DNA region containing the MYCN. Both lncUSMycN and NCYM lncRNAs were shown to bind to the RNA-binding protein NonO which negatively controls MYCN mRNA levels while lncUSMycN also upregulates NCYM expression through modulation of H3K4 trimethylation of the NCYM gene promoter [94].

In another study, NCYM was shown to physically interact with the CCCTC-binding factor (CTCF) thus facilitating the recruitment of CTCF to its binding sites within the MYCN promoter to induce chromatin remodeling and resulting in enhanced MYCN levels and altered downstream gene expression [95]. CTCF cooperated with NCYM to suppress the differentiation and promote the growth, invasion, and metastasis. CTCF thus cooperates with noncoding Cis-antisense RNA NCYM to exhibit oncogenic activity that affects the aggressiveness and progression of NB through transcriptional upregulation of MYCN.

Mondal et al. showed that a sense/antisense lncRNA pair expressed from the NB risk-associated 6p22.3 locus was implicated in a retinoic acid-induced NB differentiation gene-regulatory network [96]. Both lncRNAs regulate SOX9 expression by controlling CHD7 stability via modulating the cellular localization of the ubiquitin specific protease USP36. Given that both SOX9 and USP36 are located on 17q, these observations could point towards a regulatory nexus between 6p22.3 and 17q regions which may be exploited for drugging in future experiments [96].

5.7 MYCN, the Master Regulator of the Neuroblastoma Epigenome and Transcriptome

Given the functional redundancy of MYC and MYCN and the known role of MYC in epigenetic reprogramming, it is not surprising that MYCN also plays a crucial role in controlling and shaping the NB epigenome. Initially, MYC and MYCN were considered to act as classical transcription factors, but this dogma evolved and recent novel insights hint toward a broader function of MYC/MYCN as a regulator of global chromatin structure and transcription. In particular, MYC has been shown to be a universal transcriptional amplifier [97, 98], increasing transcriptional activation of genes transcriptionally active genes. Whether MYCN plays a similar role has not been formally investigated. However, these new findings point towards a role for MYC/MYCN in reshaping the cancer epigenome and transcriptome through site-specific, local mechanisms, as well as genome-wide effects. For the first, MYC/MYCN recruits chromatin modifying co-factors that remodel chromatin structure in the vicinity of their binding sites. Co-factors implicated in the transcriptional activation function include WDR5 [99], histone acetylases TRRAP [100], P300/CBP and GCN5 [101], and the histone demethylase KDM4B [46] for removing H3K9me3 repressive marks, while recruitment of LSD1 [102], HDACs [55], and PRC2 [29, 33, 35] are implicated in MYCN controlled gene repression.

In the context of MYC, global effects on chromatin were shown to be mediated through suppression of the SIN3 Transcription Regulator Family Member B (SIN3B), HMG-box Transcription Factor 1 (HBP1), suppressor of Variegation 4–20 Homolog 1 (SUV420H1), and B Cell Translocation Gene 1 (BTG1) through miR-17-92. SIN3B interacts with HBP1 and recruits HDACs to silence proliferation-related genes and mediate cell cycle exit and senescence [103]. We confirmed that in NB also MYCN down regulated HBP1 through miR-17-92 and that modulating HBP1 levels impact on the MYCN activity, suggesting that the previously reported repressive role for HBP1 on MYC activity is also involved in the control of MYCN [104]. Further, MYCN also causes DOTL1 overexpression through promoter binding impacting on global H3K79 methylation and gene activity [105]. A detailed description of targeting MYCN transcription by using epigenetic compounds is provided in Liu Z. et al. [106].

5.8 Drugging the Neuroblastoma Epigenome

The dynamic and reversible nature of epigenetic modifications implies that it may be possible to alter disease-associated epigenetic states through direct manipulation of the molecular factors involved in this process. Given that many chromatin remodelers and enzymes involved in DNA and histone modifications have been identified as crucial regulators of NB tumorigenesis and aggressiveness as described above, we will focus in this section on the recent advances in drugging the epigenome and their application to NB therapeutics (Table 5.1).

5.8.1 Small Molecule Inhibitors and Therapeutic Development in Neuroblastoma

Histone deacetylases (HDACs) and DNA methyltransferases (DNMTs) were the first epigenetic targets to be approved for cancer application by US Food and Drug Administration (FDA) but these compounds have broad activities. While their activities in pre-clinical in vitro and in vivo models of NB are demonstrated [49, 107], their transition and integration into therapeutic regimens have usually been in combination with agents used in the setting of minimal residual disease [108–110].

Given the success of small molecule inhibitors targeting specific mutations in the enzymatic

Table 5.1 Epigenetic inhibitors with potential clinical application in neuroblastoma and other tumors

Class	Compound	Target/mechanism of action	Clinical phase	Indication	References
HMT inhibitors					
EZH2 inhibitors	CPI-1205		Phase I	B cell lymphoma	
	GSK2816126 (GSK-126)		Phase I	DLBCL, follicular lymphoma	*[32, 110]*
	EPZ-6438		Ped. Phase I	INI-1 mutant rhabdoid tumors or synovial sarcoma	*[114]*
SETD8 inhibitors	UNC0379	Inhibition of SETD8 and p53K382me1 in NB cells and in vivo xenograft model	Preclinical		*[36]*
	SGSS05-NS3		Preclinical		*data not shown*
DOT1L inhibitors	EPZ-5676		Ped. Phase I	Pediatric leukemia with MLL mutant	*[125]*
			Phase I	Advanced hematological malignancies	
	SGC0946	Inhibition of MYCN amp NB cells proliferation in vitro	Preclinical		*[104]*
HDM inhibitors					
LSD1 inhibitors	GSK2879552		Phase I	AML, small cell lung cancer, myelodysplastic syndrome	*[127]*
HDAC inhibitors					
HDAC1-3,6	Vorinostat (SAHA)		Ped. Phase I	Refractory/recurrent NB, other cancers	*[135]*
HDAC class I and II	Valproic acid (VPA)		Ped. Phase I	Refractory solid tumors, NB	*[137]*
pan-HDAC	4-PB		Ped. Phase I	Refractory malignancies, NB	[137]
HDAC1/2	Romidepsin		Ped. Phase I, Preclinical	refractory/recurrent solid tumors, NB	*[132]*
HDAC1/2	BRD 8130		Preclinical	NB	*[48]*
HDAC8	PCI-34051	Lymphomas, NB	Preclinical		*[140,141]*
BET inhibitors					
BRD2,BRD3,BRD4,BRDT	JQ1		Preclinical		*[144,145,149]*
BRD2,BRD3,BRD4	GSK525762 (I-BET762)		Phase I-II	NUT midline carcinoma, NB, other cancers	*[150]*
DNA methylation inhibitors					
DNMT inhibitors	Decitabine	Decreases DNA methylation	Ped. Phase I	NB and other pediatric cancers	*[151]*
	Genistein	Decreases DNA methylation of CHD5	Ped. Phase II	NB and other pediatric cancers	*[137,154]*
DNMT inhibitors	Azacytidine		Ped. Phase I	AML, myelodysplastic syndrome and others	*[151]*

red=inhibitors in clinical trials for neuroblastoma; black= inhibitors that have shown a preclinical efficacy in neuroblastoma and in clinical trials for other pediatric or adult tumors
**abbreviations HMT=histone methyltransferases; HDM= histone demethylases; HDAC=histone deacetylases; DNMTi=DNA methylation inhibitors; AML=acute myelogenous leukemia; DLBCL=Diffuse large B-cell lymphoma; NB=neuroblastoma; MCL=mantle cell lymphoma; Ped.=pediatric*

activities of signaling molecules, the discovery of activating mutations in EZH2 in lymphoma [111] and translocations involving DOT1L in leukemia stimulated pharmaceutical interest in the development of similar agents that selectively targeted the enzymatic activities of epigenetic regulators. The following part will highlight some that have shown preclinical efficacy in NB cell lines in vitro and are currently in clinical trials for adult or pediatric cancers.

5.8.2 HMT Inhibitors and Their Use in NB

5.8.2.1 EZH2 Inhibitors

Given the role of EZH2 as critical enzymatic mediator of the PRC2 complex, the development of EZH2-specific inhibitors has been an area of intense research in drug discovery. Several highly potent and selective EZH2 inhibitors have been studied and Tazemetostat is in pediatric Phase I clinical trials (Table 5.1). DZNep(3-deazaneplanocin-A) selectively inhibits H3K27me3 and H4K20me3 and was the first EZH2 inhibitor widely used that reactivated PRC2 silenced genes, by promoting degradation of the PRC2 complex resulting in increased apoptosis in a number of tumor types [112–114]. In NB, DZNep induced differentiation by de-repressing tumor suppressor and differentiation genes, such as CASZ1, CLU, RUNX3, and NGFR resulting in decreased growth of NB tumor xenografts [29]. As DZNep inhibits S-adenosyl-methionine (SAM)-dependent reactions, which are carried out by many HMTs, it is not as selective as more recently developed EZH2-targeted inhibitors that compete with the methyl group donor SAM. EPZ-6438 (Tazemetostat) is the first-in-class selective inhibitor targeting EZH2's methylase activity [114] to reach the clinic and this compound is 500 times more selective for EZH2 compared with other HMTs [115]. In pediatrics, active trials are aimed at targeting INI-1 mutant, synovial sarcomas, and the relevant indications in the pediatric MATCH trial. The Pediatric Preclinical testing group evaluating Tazemetostat did not show preclinical efficacy in xenograft models of NB [116]. However, next generation EZH2 inhibitors are in the developmental pipeline [117, 118]. GSK126, which displays >1000-fold selectivity for EZH2 SET domain over 20 other HMTs and 150-fold over EZH1 [111, 118] has recently been shown to inhibit growth of NB xenografts [32]. The finding that EZH2 inhibitors synergize with HDAC inhibitors (panobinostat) indicates we have just begun to explore the potential of these agents [32].

5.8.2.2 SETD8 Inhibitors

Given its activity in regulating critical events in the G2/M transition and its ability to suppress the activity of p53, inhibitors of SETD8 (aka SET8, PR-set7, KMT5A) have been widely sought. Nahuoic acid A, a marine natural product, was first identified as a SETD8 selective SAM-competitive inhibitor that decreased tumor cell proliferation [119, 120]. UNC0379 was the first substrate competitive SETD8 inhibitor with selectivity for SETD8 over 15 other HMTs in biochemical assays (in vitro IC_{50} 7,3 μM) [121] and quickly followed by the development of SGSS05-NS3. Our chemical screen of epigenetic regulators indicated that UNC0379 had the highest IVTI (In Vitro Therapeutic Index) when comparing NB tumor to normal cells, rescued p53 pro-apoptotic functions, and reduced NB tumor xenograft growth [31]. For this reason, recent efforts have been made toward developing a potent inhibitor of SETD8 based on substrate peptide modifications [122].

5.8.2.3 DOT1L Inhibitors

DOT1L is the only known HMT that catalyzes the mono-, di- and tri-methylation of H3K79, which has been associated with active gene transcription linked to cell-cycle progression and DNA repair [123]. DOT1L has been identified as an epigenetic target in AML with mixed lineage leukemia gene translocations (MLLR) [124] and EPZ004777 was the first inhibitor identified [125]. In leukemia subtypes with mixed lineage leukemia rearranged acute leukemia (MLLr), DOT1L is recruited to the promoter of leukemia target genes facilitating active transcription of these oncogenes. The recently completed DOT1L inhibitor EPZ-5676 trial showed tolerability, safety, and modest efficacy with 2/50 patients with MLLr achieving CR indicating limited therapeutic potential as a single agent [126]. In NB, DOT1L has been reported as a crucial cofactor in transcriptional activation of MYCN target genes facilitating NB tumorigenesis with the DOT1L inhibitor SGC0946 (a brominated form of EPZ004777) inhibiting MYCN amplified NB cell proliferation in vitro [105].

5.8.3 Histone Demethylation Inhibitors and Their Use in NB

The role of HDMs in cancer renders them attractive targets as they regulate the reactivation or de-repression of oncogenic transcription and "Lysine-specific demethylase" (LSD1) and JMJD3 (or KDM6B) have both been implicated in NB tumorigenesis. LSD1 removes mono- and di- methyl groups from K4 and K9 of histone 3 and plays a key role maintaining repression of differentiation genes in neuronal cells [127]. In NB, overexpression of LSD1 has been associated with poor prognosis [45] and shown to cooperate with MYCN to repress tumor suppressor genes [102]. While levels decrease with ATRA treatment [45], LSD1 inhibitors have also been shown to reactivation of previously silenced tumor suppressor genes [117]. A selective and potent irreversible LSD1 inhibitor, GSK2879552, is in a phase I clinical trial for AML and small cell lung cancer [128].

JMJD3 removes di- and tri-methyl groups from H3K27 and in a small molecule screen. GSK-J4 had significant anti-growth activity in both MYCN-non amplified and amplified NB cell lines [36]. More recently, GSK-J4 was shown to induce differentiation and ER stress in NB cell lines and inhibit the growth of NB cell lines and PDX xenographs in vivo. Intriguingly, combinations with either FDA approved drugs, RA or venetoclax showed enhanced in vivo efficacy [129].

5.8.4 Histone Deacetylation Inhibitors and Their Application in NB

HATs and HDACs are key regulators of histone acetylation by their respective acetylation and deacetylation of lysines on a number of proteins including histones [51, 130]. The potential of HDAC inhibitors in cancer was appreciated with the finding that they could induce differentiation in leukemic cells [131] and similar results have been shown in various pre-clinical NB models [49, 132]. Vorinostat (SAHA), was the first FDA approved pan-HDAC inhibitor, targeting HDAC1–3,6 and has been used alone and in combination. Romidepsin, a pan-HDAC inhibitor with selective activity against HDAC1–3, 8 induces a caspase-dependent cell death in NB cells [133] and as a FDA-approved HDAC1/2 inhibitor was well-tolerated in Phase I study in refractory pediatric cancers [134]. HDAC1/2 inhibitors not only induce NB cell differentiation but also synergize with retinoids [135]. A clinical trial of Vorinostat on an intermittent schedule showed prolonged stable disease when combined with retinoic acid [110]. Based on the pre-clinical finding that Vorinostat increased expression of the norepinephrine transporter, a clinical study to evaluate Vorinostat as a radiosensitizer for ^{131}I-metaiodobenzylguanidine (^{131}I-MIBG) showed the combination to be safe and served as the basis for a Phase II study to test the combination compared to ^{131}I-MIBG alone [136]. Pre-clinical models have also shown Vorinostat to synergize with anti-GD2 monoclonal antibody [137], which would be an interesting trial given the clinical efficacy of dinutuximab. Two additional HDAC inhibitors that have reached Phase I clinical trials are 4 PB (4-phenylbutyrate), a pan-HDAC inhibitor, and VAP (valproic acid), selective for class I and II HDACs [138].

Pre-clinical studies of the HDAC inhibitors Entinostat (MS-275) and Panobinostat which target nuclear HDACs are entering pediatric clinical trials and have shown activity in NB [49]. Relatively low dose, continuous Panobinostat treatment of TH-MYCN mice showed marked long term survival with evidence of differentiation [139], while another study showed synergy with standard cytotoxics that are used in the treatment high-risk neuroblastoma [140]. Several compounds (PCI-34051, -48000, -48012, and -34051) have been generated that show selectivity for HDAC8 [141, 142] and either alone or with retinoids potentiate differentiation while in combination with the ALK kinase inhibitor Crizotinib, shift the response from differentiation to apoptosis [143, 144]. How to determine which combinations to prioritize for clinical development remains a challenge.

5.8.5 BET Inhibitors and Their Application in NB

JQ1 and I-BET762 were the first BET inhibitors to be characterized that specifically impede the binding between BET proteins and acetylate histone [145, 146]. Potent anti-proliferative effects of BET inhibitors have been observed in many tumor types but predominantly those with mutations of BRD4 such as NUT midline carcinoma and hematological malignancies [147–149]. In neuroblastoma, a high-throughput screen identified MYCN amplification as a vulnerability and predictor of response to a tool compound BET inhibitor [150]. I-BET762 which is currently in Phase I-II clinical trial also has been shown to be active in pre-clinical NB models [151]. We are still in the early stages of finding effective combinations, but JQ1 alone or in combination with HDAC inhibitor Panobinostat shows evidence of synergy in NB pre-clinical models.

5.8.6 DNA Methylation Inhibitors and Their Application in NB

Given the dynamic and reversible modification that they regulate, the global levels of DNA methylation, DNMTs represent a suitable target for the development of latest generation compounds. DNA methylation inhibitors (DNMTi), Decitabine and Azacytidine, the two oldest nucleoside compounds, have already been tested in clinical trials with promising results, thus they have been FDA approved for myelodysplastic syndrome and AML [152]. There are three clinical trials using Decitabine targeting refractory or recurrent NB, two of them completed but no results are currently available (http://www.cancer.gov/clinicaltrials). In NB, it was demonstrated that DNMTi as 5′-aza-2′-deoxycitidine rescue the expression of tumor suppressor genes such as THBS1 and HSP47, showing preclinical evidence of DNMTi clinical testing in NB [153, 154]. Further, Genestein is a natural compound found in soy currently in Phase II clinical trial for NB. It could work as a DNMT inhibitor and it has been demonstrated to enhance the expression of CHD5 by inhibiting its promoter methylation [155, 138].

5.9 Conclusions

Following the initial discovery of MYCN amplification and recurrent copy number alterations, our understanding of the genetic basis of NB has grown slowly compared to other tumor entities. However, in the past years we have witnessed a remarkable acceleration in discoveries into how altered gene activity and signaling pathways drive neuroblastoma. This includes implication of various components of the epigenetic regulatory machinery as summarized here. Importantly, these novel findings are also opening opportunities for innovative drugging strategies. In this respect, some important issues remain to be rigorously explored. Most pre-clinical studies have evaluated effects on primary tumors and neglected issues relevant to efficacy in the minimal residual disease setting or optimal dosing and scheduling. Furthermore, clinical studies have focused on dose intensification which may not be the optimal use of epigenetic regulators. Also, novel single drug approaches still face the inevitable problem of drug resistance thus urging for further developments in combining several drugs, some of which may act synergistically and some of which may be most potent when given sequentially (one-two punch approach). A more comprehensive study on the structure and function of the above mentioned epigenetic enzymes and their substrate interactions, along with their histone and non-histone targets has the potential to lead to a robust pipeline of new inhibitors with higher selectivity, enhanced cellular activity, and less or differing toxicities than cytotoxic agents.

Acknowledgements We are grateful to Els Janssens and other lab members for their thoughtful review of the study. We apologize to our colleagues if space constraints limited our ability to cite all relevant studies.

Financial Support: This work was supported and funded by the Intramural Research Program of the NIH, National Cancer Institute, Center for Cancer Research.'Kom op tegen Kanker' (Research grant to Frank Speleman), the European Union H2020 (OPTIMIZE-NB GOD9415N and TRANSCAN-ON THE TRRAC GOD8815N to F.S.P.), Olivia Hendrickx Research Fund, Villa Joep Neuroblastoma Research Fund, Kinderkankerfonds, Ghent University (BOF10/GOA/019 and BOF16/GOA/23).

V.V. is a research fellow funded by European Union-FESR FSE, PON Ricerca e Innovazione 2014–2020 (AIM line 1). K.D is a research fellow funded by the Research Foundation – Flanders (FWO; 12Q8322N).

References

1. Feinberg AP. The key role of epigenetics in human disease prevention and mitigation. N Engl J Med. 2018;378(14):1323–34. https://doi.org/10.1056/NEJMra1402513.
2. Flavahan WA, Gaskell E, Bernstein BE. Epigenetic plasticity and the hallmarks of cancer. Science (New York, NY). 2017;357:6348. https://doi.org/10.1126/science.aal2380.
3. Bergman Y, Cedar H. DNA methylation dynamics in health and disease. Nat Struct Mol Biol. 2013;20(3):274–81. https://doi.org/10.1038/nsmb.2518.
4. Baylin SB, Jones PA. A decade of exploring the cancer epigenome—biological and translational implications. Nat Rev Cancer. 2011;11(10):726–34. https://doi.org/10.1038/nrc3130.

5. Feinberg AP, Koldobskiy MA, Gondor A. Epigenetic modulators, modifiers and mediators in cancer aetiology and progression. Nat Rev Genet. 2016;17(5):284–99. https://doi.org/10.1038/nrg.2016.13.
6. Decock A, Ongenaert M, Vandesompele J, Speleman F. Neuroblastoma epigenetics: from candidate gene approaches to genome-wide screenings. Epigenetics. 2011;6(8):962–70. https://doi.org/10.4161/epi.6.8.16516.
7. He S, Liu Z, Oh DY, Thiele CJ. MYCN and the epigenome. Front Oncol. 2013;3:1. https://doi.org/10.3389/fonc.2013.00001.
8. Fetahu IS, Taschner-Mandl S. Neuroblastoma and the epigenome. Cancer Metastasis Rev. 2021;40(1):173–89. https://doi.org/10.1007/s10555-020-09946-y.
9. Henrich KO, Bender S, Saadati M, Dreidax D, Gartlgruber M, Shao C, Herrmann C, Wiesenfarth M, Parzonka M, Wehrmann L, Fischer M, Duffy DJ, Bell E, Torkov A, Schmezer P, Plass C, Hofer T, Benner A, Pfister SM, Westermann F. Integrative genome-scale analysis identifies epigenetic mechanisms of transcriptional deregulation in Unfavorable neuroblastomas. Cancer Res. 2016;76(18):5523–37. https://doi.org/10.1158/0008-5472.CAN-15-2507.
10. Abe M, Ohira M, Kaneda A, Yagi Y, Yamamoto S, Kitano Y, Takato T, Nakagawara A, Ushijima T. CpG Island methylator phenotype is a strong determinant of poor prognosis in neuroblastomas. Cancer Res. 2005;65(3):828–34.
11. Abe M, Westermann F, Nakagawara A, Takato T, Schwab M, Ushijima T. Marked and independent prognostic significance of the CpG Island methylator phenotype in neuroblastomas. Cancer Lett. 2007;247(2):253–8. https://doi.org/10.1016/j.canlet.2006.05.001.
12. Decock A, Ongenaert M, Cannoodt R, Verniers K, De Wilde B, Laureys G, Van Roy N, Berbegall AP, Bienertova-Vasku J, Bown N, Clement N, Combaret V, Haber M, Hoyoux C, Murray J, Noguera R, Pierron G, Schleiermacher G, Schulte JH, Stallings RL, Tweddle DA, Children's C, Leukaemia G, De Preter K, Speleman F, Vandesompele J. Methyl-CpG-binding domain sequencing reveals a prognostic methylation signature in neuroblastoma. Oncotarget. 2016;7(2):1960–72. https://doi.org/10.18632/oncotarget.6477.
13. Decock A, Ongenaert M, De Wilde B, Brichard B, Noguera R, Speleman F, Vandesompele J. Stage 4S neuroblastoma tumors show a characteristic DNA methylation portrait. Epigenetics. 2016;11(10):761–71. https://doi.org/10.1080/15592294.2016.1226739.
14. Blasco MA. The epigenetic regulation of mammalian telomeres. Nat Rev Genet. 2007;8(4):299–309. https://doi.org/10.1038/nrg2047.
15. Vera E, Canela A, Fraga MF, Esteller M, Blasco MA. Epigenetic regulation of telomeres in human cancer. Oncogene. 2008;27(54):6817–33. https://doi.org/10.1038/onc.2008.289.
16. Hertwig F, Peifer M, Fischer M. Telomere maintenance is pivotal for high-risk neuroblastoma. Cell cycle (Georgetown, Tex). 2016;15(3):311–2. https://doi.org/10.1080/15384101.2015.1125243.
17. Ackermann S, Cartolano M, Hero B, Welte A, Kahlert Y, Roderwieser A, Bartenhagen C, Walter E, Gecht J, Kerschke L, Volland R, Menon R, Heuckmann JM, Gartlgruber M, Hartlieb S, Henrich KO, Okonechnikov K, Altmuller J, Nurnberg P, Lefever S, de Wilde B, Sand F, Ikram F, Rosswog C, Fischer J, Theissen J, Hertwig F, Singhi AD, Simon T, Vogel W, Perner S, Krug B, Schmidt M, Rahmann S, Achter V, Lang U, Vokuhl C, Ortmann M, Buttner R, Eggert A, Speleman F, O'Sullivan RJ, Thomas RK, Berthold F, Vandesompele J, Schramm A, Westermann F, Schulte JH, Peifer M, Fischer M. A mechanistic classification of clinical phenotypes in neuroblastoma. Science (New York, NY). 2018;362(6419):1165–70. https://doi.org/10.1126/science.aat6768.
18. Strahl BD, Allis CD. The language of covalent histone modifications. Nature. 2000;403(6765):41–5. https://doi.org/10.1038/47412.
19. Arrowsmith CH, Bountra C, Fish PV, Lee K, Schapira M. Epigenetic protein families: a new frontier for drug discovery. Nat Rev Drug Discov. 2012;11(5):384–400. https://doi.org/10.1038/nrd3674.
20. Di Croce L, Helin K. Transcriptional regulation by Polycomb group proteins. Nat Struct Mol Biol. 2013;20(10):1147–55. https://doi.org/10.1038/nsmb.2669.
21. Gilchrist DA, Nechaev S, Lee C, Ghosh SK, Collins JB, Li L, Gilmour DS, Adelman K. NELF-mediated stalling of pol II can enhance gene expression by blocking promoter-proximal nucleosome assembly. Genes Dev. 2008;22(14):1921–33. https://doi.org/10.1101/gad.1643208.
22. Kagey JD, Kapoor-Vazirani P, McCabe MT, Powell DR, Vertino PM. Long-term stability of demethylation after transient exposure to 5-aza-2′-deoxycytidine correlates with sustained RNA polymerase II occupancy. Mol Cancer Res MCR. 2010;8(7):1048–59. https://doi.org/10.1158/1541-7786.MCR-10-0189.
23. Takeshima H, Yamashita S, Shimazu T, Niwa T, Ushijima T. The presence of RNA polymerase II, active or stalled, predicts epigenetic fate of promoter CpG islands. Genome Res. 2009;19(11):1974–82. https://doi.org/10.1101/gr.093310.109.
24. Nowak K, Kerl K, Fehr D, Kramps C, Gessner C, Killmer K, Samans B, Berwanger B, Christiansen H, Lutz W. BMI1 is a target gene of E2F-1 and is strongly expressed in primary neuroblastomas. Nucleic Acids Res. 2006;34(6):1745–54. https://doi.org/10.1093/nar/gkl119.
25. Ochiai H, Takenobu H, Nakagawa A, Yamaguchi Y, Kimura M, Ohira M, Okimoto Y, Fujimura Y, Koseki H, Kohno Y, Nakagawara A, Kamijo T. Bmi1 is a MYCN target gene that regulates tumorigenesis

through repression of KIF1Bbeta and TSLC1 in neuroblastoma. Oncogene. 2010;29(18):2681–90. https://doi.org/10.1038/onc.2010.22.
26. Cui H, Ma J, Ding J, Li T, Alam G, Ding HF. Bmi-1 regulates the differentiation and clonogenic self-renewal of I-type neuroblastoma cells in a concentration-dependent manner. J Biol Chem. 2006;281(45):34696–704. https://doi.org/10.1074/jbc.M604009200.
27. Calao M, Sekyere EO, Cui HJ, Cheung BB, Thomas WD, Keating J, Chen JB, Raif A, Jankowski K, Davies NP, Bekkum MV, Chen B, Tan O, Ellis T, Norris MD, Haber M, Kim ES, Shohet JM, Trahair TN, Liu T, Wainwright BJ, Ding HF, Marshall GM. Direct effects of Bmi1 on p53 protein stability inactivates oncoprotein stress responses in embryonal cancer precursor cells at tumor initiation. Oncogene. 2013;32(31):3616–26. https://doi.org/10.1038/onc.2012.368.
28. De Preter K, Vandesompele J, Heimann P, Yigit N, Beckman S, Schramm A, Eggert A, Stallings RL, Benoit Y, Renard M, De Paepe A, Laureys G, Pahlman S, Speleman F. Human fetal neuroblast and neuroblastoma transcriptome analysis confirms neuroblast origin and highlights neuroblastoma candidate genes. Genome Biol. 2006;7(9):R84. https://doi.org/10.1186/gb-2006-7-9-r84.
29. Wang C, Liu Z, Woo CW, Li Z, Wang L, Wei JS, Marquez VE, Bates SE, Jin Q, Khan J, Ge K, Thiele CJ. EZH2 mediates epigenetic silencing of neuroblastoma suppressor genes CASZ1, CLU, RUNX3, and NGFR. Cancer Res. 2012;72(1):315–24. https://doi.org/10.1158/0008-5472.CAN-11-0961.
30. Stallings RL, Howard J, Dunlop A, Mullarkey M, McDermott M, Breatnach F, O'Meara A. Are gains of chromosomal regions 7q and 11p important abnormalities in neuroblastoma? Cancer Genet Cytogenet. 2003;140(2):133–7. https://doi.org/10.1016/s0165-4608(02)00681-7.
31. Tsubota S, Kishida S, Shimamura T, Ohira M, Yamashita S, Cao D, Kiyonari S, Ushijima T, Kadomatsu K. PRC2-mediated transcriptomic alterations at the embryonic stage govern tumorigenesis and clinical outcome in MYCN-driven neuroblastoma. Cancer Res. 2017;77(19):5259–71. https://doi.org/10.1158/0008-5472.CAN-16-3144.
32. Chen L, Alexe G, Dharia NV, Ross L, Iniguez AB, Conway AS, Wang EJ, Veschi V, Lam N, Qi J, Gustafson WC, Nasholm N, Vazquez F, Weir BA, Cowley GS, Ali LD, Pantel S, Jiang G, Harrington WF, Lee Y, Goodale A, Lubonja R, Krill-Burger JM, Meyers RM, Tsherniak A, Root DE, Bradner JE, Golub TR, Roberts CW, Hahn WC, Weiss WA, Thiele CJ, Stegmaier K. CRISPR-Cas9 screen reveals a MYCN-amplified neuroblastoma dependency on EZH2. J Clin Invest. 2018;128(1):446–62. https://doi.org/10.1172/JCI90793.
33. Corvetta D, Chayka O, Gherardi S, D'Acunto CW, Cantilena S, Valli E, Piotrowska I, Perini G, Sala A. Physical interaction between MYCN oncogene and polycomb repressive complex 2 (PRC2) in neuroblastoma: functional and therapeutic implications. J Biol Chem. 2013;288(12):8332–41. https://doi.org/10.1074/jbc.M113.454280.
34. Bate-Eya LT, Gierman HJ, Ebus ME, Koster J, Caron HN, Versteeg R, Dolman MEM, Molenaar JJ. Enhancer of zeste homologue 2 plays an important role in neuroblastoma cell survival independent of its histone methyltransferase activity. Eur J Cancer (Oxford, England : 1990). 2017;75:63–72. https://doi.org/10.1016/j.ejca.2016.12.019.
35. Li Z, Takenobu H, Setyawati AN, Akita N, Haruta M, Satoh S, Shinno Y, Chikaraishi K, Mukae K, Akter J, Sugino RP, Nakazawa A, Nakagawara A, Aburatani H, Ohira M, Kamijo T. EZH2 regulates neuroblastoma cell differentiation via NTRK1 promoter epigenetic modifications. Oncogene. 2018;37(20):2714–27. https://doi.org/10.1038/s41388-018-0133-3.
36. Veschi V, Liu Z, Voss TC, Ozbun L, Gryder B, Yan C, Hu Y, Ma A, Jin J, Mazur SJ, Lam N, Souza BK, Giannini G, Hager GL, Arrowsmith CH, Khan J, Appella E, Thiele CJ. Epigenetic siRNA and chemical screens identify SETD8 inhibition as a therapeutic strategy for p53 activation in high-risk neuroblastoma. Cancer Cell. 2017;31(1):50–63. https://doi.org/10.1016/j.ccell.2016.12.002.
37. Schnepp RW, Khurana P, Attiyeh EF, Raman P, Chodosh SE, Oldridge DA, Gagliardi ME, Conkrite KL, Asgharzadeh S, Seeger RC, Madison BB, Rustgi AK, Maris JM, Diskin SJ. A LIN28B-RAN-AURKA signaling network promotes neuroblastoma tumorigenesis. Cancer Cell. 2015;28(5):599–609. https://doi.org/10.1016/j.ccell.2015.09.012.
38. Wolf M, Korja M, Karhu R, Edgren H, Kilpinen S, Ojala K, Mousses S, Kallioniemi A, Haapasalo H. Array-based gene expression, CGH and tissue data defines a 12q24 gain in neuroblastic tumors with prognostic implication. BMC Cancer. 2010;10:181. https://doi.org/10.1186/1471-2407-10-181.
39. Congdon LM, Houston SI, Veerappan CS, Spektor TM, Rice JC. PR-Set7-mediated monomethylation of histone H4 lysine 20 at specific genomic regions induces transcriptional repression. J Cell Biochem. 2010;110(3):609–19. https://doi.org/10.1002/jcb.22570.
40. Houston SI, McManus KJ, Adams MM, Sims JK, Carpenter PB, Hendzel MJ, Rice JC. Catalytic function of the PR-Set7 histone H4 lysine 20 monomethyltransferase is essential for mitotic entry and genomic stability. J Biol Chem. 2008;283(28):19478–88. https://doi.org/10.1074/jbc.M710579200.
41. Jorgensen S, Elvers I, Trelle MB, Menzel T, Eskildsen M, Jensen ON, Helleday T, Helin K, Sorensen CS. The histone methyltransferase SET8 is required for S-phase progression. J Cell Biol. 2007;179(7):1337–45. https://doi.org/10.1083/jcb.200706150.
42. Tardat M, Brustel J, Kirsh O, Lefevbre C, Callanan M, Sardet C, Julien E. The histone H4 Lys 20 meth-

yltransferase PR-Set7 regulates replication origins in mammalian cells. Nat Cell Biol. 2010;12(11):1086–93. https://doi.org/10.1038/ncb2113.
43. Wu S, Wang W, Kong X, Congdon LM, Yokomori K, Kirschner MW, Rice JC. Dynamic regulation of the PR-Set7 histone methyltransferase is required for normal cell cycle progression. Genes Dev. 2010;24(22):2531–42. https://doi.org/10.1101/gad.1984210.
44. Shi X, Kachirskaia I, Yamaguchi H, West LE, Wen H, Wang EW, Dutta S, Appella E, Gozani O. Modulation of p53 function by SET8-mediated methylation at lysine 382. Mol Cell. 2007;27(4):636–46. https://doi.org/10.1016/j.molcel.2007.07.012.
45. Schulte JH, Lim S, Schramm A, Friedrichs N, Koster J, Versteeg R, Ora I, Pajtler K, Klein-Hitpass L, Kuhfittig-Kulle S, Metzger E, Schule R, Eggert A, Buettner R, Kirfel J. Lysine-specific demethylase 1 is strongly expressed in poorly differentiated neuroblastoma: implications for therapy. Cancer Res. 2009;69(5):2065–71. https://doi.org/10.1158/0008-5472.CAN-08-1735.
46. Yang J, AlTahan AM, Hu D, Wang Y, Cheng PH, Morton CL, Qu C, Nathwani AC, Shohet JM, Fotsis T, Koster J, Versteeg R, Okada H, Harris AL, Davidoff AM. The role of histone demethylase KDM4B in Myc signaling in neuroblastoma. J Natl Cancer Inst. 2015;107(6):djv080. https://doi.org/10.1093/jnci/djv080.
47. Phimmachanh M, Han JZR, O'Donnell YEI, Latham SL, Croucher DR. Histone deacetylases and histone deacetylase inhibitors in neuroblastoma. Front Cell Dev Biol. 2020;8:578770. https://doi.org/10.3389/fcell.2020.578770.
48. Frumm SM, Fan ZP, Ross KN, Duvall JR, Gupta S, VerPlank L, Suh BC, Holson E, Wagner FF, Smith WB, Paranal RM, Bassil CF, Qi J, Roti G, Kung AL, Bradner JE, Tolliday N, Stegmaier K. Selective HDAC1/HDAC2 inhibitors induce neuroblastoma differentiation. Chem Biol. 2013;20(5):713–25. https://doi.org/10.1016/j.chembiol.2013.03.020.
49. Jaboin J, Wild J, Hamidi H, Khanna C, Kim CJ, Robey R, Bates SE, Thiele CJ. MS-27-275, an inhibitor of histone deacetylase, has marked in vitro and in vivo antitumor activity against pediatric solid tumors. Cancer Res. 2002;62(21):6108–15.
50. Schulte JH, Eggert A. Neuroblastoma. Crit Rev Oncog. 2015;20(3–4):245–70. https://doi.org/10.1615/critrevoncog.2015014033.
51. Oehme I, Deubzer HE, Wegener D, Pickert D, Linke JP, Hero B, Kopp-Schneider A, Westermann F, Ulrich SM, von Deimling A, Fischer M, Witt O. Histone deacetylase 8 in neuroblastoma tumorigenesis. Clin Cancer Res. 2009;15(1):91–9. https://doi.org/10.1158/1078-0432.CCR-08-0684.
52. Oehme I, Lodrini M, Brady NR, Witt O. Histone deacetylase 10-promoted autophagy as a druggable point of interference to improve the treatment response of advanced neuroblastomas. Autophagy. 2013;9(12):2163–5. https://doi.org/10.4161/auto.26450.
53. Lodrini M, Oehme I, Schroeder C, Milde T, Schier MC, Kopp-Schneider A, Schulte JH, Fischer M, De Preter K, Pattyn F, Castoldi M, Muckenthaler MU, Kulozik AE, Westermann F, Witt O, Deubzer HE. MYCN and HDAC2 cooperate to repress miR-183 signaling in neuroblastoma. Nucleic Acids Res. 2013;41(12):6018–33. https://doi.org/10.1093/nar/gkt346.
54. Fabian J, Lodrini M, Oehme I, Schier MC, Thole TM, Hielscher T, Kopp-Schneider A, Opitz L, Capper D, von Deimling A, Wiegand I, Milde T, Mahlknecht U, Westermann F, Popanda O, Roels F, Hero B, Berthold F, Fischer M, Kulozik AE, Witt O, Deubzer HE. GRHL1 acts as tumor suppressor in neuroblastoma and is negatively regulated by MYCN and HDAC3. Cancer Res. 2014;74(9):2604–16. https://doi.org/10.1158/0008-5472.CAN-13-1904.
55. Fabian J, Opitz D, Althoff K, Lodrini M, Hero B, Volland R, Beckers A, de Preter K, Decock A, Patil N, Abba M, Kopp-Schneider A, Astrahantseff K, Wunschel J, Pfeil S, Ercu M, Kunkele A, Hu J, Thole T, Schweizer L, Mechtersheimer G, Carter D, Cheung BB, Popanda O, von Deimling A, Koster J, Versteeg R, Schwab M, Marshall GM, Speleman F, Erb U, Zoeller M, Allgayer H, Simon T, Fischer M, Kulozik AE, Eggert A, Witt O, Schulte JH, Deubzer HE. MYCN and HDAC5 transcriptionally repress CD9 to trigger invasion and metastasis in neuroblastoma. Oncotarget. 2016;7(41):66344–59. https://doi.org/10.18632/oncotarget.11662.
56. Bartholomew B. Regulating the chromatin landscape: structural and mechanistic perspectives. Annu Rev Biochem. 2014;83:671–96. https://doi.org/10.1146/annurev-biochem-051810-093157.
57. Dawson MA. The cancer epigenome: concepts, challenges, and therapeutic opportunities. Science (New York, NY). 2017;355(6330):1147–52. https://doi.org/10.1126/science.aam7304.
58. Kadoch C, Hargreaves DC, Hodges C, Elias L, Ho L, Ranish J, Crabtree GR. Proteomic and bioinformatic analysis of mammalian SWI/SNF complexes identifies extensive roles in human malignancy. Nat Genet. 2013;45(6):592–601. https://doi.org/10.1038/ng.2628.
59. Jubierre L, Soriano A, Planells-Ferrer L, Paris-Coderch L, Tenbaum SP, Romero OA, Moubarak RS, Almazan-Moga A, Molist C, Roma J, Navarro S, Noguera R, Sanchez-Cespedes M, Comella JX, Palmer HG, Sanchez de Toledo J, Gallego S, Segura MF. BRG1/SMARCA4 is essential for neuroblastoma cell viability through modulation of cell death and survival pathways. Oncogene. 2016;35(39):5179–90. https://doi.org/10.1038/onc.2016.50.
60. Bellini A, Bessoltane-Bentahar N, Bhalshankar J, Clement N, Raynal V, Baulande S, Bernard V, Danzon A, Chicard M, Colmet-Daage L, Pierron G, Le Roux L, Planchon JM, Combaret V, Lapouble E, Corradini N, Thebaud E, Gambart M, Valteau-Couanet D, Michon J, Louis-Brennetot C, Janoueix-Lerosey I, Defachelles AS, Bourdeaut F, Delattre O,

Schleiermacher G. Study of chromatin remodeling genes implicates SMARCA4 as a putative player in oncogenesis in neuroblastoma. Int J Cancer. 2019;145(10):2781–91. https://doi.org/10.1002/ijc.32361.
61. De Wyn J, Zimmerman MW, Weichert-Leahey N, Nunes C, Cheung BB, Abraham BJ, Beckers A, Volders PJ, Decaesteker B, Carter DR, Look AT, De Preter K, Van Loocke W, Marshall GM, Durbin AD, Speleman F, Durinck K. MEIS2 is an Adrenergic Core Regulatory Transcription Factor involved in early initiation of TH-MYCN-Driven Neuroblastoma Formation. Cancers (Basel). 2021;13(19):4783.
62. Petrik D, Latchney SE, Masiulis I, Yun S, Zhang Z, Wu JI, Eisch AJ. Chromatin remodeling factor Brg1 supports the early maintenance and late responsiveness of nestin-lineage adult neural stem and progenitor cells. Stem Cells (Dayton, Ohio). 2015;33(12):3655–65. https://doi.org/10.1002/stem.2215.
63. Kidder BL, Palmer S, Knott JG. SWI/SNF-Brg1 regulates self-renewal and occupies core pluripotency-related genes in embryonic stem cells. Stem Cells (Dayton, Ohio). 2009;27(2):317–28. https://doi.org/10.1634/stemcells.2008-0710.
64. Matthay KK, Maris JM, Schleiermacher G, Nakagawara A, Mackall CL, Diller L, Weiss WA. Neuroblastoma. Nat Rev Dis Primers. 2016;2:16078. https://doi.org/10.1038/nrdp.2016.78.
65. Sausen M, Leary RJ, Jones S, Wu J, Reynolds CP, Liu X, Blackford A, Parmigiani G, Diaz LA Jr, Papadopoulos N, Vogelstein B, Kinzler KW, Velculescu VE, Hogarty MD. Integrated genomic analyses identify ARID1A and ARID1B alterations in the childhood cancer neuroblastoma. Nat Genet. 2013;45(1):12–7. https://doi.org/10.1038/ng.2493.
66. Ho L, Crabtree GR. Chromatin remodelling during development. Nature. 2010;463(7280):474–84. https://doi.org/10.1038/nature08911.
67. Li C, Xu ZL, Zhao Z, An Q, Wang L, Yu Y, Piao DX. ARID1A gene knockdown promotes neuroblastoma migration and invasion. Neoplasma. 2017;64(3):367–76. https://doi.org/10.4149/neo_2017_307.
68. Bui CB, Le HK, Vu DM, Truong KD, Nguyen NM, Ho MAN, Truong DQ. ARID1A-SIN3A drives retinoic acid-induced neuroblastoma differentiation by transcriptional repression of TERT. Mol Carcinog. 2019;58(11):1998–2007. https://doi.org/10.1002/mc.23091.
69. Garcia-Lopez J, Wallace K, Otero JH, Olsen R, Wang YD, Finkelstein D, Gudenas BL, Rehg JE, Northcott P, Davidoff AM, Freeman KW. Large 1p36 deletions affecting Arid1a locus facilitate Mycn-driven oncogenesis in neuroblastoma. Cell Rep. 2020;30(2):454–64. e455. https://doi.org/10.1016/j.celrep.2019.12.048.
70. Shi H, Tao T, Abraham BJ, Durbin AD, Zimmerman MW, Kadoch C, Look AT. ARID1A loss in neuroblastoma promotes the adrenergic-to-mesenchymal transition by regulating enhancer-mediated gene expression. Sci Adv. 2020;6(29):eaaz3440. https://doi.org/10.1126/sciadv.aaz3440.
71. Depuydt P, Boeva V, Hocking TD, Cannoodt R, Ambros IM, Ambros PF, Asgharzadeh S, Attiyeh EF, Combaret V, Defferrari R, Fischer M, Hero B, Hogarty MD, Irwin MS, Koster J, Kreissman S, Ladenstein R, Lapouble E, Laureys G, London WB, Mazzocco K, Nakagawara A, Noguera R, Ohira M, Park JR, Potschger U, Theissen J, Tonini GP, Valteau-Couanet D, Varesio L, Versteeg R, Speleman F, Maris JM, Schleiermacher G, De Preter K. Genomic amplifications and distal 6q loss: novel markers for poor survival in high-risk neuroblastoma patients. J Natl Cancer Inst. 2018;110(10):1084–93. https://doi.org/10.1093/jnci/djy022.
72. Krasteva V, Crabtree GR, Lessard JA. The BAF45a/PHF10 subunit of SWI/SNF-like chromatin remodeling complexes is essential for hematopoietic stem cell maintenance. Exp Hematol. 2017;48:58–71.e15. https://doi.org/10.1016/j.exphem.2016.11.008.
73. Banga SS, Peng L, Dasgupta T, Palejwala V, Ozer HL. PHF10 is required for cell proliferation in normal and SV40-immortalized human fibroblast cells. Cytogenet Genome Res. 2009;126(3):227–42. https://doi.org/10.1159/000251960.
74. Egan CM, Nyman U, Skotte J, Streubel G, Turner S, O'Connell DJ, Rraklli V, Dolan MJ, Chadderton N, Hansen K, Farrar GJ, Helin K, Holmberg J, Bracken AP. CHD5 is required for neurogenesis and has a dual role in facilitating gene expression and polycomb gene repression. Dev Cell. 2013;26(3):223–36. https://doi.org/10.1016/j.devcel.2013.07.008.
75. Kolla V, Naraparaju K, Zhuang T, Higashi M, Kolla S, Blobel GA, Brodeur GM. The tumour suppressor CHD5 forms a NuRD-type chromatin remodelling complex. Biochem J. 2015;468(2):345–52. https://doi.org/10.1042/BJ20150030.
76. Schramm A, Koster J, Assenov Y, Althoff K, Peifer M, Mahlow E, Odersky A, Beisser D, Ernst C, Henssen AG, Stephan H, Schroder C, Heukamp L, Engesser A, Kahlert Y, Theissen J, Hero B, Roels F, Altmuller J, Nurnberg P, Astrahantseff K, Gloeckner C, De Preter K, Plass C, Lee S, Lode HN, Henrich KO, Gartlgruber M, Speleman F, Schmezer P, Westermann F, Rahmann S, Fischer M, Eggert A, Schulte JH. Mutational dynamics between primary and relapse neuroblastomas. Nat Genet. 2015;47(8):872–7. https://doi.org/10.1038/ng.3349.
77. Koyama H, Zhuang T, Light JE, Kolla V, Higashi M, McGrady PW, London WB, Brodeur GM. Mechanisms of CHD5 inactivation in neuroblastomas. Clin Cancer Res. 2012;18(6):1588–97. https://doi.org/10.1158/1078-0432.CCR-11-2644.
78. Gibbons RJ, Pellagatti A, Garrick D, Wood WG, Malik N, Ayyub H, Langford C, Boultwood J, Wainscoat JS, Higgs DR. Identification of acquired somatic mutations in the gene encoding chromatin-remodeling factor ATRX in the alpha-thalassemia

myelodysplasia syndrome (ATMDS). Nat Genet. 2003;34(4):446–9. https://doi.org/10.1038/ng1213.
79. Voon HP, Wong LH. New players in heterochromatin silencing: histone variant H3.3 and the ATRX/DAXX chaperone. Nucleic Acids Res. 2016;44(4):1496–501. https://doi.org/10.1093/nar/gkw012.
80. Clynes D, Jelinska C, Xella B, Ayyub H, Scott C, Mitson M, Taylor S, Higgs DR, Gibbons RJ. Suppression of the alternative lengthening of telomere pathway by the chromatin remodelling factor ATRX. Nat Commun. 2015;6:7538. https://doi.org/10.1038/ncomms8538.
81. Peifer M, Hertwig F, Roels F, Dreidax D, Gartlgruber M, Menon R, Kramer A, Roncaioli JL, Sand F, Heuckmann JM, Ikram F, Schmidt R, Ackermann S, Engesser A, Kahlert Y, Vogel W, Altmuller J, Nurnberg P, Thierry-Mieg J, Thierry-Mieg D, Mariappan A, Heynck S, Mariotti E, Henrich KO, Gloeckner C, Bosco G, Leuschner I, Schweiger MR, Savelyeva L, Watkins SC, Shao C, Bell E, Hofer T, Achter V, Lang U, Theissen J, Volland R, Saadati M, Eggert A, de Wilde B, Berthold F, Peng Z, Zhao C, Shi L, Ortmann M, Buttner R, Perner S, Hero B, Schramm A, Schulte JH, Herrmann C, O'Sullivan RJ, Westermann F, Thomas RK, Fischer M. Telomerase activation by genomic rearrangements in high-risk neuroblastoma. Nature. 2015;526(7575):700–4. https://doi.org/10.1038/nature14980.
82. Le Magnen C, Shen MM, Abate-Shen C. Lineage plasticity in cancer progression and treatment. Annu Rev Cancer Biol. 2018;2:271–89. https://doi.org/10.1146/annurev-cancerbio-030617-050224.
83. Stallings RL, Foley NH, Bryan K, Buckley PG, Bray I. Therapeutic targeting of miRNAs in neuroblastoma. Expert Opin Ther Targets. 2010;14(9):951–62. https://doi.org/10.1517/14728222.2010.510136.
84. Althoff K, Beckers A, Odersky A, Mestdagh P, Koster J, Bray IM, Bryan K, Vandesompele J, Speleman F, Stallings RL, Schramm A, Eggert A, Sprussel A, Schulte JH. MiR-137 functions as a tumor suppressor in neuroblastoma by downregulating KDM1A. Int J Cancer. 2013;133(5):1064–73. https://doi.org/10.1002/ijc.28091.
85. Kopp F, Mendell JT. Functional classification and experimental dissection of long noncoding RNAs. Cell. 2018;172(3):393–407. https://doi.org/10.1016/j.cell.2018.01.011.
86. Bhan A, Soleimani M, Mandal SS. Long noncoding RNA and cancer: a new paradigm. Cancer Res. 2017;77(15):3965–81. https://doi.org/10.1158/0008-5472.CAN-16-2634.
87. Forrest ME, Khalil AM. Review: regulation of the cancer epigenome by long non-coding RNAs. Cancer Lett. 2017;407:106–12. https://doi.org/10.1016/j.canlet.2017.03.040.
88. Mercer TR, Mattick JS. Structure and function of long noncoding RNAs in epigenetic regulation. Nat Struct Mol Biol. 2013;20(3):300–7. https://doi.org/10.1038/nsmb.2480.
89. Zhao X, Li D, Huang D, Song H, Mei H, Fang E, Wang X, Yang F, Zheng L, Huang K, Tong Q. Risk-associated long noncoding RNA FOXD3-AS1 inhibits neuroblastoma progression by repressing PARP1-mediated activation of CTCF. Mol Ther. 2018;26(3):755–73. https://doi.org/10.1016/j.ymthe.2017.12.017.
90. Li D, Wang X, Mei H, Fang E, Ye L, Song H, Yang F, Li H, Huang K, Zheng L, Tong Q. Long noncoding RNA pancEts-1 promotes neuroblastoma progression through hnRNPK-mediated beta-catenin stabilization. Cancer Res. 2018;78(5):1169–83. https://doi.org/10.1158/0008-5472.CAN-17-2295.
91. Mazar J, Rosado A, Shelley J, Marchica J, Westmoreland TJ. The long non-coding RNA GAS5 differentially regulates cell cycle arrest and apoptosis through activation of BRCA1 and p53 in human neuroblastoma. Oncotarget. 2017;8(4):6589–607. https://doi.org/10.18632/oncotarget.14244.
92. Bevilacqua V, Gioia U, Di Carlo V, Tortorelli AF, Colombo T, Bozzoni I, Laneve P, Caffarelli E. Identification of linc-NeD125, a novel long non coding RNA that hosts miR-125b-1 and negatively controls proliferation of human neuroblastoma cells. RNA Biol. 2015;12(12):1323–37. https://doi.org/10.1080/15476286.2015.1096488.
93. Barnhill LM, Williams RT, Cohen O, Kim Y, Batova A, Mielke JA, Messer K, Pu M, Bao L, Yu AL, Diccianni MB. High expression of CAI2, a 9p21-embedded long noncoding RNA, contributes to advanced-stage neuroblastoma. Cancer Res. 2014;74(14):3753–63. https://doi.org/10.1158/0008-5472.CAN-13-3447.
94. Liu PY, Atmadibrata B, Mondal S, Tee AE, Liu T. NCYM is upregulated by lncUSMycN and modulates N-Myc expression. Int J Oncol. 2016;49(6):2464–70. https://doi.org/10.3892/ijo.2016.3730.
95. Zhao X, Li D, Pu J, Mei H, Yang D, Xiang X, Qu H, Huang K, Zheng L, Tong Q. CTCF cooperates with noncoding RNA MYCNOS to promote neuroblastoma progression through facilitating MYCN expression. Oncogene. 2016;35(27):3565–76. https://doi.org/10.1038/onc.2015.422.
96. Mondal T, Juvvuna PK, Kirkeby A, Mitra S, Kosalai ST, Traxler L, Hertwig F, Wernig-Zorc S, Miranda C, Deland L, Volland R, Bartenhagen C, Bartsch D, Bandaru S, Engesser A, Subhash S, Martinsson T, Caren H, Akyurek LM, Kurian L, Kanduri M, Huarte M, Kogner P, Fischer M, Kanduri C. Sense-antisense lncRNA pair encoded by locus 6p22.3 determines neuroblastoma susceptibility via the USP36-CHD7-SOX9 Regulatory Axis. Cancer Cell. 2018;33(3):417–34. e417. https://doi.org/10.1016/j.ccell.2018.01.020.
97. Nie Z, Hu G, Wei G, Cui K, Yamane A, Resch W, Wang R, Green DR, Tessarollo L, Casellas R, Zhao K, Levens D. c-Myc is a universal amplifier of expressed genes in lymphocytes and embryonic

stem cells. Cell. 2012;151(1):68–79. https://doi.org/10.1016/j.cell.2012.08.033.
98. Lin CY, Loven J, Rahl PB, Paranal RM, Burge CB, Bradner JE, Lee TI, Young RA. Transcriptional amplification in tumor cells with elevated c-Myc. Cell. 2012;151(1):56–67. https://doi.org/10.1016/j.cell.2012.08.026.
99. Sun Y, Bell JL, Carter D, Gherardi S, Poulos RC, Milazzo G, Wong JW, Al-Awar R, Tee AE, Liu PY, Liu B, Atmadibrata B, Wong M, Trahair T, Zhao Q, Shohet JM, Haupt Y, Schulte JH, Brown PJ, Arrowsmith CH, Vedadi M, MacKenzie KL, Huttelmaier S, Perini G, Marshall GM, Braithwaite A, Liu T. WDR5 supports an N-Myc transcriptional complex that drives a protumorigenic gene expression signature in neuroblastoma. Cancer Res. 2015;75(23):5143–54. https://doi.org/10.1158/0008-5472.CAN-15-0423.
100. Buchel G, Carstensen A, Mak KY, Roeschert I, Leen E, Sumara O, Hofstetter J, Herold S, Kalb J, Baluapuri A, Poon E, Kwok C, Chesler L, Maric HM, Rickman DS, Wolf E, Bayliss R, Walz S, Eilers M. Association with Aurora-a controls N-MYC-dependent promoter escape and pause release of RNA polymerase II during the cell cycle. Cell Rep. 2017;21(12):3483–97. https://doi.org/10.1016/j.celrep.2017.11.090.
101. Gajer JM, Furdas SD, Grunder A, Gothwal M, Heinicke U, Keller K, Colland F, Fulda S, Pahl HL, Fichtner I, Sippl W, Jung M. Histone acetyltransferase inhibitors block neuroblastoma cell growth in vivo. Oncogenesis. 2015;4:e137. https://doi.org/10.1038/oncsis.2014.51.
102. Amente S, Milazzo G, Sorrentino MC, Ambrosio S, Di Palo G, Lania L, Perini G, Majello B. Lysine-specific demethylase (LSD1/KDM1A) and MYCN cooperatively repress tumor suppressor genes in neuroblastoma. Oncotarget. 2015;6(16):14572–83. https://doi.org/10.18632/oncotarget.3990.
103. Poole CJ, van Riggelen J. MYC-master regulator of the cancer epigenome and transcriptome. Genes. 2017;8:5. https://doi.org/10.3390/genes8050142.
104. Claeys S, Denecker G, Durinck K, Decaesteker B, Mus LM, Loontiens S, Vanhauwaert S, Althoff K, Wigerup C, Bexell D, Dolman E, Henrich KO, Wehrmann L, Westerhout EM, Demoulin JB, Kumps C, Van Maerken T, Laureys G, Van Neste C, De Wilde B, De Wever O, Westermann F, Versteeg R, Molenaar JJ, Pahlman S, Schulte JH, De Preter K, Speleman F. ALK positively regulates MYCN activity through repression of HBP1 expression. Oncogene. 2019;38(15):2690–705. https://doi.org/10.1038/s41388-018-0595-3.
105. Wong M, Tee AEL, Milazzo G, Bell JL, Poulos RC, Atmadibrata B, Sun Y, Jing D, Ho N, Ling D, Liu PY, Zhang XD, Huttelmaier S, Wong JWH, Wang J, Polly P, Perini G, Scarlett CJ, Liu T. The histone methyltransferase DOT1L promotes neuroblastoma by regulating gene transcription. Cancer Res. 2017;77(9):2522–33. https://doi.org/10.1158/0008-5472.CAN-16-1663.
106. Liu Z, Chen SS, Clarke S, Veschi V, Thiele CJ. Targeting MYCN in Pediatric and adult cancers. Front Oncol. 2020;10:623679. https://doi.org/10.3389/fonc.2020.623679.
107. Coffey DC, Kutko MC, Glick RD, Swendeman SL, Butler L, Rifkind R, Marks PA, Richon VM, LaQuaglia MP. Histone deacetylase inhibitors and retinoic acids inhibit growth of human neuroblastoma in vitro. Med Pediatr Oncol. 2000;35(6):577–81. https://doi.org/10.1002/1096--911x(20001201)35:6<577::aid-mpo18>3.0.co;2-3.
108. DuBois SG, Groshen S, Park JR, Haas-Kogan DA, Yang X, Geier E, Chen E, Giacomini K, Weiss B, Cohn SL, Granger MM, Yanik GA, Hawkins R, Courtier J, Jackson H, Goodarzian F, Shimada H, Czarnecki S, Tsao-Wei D, Villablanca JG, Marachelian A, Matthay KK. Phase I study of Vorinostat as a radiation sensitizer with 131I-Metaiodobenzylguanidine (131I-MIBG) for patients with relapsed or refractory neuroblastoma. Clin Cancer Res. 2015;21(12):2715–21. https://doi.org/10.1158/1078-0432.CCR-14-3240.
109. George RE, Lahti JM, Adamson PC, Zhu K, Finkelstein D, Ingle AM, Reid JM, Krailo M, Neuberg D, Blaney SM, Diller L. Phase I study of decitabine with doxorubicin and cyclophosphamide in children with neuroblastoma and other solid tumors: a Children's Oncology Group study. Pediatr Blood Cancer. 2010;55(4):629–38. https://doi.org/10.1002/pbc.22607.
110. Pinto N, DuBois SG, Marachelian A, Diede SJ, Taraseviciute A, Glade Bender JL, Tsao-Wei D, Groshen SG, Reid JM, Haas-Kogan DA, Reynolds CP, Kang MH, Irwin MS, Macy ME, Villablanca JG, Matthay KK, Park JR. Phase I study of vorinostat in combination with isotretinoin in patients with refractory/recurrent neuroblastoma: a new approaches to Neuroblastoma Therapy (NANT) trial. Pediatr Blood Cancer. 2018;65(7):e27023. https://doi.org/10.1002/pbc.27023.
111. McCabe MT, Ott HM, Ganji G, Korenchuk S, Thompson C, Van Aller GS, Liu Y, Graves AP, Della Pietra A 3rd, Diaz E, LaFrance LV, Mellinger M, Duquenne C, Tian X, Kruger RG, McHugh CF, Brandt M, Miller WH, Dhanak D, Verma SK, Tummino PJ, Creasy CL. EZH2 inhibition as a therapeutic strategy for lymphoma with EZH2-activating mutations. Nature. 2012;492(7427):108–12. https://doi.org/10.1038/nature11606.
112. Mayr C, Wagner A, Stoecklinger A, Jakab M, Illig R, Berr F, Pichler M, Di Fazio P, Ocker M, Neureiter D, Kiesslich T. 3-deazaneplanocin a may directly target putative cancer stem cells in biliary tract cancer. Anticancer Res. 2015;35(9):4697–705.
113. Tan J, Yang X, Zhuang L, Jiang X, Chen W, Lee PL, Karuturi RK, Tan PB, Liu ET, Yu Q. Pharmacologic disruption of Polycomb-repressive complex 2-mediated gene repression selectively induces apop-

tosis in cancer cells. Genes Dev. 2007;21(9):1050–63. https://doi.org/10.1101/gad.1524107.
114. Knutson SK, Wigle TJ, Warholic NM, Sneeringer CJ, Allain CJ, Klaus CR, Sacks JD, Raimondi A, Majer CR, Song J, Scott MP, Jin L, Smith JJ, Olhava EJ, Chesworth R, Moyer MP, Richon VM, Copeland RA, Keilhack H, Pollock RM, Kuntz KW. A selective inhibitor of EZH2 blocks H3K27 methylation and kills mutant lymphoma cells. Nat Chem Biol. 2012;8(11):890–6. https://doi.org/10.1038/nchembio.1084.
115. Knutson SK, Kawano S, Minoshima Y, Warholic NM, Huang KC, Xiao Y, Kadowaki T, Uesugi M, Kuznetsov G, Kumar N, Wigle TJ, Klaus CR, Allain CJ, Raimondi A, Waters NJ, Smith JJ, Porter-Scott M, Chesworth R, Moyer MP, Copeland RA, Richon VM, Uenaka T, Pollock RM, Kuntz KW, Yokoi A, Keilhack H. Selective inhibition of EZH2 by EPZ 6438 leads to potent antitumor activity in EZH2-mutant non-Hodgkin lymphoma. Mol Cancer Ther. 2014;13(4):842–54. https://doi.org/10.1158/1535-7163.MCT-13-0773.
116. Kurmasheva RT, Sammons M, Favours E, Wu J, Kurmashev D, Cosmopoulos K, Keilhack H, Klaus CR, Houghton PJ, Smith MA. Initial testing (stage 1) of tazemetostat (EPZ-6438), a novel EZH2 inhibitor, by the pediatric preclinical testing program. Pediatr Blood Cancer. 2017;64:3. https://doi.org/10.1002/pbc.26218.
117. Kaniskan HU, Jin J. Chemical probes of histone lysine methyltransferases. ACS Chem Biol. 2015;10(1):40–50. https://doi.org/10.1021/cb500785t.
118. Kim KH, Roberts CW. Targeting EZH2 in cancer. Nat Med. 2016;22(2):128–34. https://doi.org/10.1038/nm.4036.
119. Williams DE, Dalisay DS, Li F, Amphlett J, Maneerat W, Chavez MA, Wang YA, Matainaho T, Yu W, Brown PJ, Arrowsmith CH, Vedadi M, Andersen RJ. Nahuoic acid A produced by a Streptomyces sp. isolated from a marine sediment is a selective SAM-competitive inhibitor of the histone methyltransferase SETD8. Org Lett. 2013;15(2):414–7. https://doi.org/10.1021/ol303416k.
120. Williams DE, Izard F, Arnould S, Dalisay DS, Tantapakul C, Maneerat W, Matainaho T, Julien E, Andersen RJ. Structures of nahuoic acids B-E produced in culture by a streptomyces sp. isolated from a marine sediment and evidence for the inhibition of the histone methyl transferase SETD8 in human cancer cells by nahuoic acid A. J Org Chem. 2016;81(4):1324–32. https://doi.org/10.1021/acs.joc.5b02569.
121. Ma A, Yu W, Li F, Bleich RM, Herold JM, Butler KV, Norris JL, Korboukh V, Tripathy A, Janzen WP, Arrowsmith CH, Frye SV, Vedadi M, Brown PJ, Jin J. Discovery of a selective, substrate-competitive inhibitor of the lysine methyltransferase SETD8. J Med Chem. 2014;57(15):6822–33. https://doi.org/10.1021/jm500871s.
122. Judge RA, Zhu H, Upadhyay AK, Bodelle PM, Hutchins CW, Torrent M, Marin VL, Yu W, Vedadi M, Li F, Brown PJ, Pappano WN, Sun C, Petros AM. Turning a substrate peptide into a potent inhibitor for the histone methyltransferase SETD8. ACS Med Chem Lett. 2016;7(12):1102–6. https://doi.org/10.1021/acsmedchemlett.6b00303.
123. Nguyen AT, Zhang Y. The diverse functions of Dot1 and H3K79 methylation. Genes Dev. 2011;25(13):1345–58. https://doi.org/10.1101/gad.2057811.
124. Nguyen AT, Taranova O, He J, Zhang Y. DOT1L, the H3K79 methyltransferase, is required for MLL-AF9-mediated leukemogenesis. Blood. 2011;117(25):6912–22. https://doi.org/10.1182/blood-2011-02-334359.
125. Yu W, Chory EJ, Wernimont AK, Tempel W, Scopton A, Federation A, Marineau JJ, Qi J, Barsyte-Lovejoy D, Yi J, Marcellus R, Iacob RE, Engen JR, Griffin C, Aman A, Wienholds E, Li F, Pineda J, Estiu G, Shatseva T, Hajian T, Al-Awar R, Dick JE, Vedadi M, Brown PJ, Arrowsmith CH, Bradner JE, Schapira M. Catalytic site remodelling of the DOT1L methyltransferase by selective inhibitors. Nat Commun. 2012;3:1288. https://doi.org/10.1038/ncomms2304.
126. Stein EM, Garcia-Manero G, Rizzieri DA, Tibes R, Berdeja JG, Savona MR, Jongen-Lavrenic M, Altman JK, Thomson B, Blakemore SJ, Daigle SR, Waters NJ, Suttle AB, Clawson A, Pollock R, Krivtsov A, Armstrong SA, DiMartino J, Hedrick E, Lowenberg B, Tallman MS. The DOT1L inhibitor pinometostat reduces H3K79 methylation and has modest clinical activity in adult acute leukemia. Blood. 2018;131(24):2661–9. https://doi.org/10.1182/blood-2017-12-818948.
127. Amente S, Lania L, Majello B. The histone LSD1 demethylase in stemness and cancer transcription programs. Biochim Biophys Acta. 2013;1829(10):981–6. https://doi.org/10.1016/j.bbagrm.2013.05.002.
128. Mohammad HP, Smitheman KN, Kamat CD, Soong D, Federowicz KE, Van Aller GS, Schneck JL, Carson JD, Liu Y, Butticello M, Bonnette WG, Gorman SA, Degenhardt Y, Bai Y, McCabe MT, Pappalardi MB, Kasparec J, Tian X, McNulty KC, Rouse M, McDevitt P, Ho T, Crouthamel M, Hart TK, Concha NO, McHugh CF, Miller WH, Dhanak D, Tummino PJ, Carpenter CL, Johnson NW, Hann CL, Kruger RG. A DNA hypomethylation signature predicts antitumor activity of LSD1 inhibitors in SCLC. Cancer Cell. 2015;28(1):57–69. https://doi.org/10.1016/j.ccell.2015.06.002.
129. Lochmann TL, Powell KM, Ham J, Floros KV, Heisey DAR, Kurupi RIJ, Calbert ML, Ghotra MS, Greninger P, Dozmorov M, Gowda M, Souers AJ, Reynolds CP, Benes CH, Faber AC. Targeted inhibition of histone H3K27 demethylation is effective in high-risk neuroblastoma. Sci Transl Med. 2018;10:441. https://doi.org/10.1126/scitranslmed.aao4680.

130. West AC, Johnstone RW. New and emerging HDAC inhibitors for cancer treatment. J Clin Invest. 2014;124(1):30–9. https://doi.org/10.1172/JCI69738.
131. Richon VM, Emiliani S, Verdin E, Webb Y, Breslow R, Rifkind RA, Marks PA. A class of hybrid polar inducers of transformed cell differentiation inhibits histone deacetylases. Proc Natl Acad Sci U S A. 1998;95(6):3003–7. https://doi.org/10.1073/pnas.95.6.3003.
132. Glick RD, Swendeman SL, Coffey DC, Rifkind RA, Marks PA, Richon VM, La Quaglia MP. Hybrid polar histone deacetylase inhibitor induces apoptosis and CD95/CD95 ligand expression in human neuroblastoma. Cancer Res. 1999;59(17):4392–9.
133. Panicker J, Li Z, McMahon C, Sizer C, Steadman K, Piekarz R, Bates SE, Thiele CJ. Romidepsin (FK228/depsipeptide) controls growth and induces apoptosis in neuroblastoma tumor cells. Cell Cycle (Georgetown, Tex). 2010;9(9):1830–8. https://doi.org/10.4161/cc.9.9.11543.
134. Children's Oncology G, Fouladi M, Furman WL, Chin T, Freeman BB 3rd, Dudkin L, Stewart CF, Krailo MD, Speights R, Ingle AM, Houghton PJ, Wright J, Adamson PC, Blaney SM. Phase I study of depsipeptide in pediatric patients with refractory solid tumors: a Children's Oncology Group report. J Clin Oncol. 2006;24(22):3678–85. https://doi.org/10.1200/JCO.2006.06.4964.
135. Hahn CK, Ross KN, Warrington IM, Mazitschek R, Kanegai CM, Wright RD, Kung AL, Golub TR, Stegmaier K. Expression-based screening identifies the combination of histone deacetylase inhibitors and retinoids for neuroblastoma differentiation. Proc Natl Acad Sci U S A. 2008;105(28):9751–6. https://doi.org/10.1073/pnas.0710413105.
136. DuBois SG, Chesler L, Groshen S, Hawkins R, Goodarzian F, Shimada H, Yanik G, Tagen M, Stewart C, Mosse YP, Maris JM, Tsao-Wei D, Marachelian A, Villablanca JG, Matthay KK. Phase I study of vincristine, irinotecan, and (1)(3)(1)I-metaiodobenzylguanidine for patients with relapsed or refractory neuroblastoma: a new approaches to neuroblastoma therapy trial. Clin Cancer Res. 2012;18(9):2679–86. https://doi.org/10.1158/1078-0432.CCR-11-3201.
137. Kroesen M, Bull C, Gielen PR, Brok IC, Armandari I, Wassink M, Looman MW, Boon L, den Brok MH, Hoogerbrugge PM, Adema GJ. Anti-GD2 mAb and Vorinostat synergize in the treatment of neuroblastoma. Onco Targets Ther. 2016;5(6):e1164919. https://doi.org/10.1080/2162402X.2016.1164919.
138. Jubierre L, Jimenez C, Rovira E, Soriano A, Sabado C, Gros L, Llort A, Hladun R, Roma J, Toledo JS, Gallego S, Segura MF. Targeting of epigenetic regulators in neuroblastoma. Exp Mol Med. 2018;50(4):1–12. https://doi.org/10.1038/s12276-018-0077-2.
139. Waldeck K, Cullinane C, Ardley K, Shortt J, Martin B, Tothill RW, Li J, Johnstone RW, McArthur GA, Hicks RJ, Wood PJ. Long term, continuous exposure to panobinostat induces terminal differentiation and long term survival in the TH-MYCN neuroblastoma mouse model. Int J Cancer. 2016;139(1):194–204. https://doi.org/10.1002/ijc.30056.
140. Wang G, Edwards H, Caldwell JT, Buck SA, Qing WY, Taub JW, Ge Y, Wang Z. Panobinostat synergistically enhances the cytotoxic effects of cisplatin, doxorubicin or etoposide on high-risk neuroblastoma cells. PLoS One. 2013;8(9):e76662. https://doi.org/10.1371/journal.pone.0076662.
141. Balasubramanian S, Ramos J, Luo W, Sirisawad M, Verner E, Buggy JJ. A novel histone deacetylase 8 (HDAC8)-specific inhibitor PCI-34051 induces apoptosis in T-cell lymphomas. Leukemia. 2008;22(5):1026–34. https://doi.org/10.1038/leu.2008.9.
142. Shen J, Najafi S, Stable S, Fabian J, Koeneke E, Kolbinger FR, Wrobel JK, Meder B, Distel M, Heimburg T, Sippl W, Jung M, Peterziel H, Kranz D, Boutros M, Westermann F, Witt O, Oehme I. A kinome-wide RNAi screen identifies ALK as a target to sensitize neuroblastoma cells for HDAC8-inhibitor treatment. Cell Death Differ. 2018;25(12):2053–70. https://doi.org/10.1038/s41418-018-0080-0.
143. Oehme I, Deubzer HE, Lodrini M, Milde T, Witt O. Targeting of HDAC8 and investigational inhibitors in neuroblastoma. Expert Opin Investig Drugs. 2009;18(11):1605–17. https://doi.org/10.1517/14728220903241658.
144. Rettig I, Koeneke E, Trippel F, Mueller WC, Burhenne J, Kopp-Schneider A, Fabian J, Schober A, Fernekorn U, von Deimling A, Deubzer HE, Milde T, Witt O, Oehme I. Selective inhibition of HDAC8 decreases neuroblastoma growth in vitro and in vivo and enhances retinoic acid-mediated differentiation. Cell Death Dis. 2015;6:e1657. https://doi.org/10.1038/cddis.2015.24.
145. Filippakopoulos P, Knapp S. Targeting bromodomains: epigenetic readers of lysine acetylation. Nat Rev Drug Discov. 2014;13(5):337–56. https://doi.org/10.1038/nrd4286.
146. Filippakopoulos P, Qi J, Picaud S, Shen Y, Smith WB, Fedorov O, Morse EM, Keates T, Hickman TT, Felletar I, Philpott M, Munro S, McKeown MR, Wang Y, Christie AL, West N, Cameron MJ, Schwartz B, Heightman TD, La Thangue N, French CA, Wiest O, Kung AL, Knapp S, Bradner JE. Selective inhibition of BET bromodomains. Nature. 2010;468(7327):1067–73. https://doi.org/10.1038/nature09504.
147. French CA. NUT midline carcinoma. Cancer Genet Cytogenet. 2010;203(1):16–20. https://doi.org/10.1016/j.cancergencyto.2010.06.007.
148. Dohner H, Weisdorf DJ, Bloomfield CD. Acute Myeloid Leukemia. N Engl J Med. 2015;373(12):1136–52. https://doi.org/10.1056/NEJMra1406184.
149. Lee YS, Lee JW, Jang JW, Chi XZ, Kim JH, Li YH, Kim MK, Kim DM, Choi BS, Kim EG, Chung JH, Lee OJ, Lee YM, Suh JW, Chuang LS, Ito Y, Bae SC. Runx3 inactivation is a crucial early event in

the development of lung adenocarcinoma. Cancer Cell. 2013;24(5):603–16. https://doi.org/10.1016/j.ccr.2013.10.003.

150. Puissant A, Frumm SM, Alexe G, Bassil CF, Qi J, Chanthery YH, Nekritz EA, Zeid R, Gustafson WC, Greninger P, Garnett MJ, McDermott U, Benes CH, Kung AL, Weiss WA, Bradner JE, Stegmaier K. Targeting MYCN in neuroblastoma by BET bromodomain inhibition. Cancer Discov. 2013;3(3):308–23. https://doi.org/10.1158/2159-8290.CD-12-0418.

151. Wyce A, Ganji G, Smitheman KN, Chung CW, Korenchuk S, Bai Y, Barbash O, Le B, Craggs PD, McCabe MT, Kennedy-Wilson KM, Sanchez LV, Gosmini RL, Parr N, McHugh CF, Dhanak D, Prinjha RK, Auger KR, Tummino PJ. BET inhibition silences expression of MYCN and BCL2 and induces cytotoxicity in neuroblastoma tumor models. PLoS One. 2013;8(8):e72967. https://doi.org/10.1371/journal.pone.0072967.

152. Derissen EJ, Beijnen JH, Schellens JH. Concise drug review: azacitidine and decitabine. Oncologist. 2013;18(5):619–24. https://doi.org/10.1634/theoncologist.2012-0465.

153. Yang Q, Liu S, Tian Y, Hasan C, Kersey D, Salwen HR, Chlenski A, Perlman EJ, Cohn SL. Methylation-associated silencing of the heat shock protein 47 gene in human neuroblastoma. Cancer Res. 2004;64(13):4531–8. https://doi.org/10.1158/0008-5472.CAN-04-0956.

154. Yang QW, Liu S, Tian Y, Salwen HR, Chlenski A, Weinstein J, Cohn SL. Methylation-associated silencing of the thrombospondin-1 gene in human neuroblastoma. Cancer Res. 2003;63(19):6299–310.

155. Li H, Xu W, Huang Y, Huang X, Xu L, Lv Z. Genistein demethylates the promoter of CHD5 and inhibits neuroblastoma growth in vivo. Int J Mol Med. 2012;30(5):1081–6. https://doi.org/10.3892/ijmm.2012.1118.

6 The Genetic Basis of the Divergent Clinical Courses in Neuroblastoma

Carolina Rosswog and Matthias Fischer

6.1 Introduction

The molecular basis underlying the highly divergent clinical courses of neuroblastoma has been a major focus of neuroblastoma research since many decades. It has been proposed that a better understanding of the mechanisms of spontaneous regression, differentiation, metastasis, and disease progression would identify factors that are crucial for driving malignant transformation of neuroblastoma and other tumors. In addition, detailed knowledge on the alterations specific for the distinct neuroblastoma subtypes might improve risk assessment and treatment stratification of patients and may provide starting points for the development of targeted therapies in high-risk neuroblastoma. Indeed, various chromosomal aberrations have been discovered already in the late-seventies and early eighties of the last century, including deletions of the short arm of chromosome 1, copy number gains of the long arm of chromosome 17, and amplification of a genomic region of chromosome 2 covering the *MYCN* gene locus [1–3]. It became soon clear that 1p deletion and *MYCN* amplification do not randomly occur in neuroblastoma but are associated with advanced disease stages and poor patient outcome [4–7]. Additional chromosomal alterations with prognostic impact, such as loss of 11q, were identified a few years later [8, 9]. In-depth characterization of the landscape of genomic copy number alterations was further advanced by the advent of microarray-based comparative genomic hybridization, which revealed that the presence of segmental copy number alterations was associated with high risk of relapse and poor outcome [10, 11]. The relevant genes within affected genomic regions and the mechanistic consequences of these alterations, however, have remained largely uncertain, except for proto-oncogenes with high-level amplification, such as *MYCN*. Apart from copy number alterations, gene expression profiling studies uncovered substantially differing transcriptional patterns of high- and low-risk tumors [12–18]. While gene expression analyses were able to accurately predict patient outcome, only modest knowledge was inferred on the mechanistic principles that discriminate the distinct biological phenotypes of neuroblastoma. Nevertheless, these findings strongly indicated that unfavorable neuroblastomas differ from those with favorable clinical courses in their genomic and transcriptional profiles, suggesting that distinct molecular programs are active in the various disease subtypes. High hopes were therefore raised by the development of massively par-

C. Rosswog · M. Fischer (✉)
Department of Experimental Pediatric Oncology, University Children's Hospital of Cologne, Cologne, Germany

Faculty of Medicine, University of Cologne, Cologne, Germany
e-mail: matthias.fischer@uk-koeln.de

S. Asgharzadeh, F. Westermann (eds.), *Neuroblastoma*, Pediatric Oncology,
https://doi.org/10.1007/978-3-031-51292-6_6

allel sequencing technologies. Early sequencing studies mostly focused on the detection of single nucleotide variants, however, only few recurrent somatic mutations were discovered [19, 20]. By contrast, more recent studies examined alterations across the entire genome, which revealed that—in addition to copy number alterations—structural variations of genomic regions significantly contribute to malignant transformation in this disease [21–24].

In the following chapter, we review the current knowledge on recurrent genomic alterations that are key to neuroblastoma pathogenesis and their supposed mechanistic consequences in determining the biological and clinical phenotype of neuroblastoma.

6.2 *MYCN* Amplification

MYCN was the first oncogene that had been associated with aggressive disease and poor outcome in neuroblastoma [4, 5] and is a well-established molecular marker of high-risk disease today. The proto-oncogene *MYCN* encodes the protein N-myc that belongs to a family of transcription factors which regulate the expression of genes involved in cell proliferation, differentiation, and metabolism as well as apoptosis and senescence [25]. While the family member c-Myc is a main regulator in early pluripotent embryonic stem cells and is ubiquitously expressed, N-myc is highly expressed in multipotent cells of the migratory neural crest and is essential for neuronal development and differentiation [26]. Myc proteins have central functions during malignant transformation, tumor initiation, and tumor maintenance [27]. The ability of cancer cells bearing oncogenic c-Myc to proliferate infinitely may be due to its role in activating telomerase [28], and also N-Myc is known to induce *TERT*, the gene encoding the catalytic subunit of telomerase, via direct binding to its promoter region [29]. Similar to c-Myc, the functions of N-Myc are diverse and depend on cooperating factors, like BCL2 or p53. Expression of a *MYCN* transgene under the tyrosine hydroxylase promoter led to development of neuroblastoma in genetically engineered mice, thus validating its crucial role in malignant transformation [30].

N-Myc is primarily activated via genomic amplification in neuroblastoma and is associated with chemoresistance and poor patient outcome [31, 32]. Amplification of *MYCN* is defined as greater than four-fold increase of *MYCN* signals in comparison to the centromere reference signal [33], and usually appears as narrow but high-level increase in chromosome 2p24 copy numbers. Amplification of *MYCN* in neuroblastoma may occur as extra-chromosomal circular DNA, so-called double minutes, or as intra-chromosomal homogeneously staining regions [34]. Both extra- and intra-chromosomal *MYCN* amplicons frequently appear as highly complex genomic structures accompanied by dozens to hundreds of genomic rearrangements. These highly complex amplifications have been termed seismic amplification and develop through chromothripsis followed by circular recombination of extra-chromosomal DNA circles, which may re-integrate into a chromosome later [35]. It has been suggested that the process of seismic amplification is massively increasing copy number levels and thus may drive gene expression of proto-oncogenes, such as *MYCN*, thereby boosting the malignant potential of cancer [35]. In neuroblastoma, *MYCN* amplification affects roughly 20% of all neuroblastoma cases and accounts for 40–50% of high-risk tumors [36]. In addition to clinical variables, such as stage of disease or age at diagnosis, assessment of the copy number status of *MYCN* is part of clinical routine for risk stratification and treatment allocation. While the biological and clinical significance of *MYCN* amplification is well established since many years, it has remained less clear until recently which events drive tumor development and progression in the remaining 50–60% of high-risk neuroblastomas lacking *MYCN* amplification.

6.3 *TERT* Rearrangements

The gene *telomerase reverse transcriptase (TERT)* is located on chromosome 5p and encodes for the catalytic protein subunit of human telomerase reverse transcriptase (hTERT), an enzyme with reverse transcriptase activity. Together with the human telomerase RNA component, encoded by *TERC* on chromosome 3q, hTERT contributes to the telomerase enzymatic complex [27] that is capable of extending telomeric repeat sequences [37]. Recurrent genomic rearrangements of the *TERT* locus have been discovered as an independent prognostic marker of aggressive phenotypes and poor outcome in neuroblastoma [23, 24]. The genomic rearrangements mostly cluster within 50 kb upstream of *TERT* without affecting the gene itself and show diverse rearrangement partners originating from regions across the entire genome. It has been demonstrated that such rearrangements lead to juxtaposition of super-enhancers in close proximity to the *TERT* locus, which in turn transcriptionally activate *TERT*, which is silenced in most somatic cells. Thus, *TERT* rearrangements are accompanied by upregulation of *TERT* expression, leading to a massive increase of telomerase activity [23]. Rearrangements of the *TERT* locus occur in roughly 10% of all neuroblastomas and in 20% of the high-risk cases [38]. *MYCN* amplification and *TERT* rearrangements occur mostly in a mutually exclusive fashion, and, thus, each account for substantial fractions of high-risk tumors.

6.4 Genomic Alterations of *ATRX*

About 8% of all neuroblastomas harbor loss of function mutations of the gene *ATRX* (*alpha-thalassemia/mental retardation syndrome X-linked*) [39]. The protein encoded by *ATRX* has been attributed to multiple biological processes, including regulation of chromatin compaction and maintenance of telomeric and subtelomeric chromatin [40, 41]. *ATRX* is located on the long arm of chromosome X and consists of 36 exons with a length of >300 kb [42]. Hypomorphic germline mutations of *ATRX* are associated with X-linked mental retardation and alpha-thalassemia. In cancer, somatic mutations of *ATRX* include single nucleotide variants in the coding region as well as deletions and insertion-induced frameshifts, all of which lead to loss of function [42]. Inactivating genomic alterations of *ATRX* have been associated with alternative lengthening of telomeres (ALT) in various cancer types [43, 44], and intact ATRX acts as suppressor of ALT [45, 46]. In neuroblastoma, *ATRX* alterations are predominantly found in high-risk cases, however, such mutations do not affect tumors bearing *MYCN* amplification or *TERT* rearrangements [22, 38, 47]. Mutations of *ATRX* occur at roughly 8% in neuroblastoma [38] and are found at increasing frequencies in adolescent and adult patients [48]. As the incidence of neuroblastoma among children with X-linked mental retardation is not increased, it is unlikely that *ATRX* mutations alone are sufficient to drive neuroblastoma development [49]. In addition to loss of function mutations, epigenetic changes mediated by ATRX are discussed to play a role in neuroblast differentiation, however, the exact impact of ATRX on epigenetic regulation still has to be determined [50].

6.5 Telomere Maintenance in Neuroblastoma

Telomeres are repetitive nucleotide sequences located at the ends of each chromosome. Telomeres consist of repetitive hexamer sequences arranged in tandem repeats, which constitute 5–15 kb of double stranded DNA, followed by a single-stranded G-rich overhang [51]. In addition to the DNA component, telomere-binding proteins, termed the shelterin complex, are located at the chromosomal ends [52]. Telomeres protect the termini of the linear chromosomal DNA strands from being recognized as damaged DNA and are thus essential for genome stability and control of cell proliferation [53]. The telomeres physiologically shorten with each cell division, due to the end replication problem, until they reach a critical length, which then induces permanent proliferation arrest by senescence or – if telomeres continue to shorten—programmed cell death [54]. In contrast to most somatic cells, cancer cells gain unlimited proliferative capacity through activation of mechanisms that enable maintenance of the telomere length. Due to its essential role in acquiring limitless replicative potential of malignant cells, telomere maintenance has been considered a hallmark of cancer [55]. In neuroblastoma, telomere maintenance has recently been shown to form the molecular basis of the divergent biological and clinical courses of the disease [56].

6.5.1 Telomerase Dependent Telomere Maintenance

Telomere maintenance is mostly achieved by induction of telomerase, a reverse transcriptase that is specialized for synthesis of telomeric DNA [57], which can keep the length of telomeres above a critical threshold in replicating cells [58]. Consisting of a catalytic subunit together with an RNA component, telomerase is activated in the majority of malignancies across many cancer types [44, 59]. Induction of *TERT* expression in cancer cells can result from structural variations of the *TERT* locus (including amplification and rearrangements), mutations of the *TERT* promoter, or *TERT* promoter methylation [44]. Overall, telomerase is considered to be activated in more than 70 to 80% of all malignancies [44]. In neuroblastoma, telomerase is transcriptionally induced predominantly by elevated N-myc levels, caused by genomic *MYCN* amplification, or by translocation of strong enhancer elements in proximity to the *TERT* locus through genomic rearrangements (Fig. 6.1) [23, 24]. However, not all cases with high *TERT* expression harbor *TERT* rearrangements or *MYCN* amplification: In roughly 5% of the tumors, high levels of *TERT* expression have been found without evidence for causal genomic alterations [38]. Elevated expression of *TERT* and high telomerase activity is associated with unfavorable prognostic markers, high-risk disease, and poor patient outcome in neuroblastoma [23, 24, 38, 60].

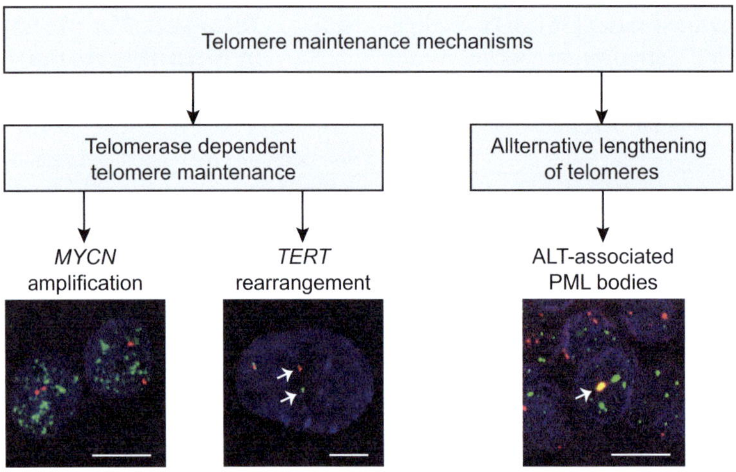

Fig. 6.1 Telomere maintenance mechanisms in neuroblastoma. Telomerase dependent telomere maintenance is mediated by induction of *TERT* expression through amplification of *MYCN* or rearrangements of the *TERT* locus, as illustrated by fluorescence in situ hybridization (FISH) in interphase nuclei. Left panel, amplification of *MYCN* (green signals, *MYCN* probe; red signals, control probe). Middle panel, rearrangement of the *TERT* locus (white arrows indicate split probes of the *TERT* locus by break-apart FISH). Alternative Lengthening of Telomeres can be determined by detection of ALT-associated PML nuclear bodies (APB) using a combination of telomere FISH with immunofluorescence staining of the protein PML. Right panel, FISH analysis of telomeres (green signals) and PML nuclear bodies (red signals). In ALT positive cells, telomeres show typically heterogeneous and bright signals and co-localize with PML nuclear bodies, giving rise to APBs (indicated by white arrow). Scale bars, 10 μm

6.5.2 Alternative Lengthening of Telomeres

Telomere maintenance in the absence of telomerase activity is defined as Alternative Lengthening of Telomeres (ALT), a mechanism leading to replication of telomeric DNA by homologous recombination [61, 62]. In neuroblastoma, ALT is activated in roughly 10–15% of all cases and in 10–25% of high-risk tumors [19, 38, 40, 47]. While event-free survival of patients whose tumors harbored ALT was found to be as poor as that of patients with telomerase-positive tumors, overall survival was significantly better, pointing towards a more indolent course of disease [38, 47]. In addition, ALT is associated with elevated patient age at diagnosis [38, 47, 48]. Activation of ALT can be detected by assessment of phenotypic characteristics that have been associated with this pathway, however, none of these features is unambiguously diagnostic for ALT [63, 64]. To determine ALT in cells or tissues, the C-circle assay, which detects single-stranded telomeric DNA circles, is widely used, or—alternatively—detection of ALT-associated promyelocytic nuclear bodies (APB) by a combination of telomere fluorescence in situ hybridization with immunofluorescence staining of the protein PML (Fig. 6.1). In addition, genomic alterations that are associated with ALT, such as *ATRX* mutations, are examined in order to assess the ALT status of tumor samples [64]. About 50–60% of ALT-positive neuroblastomas harbor alterations of *ATRX* [38, 47, 65]. The protein ATRX forms complexes with the death domain-associated protein DAXX, which colocalize with the replication-independent histone 3 variant H3.3 [66]. Molecular alterations of *DAXX* [43] and *H3F3A*, which encodes H3.3 [67], have also been associated with an ALT phenotype, however, mutations in these genes are extremely rare in neuroblastoma [47]. Although none of these alterations alone is sufficient to induce an ALT phenotype in vitro, genomic alterations of each of these genes have been associated with abnormal telomeres and other features indicating ALT in cancer cells [47, 66–68].

6.6 Mutations in Genes of the RAS/MAPK and the P53 Pathways

Pediatric cancers in general have a low overall mutational burden [22, 69]. In neuroblastoma, the overall exonic mutation frequency at diagnosis is about 0.6 per megabase in high-risk disease [19] and 0.4 per megabase across all risk groups [70]. In addition, only few genes have been found to be recurrently mutated [19]. Mechanistically, recurrent somatic mutations frequently affect genes of the RAS/MAPK and the p53 pathway. Genes related to these pathways harbored somatic mutations in 21% of high-risk and 13% non-high-risk patients in a large sequencing study [56].

The *anaplastic lymphoma kinase* (*ALK*) gene, encoding for a receptor tyrosine kinase, is one of the most frequently mutated genes in neuroblastoma [71–74]. While the vast majority of *ALK* alterations in neuroblastoma present as somatic mutations, single nucleotide variants can also occur in germline, and *ALK* is the most frequently mutated predisposition gene in familial neuroblastoma [75]. Somatic mutations in *ALK* are observed in 8 to 10% of primary neuroblastomas and mostly affect the tyrosine kinase domain, predominantly at three hotspot amino acid positions, i.e., F1174, R1275, and F1245 [71–74]. Oncogenic mutations of *ALK* lead to hyperphosphorylation of the receptor kinase and activation of multiple signaling pathways, including the RAS/MAPK and the PI3K/AKT pathways [76]. In mouse and zebrafish models, oncogenic ALK has been shown to efficiently induce neuroblastoma development in combination with N-myc overexpression [77–79]. By contrast, neuroblastoma did not or rarely develop in these models when activated ALK was expressed in the absence of a *MYCN* transgene. In relapsed disease, even higher mutation frequencies are observed, which may be due to a high de novo mutation rate during the course of disease [80]. Despite the increased mutation frequency at relapse, the impact of *ALK* mutations on patient outcome is not entirely clear: Some studies reported a significant association with unfavorable outcome in the high- and intermediate-risk groups [81], whereas others did not report on differences of survival between patients with and without *ALK* mutated tumors [72, 82]. In addition to oncogenic single nucleotide variants, genomic amplification of the *ALK* locus is observed in 2–5% of neuroblastoma [71, 72, 74, 81]. *ALK* amplification occurs exclusively in high-risk tumors bearing amplification of *MYCN*, with few exceptions [71, 72]. *ALK* is located on chromosome 2p23 in proximity to *MYCN* and is frequently co-amplified within the same amplicon. Unlike *ALK* single nucleotide variants, amplification of *ALK* is associated with dismal outcome [81]. Therapeutic targeting of oncogenic ALK by small molecule inhibitors has demonstrated anti-tumor activity in a fraction of relapsed or progressive neuroblastoma patients [83–85], and implementation of ALK inhibitors in first-line treatment is currently in preparation.

The identification of oncogenic N-Ras, a member of the RAS gene family, in the neuroblastoma cell line SK-N-SH in the early 1980s [86] suggested that RAS signaling may be involved in neuroblastoma pathogenesis. The RAS/MAPK pathway plays a central role in tumorigenesis and malignant transformation [87–89]. RAS proteins are small GTPases that transmit signals within cells. The downstream components ERK1 and ERK2 belong to the family of mitogen-activated kinases (MAPKs) that regulate the transcription of hundreds of different genes by phosphorylation of various proteins [90]. The RAS/MAPK pathway is pivotal not only for the regulation of cell cycle progression from G1 to S phase, but also for cell growth, metabolism, migration, and differentiation [91]. Oncogenic alterations of genes of the RAS/MAKP pathway occur recurrently in neuroblastoma and affect 4–10% of all cases [39, 92], with significantly higher frequencies in relapsed disease [56, 93, 94]. Genes of the RAS/MAPK pathway that were found to be affected by oncogenic mutations in neuroblastoma are *PTPN11*, *NF1*, *HRAS, NRAS, KRAS*, and *BRAF* [56]. Oncogenic mutations of genes of the RAS/MAPK pathway have been suggested to provide a rationale for therapeutic intervention by MEK inhibitors [93]. However, recent studies showed limited efficacy of such compounds in neuroblastoma and other pediatric cancers [95, 96], indicating that inhibition of aberrant MAPK signaling may not be sufficient for effective neuroblastoma treatment.

TP53 encodes for the tumor suppressor protein p53 and is frequently affected by inactivating alterations in many pediatric and adult cancer types [70]. The nuclear phosphoprotein p53 is activated in response to cellular stress, which facilitates its binding to DNA and subsequently the transcription of multiple genes involved in cell cycle control, genomic stability, and apoptosis [97, 98]. Mutations of *TP53* itself are rare in neuroblastoma and affect less than 2% of all tumors [39, 99–102]. Thus, most neuroblastomas harbor wild-type p53 with intact target gene regulation [103, 104]. However, oncogenic alterations of genes up- or downstream in the p53 signaling cascade can also account for escape from p53 control [101, 105]. Genes of the p53 pathway that are recurrently affected by genomic alterations in neuroblastoma are *MDM2* and *CDKN2A*, amongst others [106, 107]. It has been suggested that alterations in genes of the p53 pathway are increasingly acquired during the course of disease under chemotherapy and thereby contribute to neuroblastoma relapse and progression [108–110]. A major negative regulator of p53 is the proto-oncogene *MDM2*, which counteracts p53 activation on various levels [111]. In neuroblastoma, *MDM2* is recurrently upregulated by genomic amplification, often within seismic amplicons that also harbor the *CDK4* locus, both of which are located on chromosome 12q [35].

6.7 A Mechanistic Classification of Neuroblastoma

The strong association of genomic alterations affecting *MYCN*, *TERT*, and *ATRX* with advanced stage and poor outcome as well as their almost complete mutually exclusive occurrence suggested that these mutations converge on a common mechanism that discriminates high- from low-risk neuroblastoma. This hypothesis was confirmed by analysis of large primary neuro-

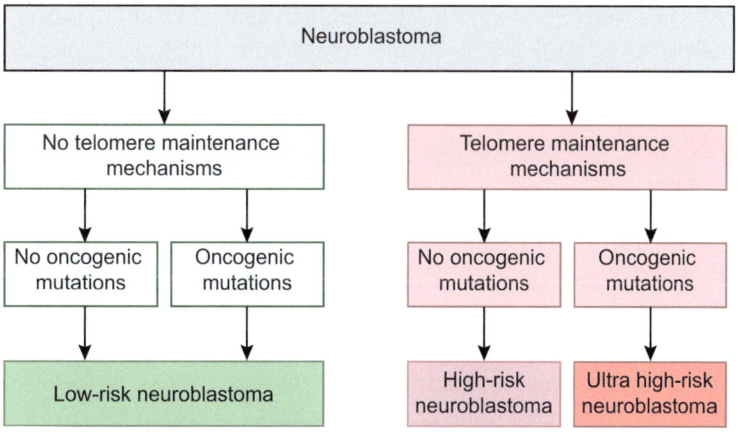

Fig. 6.2 Mechanistic classification of clinical neuroblastoma subtypes according to telomere maintenance status and oncogenic mutations in genes of the RAS/MAPK and p53 pathways [56]

blastoma cohorts and neuroblastoma cell lines, in which the presence of *MYCN* and *TERT* alterations was strongly associated with induction of *TERT* expression and telomerase activity, whereas *ATRX* mutations were exclusively found in ALT-positive tumors and cell lines [56, 64]. While most high-risk tumors bear either of these genomic alterations, they have not been detected in a fraction of roughly 20% of this clinical subtype [38, 56]. It has to be noted, though, that elevated *TERT* expression accompanied by telomerase activation or evidence of ALT has been found in almost all of the high-risk cases lacking such genomic alterations [38, 56]. By contrast, the vast majority of low- and intermediate-risk tumors lacked telomere maintenance activation. Moreover, the clinical outcome of those few non-high-risk patients whose tumors harbored telomerase or ALT was as poor as that of high-risk patients [56]. Together, these findings strongly suggest that induction of telomere maintenance is the key hallmark of high-risk neuroblastoma, representing the molecular switch that drives tumor cells to the fully malignant state [23, 56]. By contrast, lack of telomere maintenance and consequently the inability to proliferate infinitely may represent the basis for growth arrest, differentiation, and spontaneous regression occurring regularly in low-risk neuroblastoma.

Given the fundamental significance of telomere maintenance mechanisms in determining the clinical phenotype of neuroblastoma, the question arose in which way other recurrent genomic alterations contribute to the development of the distinct subtypes. Integration of information on telomere maintenance and genomic alterations of other genes in a large neuroblastoma cohort revealed that mutations in genes of the RAS/MAPK and the p53 pathways affected patient outcome only if telomere maintenance mechanisms were present [56]. Patients with tumors that were positive for telomere maintenance had significantly worse outcome if tumors also harbored mutations in genes of these pathways [56]. By contrast, outcome of patients with tumors that lacked mechanisms of telomere maintenance was not affected by presence or absence of such mutations and was favorable in general. Together, these findings suggest a mechanistic classification of neuroblastoma based on molecular alterations (Fig. 6.2): Low-risk disease is defined by the absence of telomere maintenance mechanisms, independent of the occurrence of other genomic alterations. On the other hand, high-risk disease is defined by the presence of telomere maintenance mechanisms. In case of additional mutations in genes of the RAS/MAPK or p53 pathway, clinical outcome is dismal, and these patients are therefore considered as ultra-high-risk patients [56].

6.8 Conclusion and Perspectives

In-depth characterization of genomic alterations in large neuroblastoma cohorts and their integration with gene expression and epigenetics data have uncovered key aspects of neuroblastoma pathogenesis, particularly on the mechanisms underlying the fundamentally distinct clinical phenotypes. Mechanisms of telomere maintenance were demonstrated to play a crucial role in neuroblastoma pathogenesis. Their presence and absence define high-risk and low-risk disease, respectively, and may thus explain the extreme diversity of clinical courses. Oncogenic mutations in genes of the RAS/MAPK and p53 pathways also occur recurrently in neuroblastoma, however, their clinical impact depends on the telomere maintenance status of the tumor cells.

Despite the advancements in our understanding of the molecular pathogenesis of neuroblastoma, however, a number of important questions still remain. It is not known, for instance, which factors lead to massive proliferation and clonal expansion of low-risk neuroblastoma. Although low-risk tumors have a high likelihood to undergo growth arrest, differentiation, and spontaneous regression, some children die from the disease due to massive initial tumor progression. It is not entirely clear so far, which molecular alterations cause such massive tumor progression in the absence of telomere maintenance. In addition, while lack of telomere maintenance is likely to be the cause of the benign phenotype of low-risk neuroblastoma, this hypothesis has not been experimentally proven, yet, and the molecular mechanisms underlying tumor differentiation and regression are still uncertain.

Even more important, it has remained largely unclear, which transforming events contribute to the pathogenesis of high-risk neuroblastoma in the majority of cases. While activation of telomere maintenance is obviously required for development of high-risk tumors, it is certainly not sufficient for full malignant transformation [112, 113]. In a fraction of cases, oncogenic mutations in genes of the RAS/MAPK or the p53 pathway account for the malignant phenotype, however, such alterations are absent in the majority of high-risk tumors. It has to be determined, therefore, which transforming events contribute to high-risk neuroblastoma development in these cases. In this context, the mechanistic consequences of large copy number alterations, such as 1p and 11q loss or 17q gain, are still unclear. The high prevalence of these alterations in high-risk neuroblastoma strongly supports their mechanistic relevance. It will be thus important to find out which gene or genes are essential in these genomic regions, and which molecular mechanisms (e.g., gene dosage effects or enhancer hijacking) are responsible for the phenotypic effects they are associated with.

Taken together, telomere maintenance mechanisms are a key hallmark of high-risk neuroblastoma. Assessment of telomere maintenance therefore seems to be a promising novel approach for accurate risk stratification, however, its exact value in risk assessment and treatment stratification has to be evaluated retro- and prospectively in more detail. In addition, improved knowledge on the molecular mechanisms that are essentially driving high-risk neuroblastoma pathogenesis may provide a starting point for the development of targeted therapies in the future.

References

1. Brodeur GM, Sekhon G, Goldstein MN. Chromosomal aberrations in human neuroblastomas. Cancer. 1977;40(5):2256–63. https://doi.org/10.1002/1097-0142(197711)40:5<2256::aid-cncr2820400536>3.0.co;2-1.
2. Gilbert F, Feder M, Balaban G, Brangman D, Lurie DK, Podolsky R, et al. Human neuroblastomas and abnormalities of chromosomes 1 and 17. Cancer Res. 1984;44(11):5444–9.
3. Schwab M, Alitalo K, Klempnauer KH, Varmus HE, Bishop JM, Gilbert F, et al. Amplified DNA with limited homology to myc cellular oncogene is shared by human neuroblastoma cell lines and a neuroblastoma tumour. Nature. 1983;305(5931):245–8. https://doi.org/10.1038/305245a0.
4. Brodeur GM, Seeger RC, Schwab M, Varmus HE, Bishop JM. Amplification of N-myc in untreated human neuroblastomas correlates with advanced disease stage. Science. 1984;224(4653):1121–4. https://doi.org/10.1126/science.6719137.
5. Seeger RC, Brodeur GM, Sather H, Dalton A, Siegel SE, Wong KY, et al. Association of multiple copies of the N-myc oncogene with rapid progression of neuroblastomas. N Engl J Med. 1985;313(18):1111–6. https://doi.org/10.1056/NEJM198510313131802.
6. Fong CT, Dracopoli NC, White PS, Merrill PT, Griffith RC, Housman DE, et al. Loss of heterozygosity for the short arm of chromosome 1 in human

neuroblastomas: correlation with N-myc amplification. Proc Natl Acad Sci U S A. 1989;86(10):3753–7. https://doi.org/10.1073/pnas.86.10.3753.
7. Caron H, van Sluis P, de Kraker J, Bokkerink J, Egeler M, Laureys G, et al. Allelic loss of chromosome 1p as a predictor of unfavorable outcome in patients with neuroblastoma. N Engl J Med. 1996;334(4):225–30. https://doi.org/10.1056/NEJM199601253340404.
8. Srivatsan ES, Ying KL, Seeger RC. Deletion of chromosome 11 and of 14q sequences in neuroblastoma. Genes Chromosomes Cancer. 1993;7(1):32–7. https://doi.org/10.1002/gcc.2870070106.
9. Attiyeh EF, London WB, Mosse YP, Wang Q, Winter C, Khazi D, et al. Chromosome 1p and 11q deletions and outcome in neuroblastoma. N Engl J Med. 2005;353(21):2243–53. https://doi.org/10.1056/NEJMoa052399.
10. Janoucix-Lerosey I, Schleiermacher G, Michels E, Mosseri V, Ribeiro A, Lequin D, et al. Overall genomic pattern is a predictor of outcome in neuroblastoma. J Clin Oncol. 2009;27(7):1026–33. https://doi.org/10.1200/JCO.2008.16.0630.
11. Fischer M, Berthold F. The role of complex genomic alterations in neuroblastoma risk estimation. Genome Med. 2010;2(5):31. https://doi.org/10.1186/gm152.
12. Oberthuer A, Hero B, Berthold F, Juraeva D, Faldum A, Kahlert Y, et al. Prognostic impact of gene expression-based classification for neuroblastoma. J Clin Oncol. 2010;28(21):3506–15. https://doi.org/10.1200/JCO.2009.27.3367.
13. De Preter K, Vermeulen J, Brors B, Delattre O, Eggert A, Fischer M, et al. Accurate outcome prediction in neuroblastoma across independent data sets using a multigene signature. Clin Cancer Res. 2010;16(5):1532–41. https://doi.org/10.1158/1078-0432.CCR-09-2607.
14. Oberthuer A, Berthold F, Warnat P, Hero B, Kahlert Y, Spitz R, et al. Customized oligonucleotide microarray gene expression-based classification of neuroblastoma patients outperforms current clinical risk stratification. J Clin Oncol. 2006;24(31):5070–8. https://doi.org/10.1200/JCO.2006.06.1879.
15. Ohira M, Oba S, Nakamura Y, Isogai E, Kaneko S, Nakagawa A, et al. Expression profiling using a tumor-specific cDNA microarray predicts the prognosis of intermediate risk neuroblastomas. Cancer Cell. 2005;7(4):337–50. https://doi.org/10.1016/j.ccr.2005.03.019.
16. Asgharzadeh S, Pique-Regi R, Sposto R, Wang H, Yang Y, Shimada H, et al. Prognostic significance of gene expression profiles of metastatic neuroblastomas lacking MYCN gene amplification. J Natl Cancer Inst. 2006;98(17):1193–203. https://doi.org/10.1093/jnci/djj330.
17. Vermeulen J, De Preter K, Laureys G, Speleman F, Vandesompele J. 59-gene prognostic signature substratifies high-risk neuroblastoma patients. Lancet Oncol. 2009;10(11):1030. https://doi.org/10.1016/S1470-2045(09)70325-0.
18. Oberthuer A, Juraeva D, Hero B, Volland R, Sterz C, Schmidt R, et al. Revised risk estimation and treatment stratification of low- and intermediate-risk neuroblastoma patients by integrating clinical and molecular prognostic markers. Clin Cancer Res. 2015;21(8):1904–15. https://doi.org/10.1158/1078-0432.CCR-14-0817.
19. Pugh TJ, Morozova O, Attiyeh EF, Asgharzadeh S, Wei JS, Auclair D, et al. The genetic landscape of high-risk neuroblastoma. Nat Genet. 2013;45(3):279–84. https://doi.org/10.1038/ng.2529.
20. Sausen M, Leary RJ, Jones S, Wu J, Reynolds CP, Liu X, et al. Integrated genomic analyses identify ARID1A and ARID1B alterations in the childhood cancer neuroblastoma. Nat Genet. 2013;45(1):12–7. https://doi.org/10.1038/ng.2493.
21. Lopez G, Conkrite KL, Doepner M, Rathi KS, Modi A, Vaksman Z, et al. Somatic structural variation targets neurodevelopmental genes and identifies SHANK2 as a tumor suppressor in neuroblastoma. Genome Res. 2020;30(9):1228–42. https://doi.org/10.1101/gr.252106.119.
22. Molenaar JJ, Koster J, Zwijnenburg DA, van Sluis P, Valentijn LJ, van der Ploeg I, et al. Sequencing of neuroblastoma identifies chromothripsis and defects in neuritogenesis genes. Nature. 2012;483(7391):589–93. https://doi.org/10.1038/nature10910.
23. Peifer M, Hertwig F, Roels F, Dreidax D, Gartlgruber M, Menon R, et al. Telomerase activation by genomic rearrangements in high-risk neuroblastoma. Nature. 2015;526(7575):700–4. https://doi.org/10.1038/nature14980.
24. Valentijn LJ, Koster J, Zwijnenburg DA, Hasselt NE, van Sluis P, Volckmann R, et al. TERT rearrangements are frequent in neuroblastoma and identify aggressive tumors. Nat Genet. 2015;47(12):1411–4. https://doi.org/10.1038/ng.3438.
25. Dang CV. MYC on the path to cancer. Cell. 2012;149(1):22–35. https://doi.org/10.1016/j.cell.2012.03.003.
26. Otte J, Dyberg C, Pepich A, Johnsen JI. MYCN function in neuroblastoma development. Front Oncol. 2020;10:624079. https://doi.org/10.3389/fonc.2020.624079.
27. Meyer N, Penn LZ. Reflecting on 25 years with MYC. Nat Rev Cancer. 2008;8(12):976–90. https://doi.org/10.1038/nrc2231.
28. Wang J, Xie LY, Allan S, Beach D, Hannon GJ. Myc activates telomerase. Genes Dev. 1998;12(12):1769–74. https://doi.org/10.1101/gad.12.12.1769.
29. Yuan X, Larsson C, Xu D. Mechanisms underlying the activation of TERT transcription and telomerase activity in human cancer: old actors and new players. Oncogene. 2019;38(34):6172–83. https://doi.org/10.1038/s41388-019-0872-9.
30. Weiss WA, Aldape K, Mohapatra G, Feuerstein BG, Bishop JM. Targeted expression of MYCN

causes neuroblastoma in transgenic mice. EMBO J. 1997;16(11):2985–95. https://doi.org/10.1093/emboj/16.11.2985.
31. Huang M, Weiss WA. Neuroblastoma and MYCN. Cold Spring Harb Perspect Med. 2013;3(10):a014415. https://doi.org/10.1101/cshperspect.a014415.
32. Baluapuri A, Wolf E, Eilers M. Target gene-independent functions of MYC oncoproteins. Nat Rev Mol Cell Biol. 2020;21(5):255–67. https://doi.org/10.1038/s41580-020-0215-2.
33. Theissen J, Boensch M, Spitz R, Betts D, Stegmaier S, Christiansen H, et al. Heterogeneity of the MYCN oncogene in neuroblastoma. Clin Cancer Res. 2009;15(6):2085–90. https://doi.org/10.1158/1078-0432.CCR-08-1648.
34. Storlazzi CT, Lonoce A, Guastadisegni MC, Trombetta D, D'Addabbo P, Daniele G, et al. Gene amplification as double minutes or homogeneously staining regions in solid tumors: origin and structure. Genome Res. 2010;20(9):1198–206. https://doi.org/10.1101/gr.106252.110.
35. Rosswog C, Bartenhagen C, Welte A, Kahlert Y, Hemstedt N, Lorenz W, et al. Chromothripsis followed by circular recombination drives oncogene amplification in human cancer. Nat Genet. 2021;53(12):1673–85. https://doi.org/10.1038/s41588-021-00951-7.
36. Maris JM. Recent advances in neuroblastoma. N Engl J Med. 2010;362(23):2202–11. https://doi.org/10.1056/NEJMra0804577.
37. Greider CW, Blackburn EH. A telomeric sequence in the RNA of tetrahymena telomerase required for telomere repeat synthesis. Nature. 1989;337(6205):331–7. https://doi.org/10.1038/337331a0.
38. Roderwieser A, Sand F, Walter E, Fischer J, Gecht J, Bartenhagen C, et al. Telomerase is a prognostic marker of poor outcome and a therapeutic target in neuroblastoma. JCO Precis Oncol. 2019;3:1–20. https://doi.org/10.1200/PO.19.00072.
39. Brady SW, Liu Y, Ma X, Gout AM, Hagiwara K, Zhou X, et al. Pan-neuroblastoma analysis reveals age- and signature-associated driver alterations. Nat Commun. 2020;11(1):5183. https://doi.org/10.1038/s41467-020-18987-4.
40. Koneru B, Lopez G, Farooqi A, Conkrite KL, Nguyen TH, Macha SJ, et al. Telomere maintenance mechanisms define clinical outcome in high-risk neuroblastoma. Cancer Res. 2020;80(12):2663–75. https://doi.org/10.1158/0008-5472.CAN-19-3068.
41. Cai J, Chen J, Zhang W, Yang P, Zhang C, Li M, et al. Loss of ATRX, associated with DNA methylation pattern of chromosome end, impacted biological behaviors of astrocytic tumors. Oncotarget. 2015;6(20):18105–15. https://doi.org/10.18632/oncotarget.3906.
42. Watson LA, Goldberg H, Berube NG. Emerging roles of ATRX in cancer. Epigenomics. 2015;7(8):1365–78. https://doi.org/10.2217/epi.15.82.
43. Heaphy CM, de Wilde RF, Jiao Y, Klein AP, Edil BH, Shi C, et al. Altered telomeres in tumors with ATRX and DAXX mutations. Science. 2011;333(6041):425. https://doi.org/10.1126/science.1207313.
44. Barthel FP, Wei W, Tang M, Martinez-Ledesma E, Hu X, Amin SB, et al. Systematic analysis of telomere length and somatic alterations in 31 cancer types. Nat Genet. 2017;49(3):349–57. https://doi.org/10.1038/ng.3781.
45. Clynes D, Jelinska C, Xella B, Ayyub H, Scott C, Mitson M, et al. Suppression of the alternative lengthening of telomere pathway by the chromatin remodelling factor ATRX. Nat Commun. 2015;6:7538. https://doi.org/10.1038/ncomms8538.
46. Napier CE, Huschtscha LI, Harvey A, Bower K, Noble JR, Hendrickson EA, et al. ATRX represses alternative lengthening of telomeres. Oncotarget. 2015;6(18):16543–58. https://doi.org/10.18632/oncotarget.3846.
47. Hartlieb SA, Sieverling L, Nadler-Holly M, Ziehm M, Toprak UH, Herrmann C, et al. Alternative lengthening of telomeres in childhood neuroblastoma from genome to proteome. Nat Commun. 2021;12(1):1269. https://doi.org/10.1038/s41467-021-21247-8.
48. Cheung NK, Zhang J, Lu C, Parker M, Bahrami A, Tickoo SK, et al. Association of age at diagnosis and genetic mutations in patients with neuroblastoma. JAMA. 2012;307(10):1062–71. https://doi.org/10.1001/jama.2012.228.
49. Duan XF, Zhao Q. TERT-mediated and ATRX-mediated telomere maintenance and neuroblastoma. J Pediatr Hematol Oncol. 2018;40(1):1–6. https://doi.org/10.1097/MPH.0000000000000840.
50. Qadeer ZA, Valle-Garcia D, Hasson D, Sun Z, Cook A, Nguyen C, et al. ATRX in-frame fusion neuroblastoma is sensitive to EZH2 inhibition via modulation of neuronal gene signatures. Cancer Cell. 2019;36(5):512–27. e9. https://doi.org/10.1016/j.ccell.2019.09.002.
51. Makarov VL, Hirose Y, Langmore JP. Long G tails at both ends of human chromosomes suggest a C strand degradation mechanism for telomere shortening. Cell. 1997;88(5):657–66. https://doi.org/10.1016/s0092-8674(00)81908-x.
52. Nandakumar J, Cech TR. Finding the end: recruitment of telomerase to telomeres. Nat Rev Mol Cell Biol. 2013;14(2):69–82. https://doi.org/10.1038/nrm3505.
53. Blackburn EH, Epel ES, Lin J. Human telomere biology: a contributory and interactive factor in aging, disease risks, and protection. Science. 2015;350(6265):1193–8. https://doi.org/10.1126/science.aab3389.
54. Blackburn EH. Switching and signaling at the telomere. Cell. 2001;106(6):661–73. https://doi.org/10.1016/s0092-8674(01)00492-5.
55. Hanahan D, Weinberg RA. The hallmarks of cancer. Cell. 2000;100(1):57–70. https://doi.org/10.1016/s0092-8674(00)81683-9.

56. Ackermann S, Cartolano M, Hero B, Welte A, Kahlert Y, Roderwieser A, et al. A mechanistic classification of clinical phenotypes in neuroblastoma. Science. 2018;362(6419):1165–70. https://doi.org/10.1126/science.aat6768.
57. Wong JM, Collins K. Telomere maintenance and disease. Lancet. 2003;362(9388):983–8. https://doi.org/10.1016/S0140-6736(03)14369-3.
58. Morin GB. The human telomere terminal transferase enzyme is a ribonucleoprotein that synthesizes TTAGGG repeats. Cell. 1989;59(3):521–9. https://doi.org/10.1016/0092-8674(89)90035-4.
59. Lingner J, Cooper JP, Cech TR. Telomerase and DNA end replication: no longer a lagging strand problem? Science. 1995;269(5230):1533–4. https://doi.org/10.1126/science.7545310.
60. Onitake Y, Hiyama E, Kamei N, Yamaoka H, Sueda T, Hiyama K. Telomere biology in neuroblastoma: telomere binding proteins and alternative strengthening of telomeres. J Pediatr Surg. 2009;44(12):2258–66. https://doi.org/10.1016/j.jpedsurg.2009.07.046.
61. Bryan TM, Englezou A, Gupta J, Bacchetti S, Reddel RR. Telomere elongation in immortal human cells without detectable telomerase activity. EMBO J. 1995;14(17):4240–8.
62. Bryan TM, Englezou A, Dalla-Pozza L, Dunham MA, Reddel RR. Evidence for an alternative mechanism for maintaining telomere length in human tumors and tumor-derived cell lines. Nat Med. 1997;3(11):1271–4. https://doi.org/10.1038/nm1197-1271.
63. Henson JD, Reddel RR. Assaying and investigating alternative lengthening of telomeres activity in human cells and cancers. FEBS Lett. 2010;584(17):3800–11. https://doi.org/10.1016/j.febslet.2010.06.009.
64. Meeser A, Bartenhagen C, Werr L, Hellmann A-M, Kahlert Y, Hemstedt N, et al. Reliable assessment of telomere maintenance mechanisms in neuroblastoma. Cell Biosci. 2022;12(1):160. https://doi.org/10.1186/s13578-022-00896-2.
65. Farooqi AS, Dagg RA, Choi LM, Shay JW, Reynolds CP, Lau LM. Alternative lengthening of telomeres in neuroblastoma cell lines is associated with a lack of MYCN genomic amplification and with p53 pathway aberrations. J Neuro-Oncol. 2014;119(1):17–26. https://doi.org/10.1007/s11060-014-1456-8.
66. Drane P, Ouararhni K, Depaux A, Shuaib M, Hamiche A. The death-associated protein DAXX is a novel histone chaperone involved in the replication-independent deposition of H3.3. Genes Dev. 2010;24(12):1253–65. https://doi.org/10.1101/gad.566910.
67. Schwartzentruber J, Korshunov A, Liu XY, Jones DT, Pfaff E, Jacob K, et al. Driver mutations in histone H3.3 and chromatin remodelling genes in paediatric glioblastoma. Nature. 2012;482(7384):226–31. https://doi.org/10.1038/nature10833.
68. Sieverling L, Hong C, Koser SD, Ginsbach P, Kleinheinz K, Hutter B, et al. Genomic footprints of activated telomere maintenance mechanisms in cancer. Nat Commun. 2020;11(1):733. https://doi.org/10.1038/s41467-019-13824-9.
69. Hwang WL, Wolfson RL, Niemierko A, Marcus KJ, DuBois SG, Haas-Kogan D. Clinical impact of tumor mutational burden in neuroblastoma. J Natl Cancer Inst. 2019;111(7):695–9. https://doi.org/10.1093/jnci/djy157.
70. Ma X, Liu Y, Liu Y, Alexandrov LB, Edmonson MN, Gawad C, et al. Pan-cancer genome and transcriptome analyses of 1,699 paediatric leukaemias and solid tumours. Nature. 2018;555(7696):371–6. https://doi.org/10.1038/nature25795.
71. Janoueix-Lerosey I, Lequin D, Brugieres L, Ribeiro A, de Pontual L, Combaret V, et al. Somatic and germline activating mutations of the ALK kinase receptor in neuroblastoma. Nature. 2008;455(7215):967–70. https://doi.org/10.1038/nature07398.
72. Chen Y, Takita J, Choi YL, Kato M, Ohira M, Sanada M, et al. Oncogenic mutations of ALK kinase in neuroblastoma. Nature. 2008;455(7215):971–4. https://doi.org/10.1038/nature07399.
73. George RE, Sanda T, Hanna M, Frohling S, Luther W 2nd, Zhang J, et al. Activating mutations in ALK provide a therapeutic target in neuroblastoma. Nature. 2008;455(7215):975–8. https://doi.org/10.1038/nature07397.
74. Mosse YP, Laudenslager M, Longo L, Cole KA, Wood A, Attiyeh EF, et al. Identification of ALK as a major familial neuroblastoma predisposition gene. Nature. 2008;455(7215):930–5. https://doi.org/10.1038/nature07261.
75. Tolbert VP, Coggins GE, Maris JM. Genetic susceptibility to neuroblastoma. Curr Opin Genet Dev. 2017;42:81–90. https://doi.org/10.1016/j.gde.2017.03.008.
76. Janoueix-Lerosey I, Lopez-Delisle L, Delattre O, Rohrer H. The ALK receptor in sympathetic neuron development and neuroblastoma. Cell Tissue Res. 2018;372(2):325–37. https://doi.org/10.1007/s00441-017-2784-8.
77. Heukamp LC, Thor T, Schramm A, De Preter K, Kumps C, De Wilde B, et al. Targeted expression of mutated ALK induces neuroblastoma in transgenic mice. Sci Transl Med. 2012;4(141):141ra91. https://doi.org/10.1126/scitranslmed.3003967.
78. Berry T, Luther W, Bhatnagar N, Jamin Y, Poon E, Sanda T, et al. The ALK(F1174L) mutation potentiates the oncogenic activity of MYCN in neuroblastoma. Cancer Cell. 2012;22(1):117–30. https://doi.org/10.1016/j.ccr.2012.06.001.
79. Zhu S, Lee JS, Guo F, Shin J, Perez-Atayde AR, Kutok JL, et al. Activated ALK collaborates with MYCN in neuroblastoma pathogenesis. Cancer Cell. 2012;21(3):362–73. https://doi.org/10.1016/j.ccr.2012.02.010.

80. Schleiermacher G, Javanmardi N, Bernard V, Leroy Q, Cappo J, Rio Frio T, et al. Emergence of new ALK mutations at relapse of neuroblastoma. J Clin Oncol. 2014;32(25):2727–34. https://doi.org/10.1200/JCO.2013.54.0674.
81. Bresler SC, Weiser DA, Huwe PJ, Park JH, Krytska K, Ryles H, et al. ALK mutations confer differential oncogenic activation and sensitivity to ALK inhibition therapy in neuroblastoma. Cancer Cell. 2014;26(5):682–94. https://doi.org/10.1016/j.ccell.2014.09.019.
82. De Brouwer S, De Preter K, Kumps C, Zabrocki P, Porcu M, Westerhout EM, et al. Meta-analysis of neuroblastomas reveals a skewed ALK mutation spectrum in tumors with MYCN amplification. Clin Cancer Res. 2010;16(17):4353–62. https://doi.org/10.1158/1078-0432.CCR-09-2660.
83. Mosse YP, Lim MS, Voss SD, Wilner K, Ruffner K, Laliberte J, et al. Safety and activity of crizotinib for paediatric patients with refractory solid tumours or anaplastic large-cell lymphoma: a Children's oncology group phase 1 consortium study. Lancet Oncol. 2013;14(6):472–80. https://doi.org/10.1016/S1470-2045(13)70095-0.
84. Fischer M, Moreno L, Ziegler DS, Marshall LV, Zwaan CM, Irwin MS, et al. Ceritinib in paediatric patients with anaplastic lymphoma kinase-positive malignancies: an open-label, multicentre, phase 1, dose-escalation and dose-expansion study. Lancet Oncol. 2021;22(12):1764–76. https://doi.org/10.1016/S1470-2045(21)00536-2.
85. Foster JH, Voss SD, Hall DC, Minard CG, Balis FM, Wilner K, et al. Activity of Crizotinib in patients with ALK-aberrant relapsed/refractory neuroblastoma: a Children's Oncology Group Study (ADVL0912). Clin Cancer Res. 2021;27(13):3543–8. https://doi.org/10.1158/1078-0432.CCR-20-4224.
86. Shimizu K, Goldfarb M, Suard Y, Perucho M, Li Y, Kamata T, et al. Three human transforming genes are related to the viral ras oncogenes. Proc Natl Acad Sci U S A. 1983;80(8):2112–6. https://doi.org/10.1073/pnas.80.8.2112.
87. Braicu C, Buse M, Busuioc C, Drula R, Gulei D, Raduly L, et al. A comprehensive review on MAPK: a promising therapeutic target in cancer. Cancers (Basel). 2019;11(10) https://doi.org/10.3390/cancers11101618.
88. Santarpia L, Lippman SM, El-Naggar AK. Targeting the MAPK-RAS-RAF signaling pathway in cancer therapy. Expert Opin Ther Targets. 2012;16(1):103–19. https://doi.org/10.1517/14728222.2011.645805.
89. Punekar SR, Velcheti V, Neel BG, Wong KK. The current state of the art and future trends in RAS-targeted cancer therapies. Nat Rev Clin Oncol. 2022;19(10):637–55. https://doi.org/10.1038/s41571-022-00671-9.
90. Unal EB, Uhlitz F, Bluthgen N. A compendium of ERK targets. FEBS Lett. 2017;591(17):2607–15. https://doi.org/10.1002/1873-3468.12740.
91. Lavoie H, Gagnon J, Therrien M. ERK signalling: a master regulator of cell behaviour, life and fate. Nat Rev Mol Cell Biol. 2020;21(10):607–32. https://doi.org/10.1038/s41580-020-0255-7.
92. Mlakar V, Morel E, Mlakar SJ, Ansari M, Gumy-Pause F. A review of the biological and clinical implications of RAS-MAPK pathway alterations in neuroblastoma. J Exp Clin Cancer Res. 2021;40(1):189. https://doi.org/10.1186/s13046-021-01967-x.
93. Eleveld TF, Oldridge DA, Bernard V, Koster J, Colmet Daage L, Diskin SJ, et al. Relapsed neuroblastomas show frequent RAS-MAPK pathway mutations. Nat Genet. 2015;47(8):864–71. https://doi.org/10.1038/ng.3333.
94. Schramm A, Koster J, Assenov Y, Althoff K, Peifer M, Mahlow E, et al. Mutational dynamics between primary and relapse neuroblastomas. Nat Genet. 2015;47(8):872–7. https://doi.org/10.1038/ng.3349.
95. Johnson DB, Zhao F, Noel M, Riely GJ, Mitchell EP, Wright JJ, et al. Trametinib activity in patients with solid tumors and lymphomas Harboring BRAF non-V600 mutations or fusions: results from NCI-MATCH (EAY131). Clin Cancer Res. 2020;26(8):1812–9. https://doi.org/10.1158/1078-0432.CCR-19-3443.
96. Eckstein OS, Allen CE, Williams PM, Roy-Chowdhuri S, Patton DR, Coffey B, et al. Phase II study of selumetinib in children and young adults with tumors harboring activating mitogen-activated protein kinase pathway genetic alterations: arm E of the NCI-COG Pediatric MATCH trial. J Clin Oncol. 2022:JCO2102840. https://doi.org/10.1200/JCO.21.02840.
97. Mantovani F, Collavin L, Del Sal G. Mutant p53 as a guardian of the cancer cell. Cell Death Differ. 2019;26(2):199–212. https://doi.org/10.1038/s41418-018-0246-9.
98. Munoz-Fontela C, Mandinova A, Aaronson SA, Lee SW. Emerging roles of p53 and other tumour-suppressor genes in immune regulation. Nat Rev Immunol. 2016;16(12):741–50. https://doi.org/10.1038/nri.2016.99.
99. Hosoi G, Hara J, Okamura T, Osugi Y, Ishihara S, Fukuzawa M, et al. Low frequency of the p53 gene mutations in neuroblastoma. Cancer. 1994;73(12):3087–93. https://doi.org/10.1002/1097-0142(19940615)73:12<3087::aid-cncr2820731230>3.0.co;2-9.
100. Imamura J, Bartram CR, Berthold F, Harms D, Nakamura H, Koeffler HP. Mutation of the p53 gene in neuroblastoma and its relationship with N-myc amplification. Cancer Res. 1993;53(17):4053–8.
101. Van Maerken T, Vandesompele J, Rihani A, De Paepe A, Speleman F. Escape from p53-mediated tumor surveillance in neuroblastoma: switching off the p14(ARF)-MDM2-p53 axis. Cell Death Differ. 2009;16(12):1563–72. https://doi.org/10.1038/cdd.2009.138.

102. Tweddle DA, Pearson AD, Haber M, Norris MD, Xue C, Flemming C, et al. The p53 pathway and its inactivation in neuroblastoma. Cancer Lett. 2003;197(1–2):93–8. https://doi.org/10.1016/s0304-3835(03)00088-0.
103. Vogan K, Bernstein M, Leclerc JM, Brisson L, Brossard J, Brodeur GM, et al. Absence of p53 gene mutations in primary neuroblastomas. Cancer Res. 1993;53(21):5269–73.
104. Chen L, Malcolm AJ, Wood KM, Cole M, Variend S, Cullinane C, et al. p53 is nuclear and functional in both undifferentiated and differentiated neuroblastoma. Cell Cycle. 2007;6(21):2685–96. https://doi.org/10.4161/cc.6.21.4853.
105. Tweddle DA, Malcolm AJ, Cole M, Pearson AD, Lunec J. p53 cellular localization and function in neuroblastoma: evidence for defective G(1) arrest despite WAF1 induction in MYCN-amplified cells. Am J Pathol. 2001;158(6):2067–77. https://doi.org/10.1016/S0002-9440(10)64678-0.
106. Martinez-Monleon A, Kryh Oberg H, Gaarder J, Berbegall AP, Javanmardi N, Djos A, et al. Amplification of CDK4 and MDM2: a detailed study of a high-risk neuroblastoma subgroup. Sci Rep. 2022;12(1):12420. https://doi.org/10.1038/s41598-022-16455-1.
107. Sorteberg AL, Halipi V, Wickstrom M, Shirazi FS. The cyclin dependent kinase inhibitor p21(Cip1/Waf1) is a therapeutic target in high-risk neuroblastoma. Front Oncol. 2022;12:906194. https://doi.org/10.3389/fonc.2022.906194.
108. Kotchetkov R, Driever PH, Cinatl J, Michaelis M, Karaskova J, Blaheta R, et al. Increased malignant behavior in neuroblastoma cells with acquired multi-drug resistance does not depend on P-gp expression. Int J Oncol. 2005;27(4):1029–37.
109. Xue C, Haber M, Flemming C, Marshall GM, Lock RB, MacKenzie KL, et al. p53 determines multidrug sensitivity of childhood neuroblastoma. Cancer Res. 2007;67(21):10351–60. https://doi.org/10.1158/0008-5472.CAN-06-4345.
110. Carr-Wilkinson J, O'Toole K, Wood KM, Challen CC, Baker AG, Board JR, et al. High frequency of p53/MDM2/p14ARF pathway abnormalities in relapsed neuroblastoma. Clin Cancer Res. 2010;16(4):1108–18. https://doi.org/10.1158/1078-0432.CCR-09-1865.
111. Oliner JD, Pietenpol JA, Thiagalingam S, Gyuris J, Kinzler KW, Vogelstein B. Oncoprotein MDM2 conceals the activation domain of tumour suppressor p53. Nature. 1993;362(6423):857–60. https://doi.org/10.1038/362857a0.
112. Morales CP, Holt SE, Ouellette M, Kaur KJ, Yan Y, Wilson KS, et al. Absence of cancer-associated changes in human fibroblasts immortalized with telomerase. Nat Genet. 1999;21(1):115–8. https://doi.org/10.1038/5063.
113. Hahn WC, Counter CM, Lundberg AS, Beijersbergen RL, Brooks MW, Weinberg RA. Creation of human tumour cells with defined genetic elements. Nature. 1999;400(6743):464–8. https://doi.org/10.1038/22780.

7 Developmental Programs in Neuroblastoma

Selina Jansky and Frank Westermann

7.1 Normal Development of Human Neural Crest-Derived Sympathoadrenal Cells

7.1.1 Schwann Cell Progenitors Are Common Progenitors of Chromaffin Cells and Sympathetic Neuroblasts in the Developing Human Adrenal Gland

Sympathetic neurons and chromaffin cells originate from the trunk neural crest during development and share many characteristics, including the secretion of catecholamines. Therefore, it has been suggested that these cell types are closely related, arise from a common progenitor cell and together represent the sympathoadrenal lineage of the neural crest [1, 2]. However, this view has recently been challenged by lineage tracing and scRNA-seq experiments in mice, which identified the majority of chromaffin cells in the adrenal gland to originate from late migrating Schwann Cell Precursors (SCPs), whereas neuroblasts in sympathetic ganglia were shown to arise from early migrating neural crest cells [3]. These data suggest that the sympathetic and the adrenal chromaffin cell lineages split earlier than previously thought.

Single cell transcript profiling of human adrenal glands using snRNA-seq/scRNA-seq at various time points during embryonic and fetal development resolved the cell types and differentiation trajectories within the developing adrenal medulla [4–6]. Notably, SCPs were identified to give rise to sympathetic neuroblasts and chromaffin cells. These results are consistent with earlier studies suggesting sympathetic neurons and chromaffin cells to originate from a common progenitor and contradictory to the early lineage split proposed by Furlan et al. [3]. Similar to Furlan et al. in the mouse, and Kildisiute et al. and Kameneva et al., adrenal medullas comprise SCPs, bridge cells, sympathetic neuroblasts, and chromaffin cells. Jansky et al. included many samples covering a broad range of developmental stages and made a more fine-grained analysis possible. Hence, adrenal medullary cell types could be further subdivided into early cells, which were detected at 7 and 8 post conception week (pcw), and late cells, which were more differentiated and observed between 11 and 17 pcw.

S. Jansky
Division of Neuroblastoma Genomics, German Cancer Research Center (DKFZ), Heidelberg, Germany

Hopp Children's Cancer Center (KiTZ), Heidelberg, Germany

F. Westermann (✉)
Division of Neuroblastoma Genomics, German Cancer Research Center (DKFZ), Heidelberg, Germany
e-mail: frank.westermann@dkfz.de

S. Asgharzadeh, F. Westermann (eds.), *Neuroblastoma*, Pediatric Oncology,
https://doi.org/10.1007/978-3-031-51292-6_7

Moreover, an additional cell population that connected neuroblasts, bridge and chromaffin cells and that was termed connecting progenitor cells, was identified. Bridge and connecting progenitor cells were transient cell populations, thus, only present during a specific time during development. From 11 pcw on, almost no bridge and connecting progenitor cells were detected in adrenal glands by snRNA-seq or single molecule (sm)FISH anymore. RNA velocity and pseudotime analyses support SCPs to give rise to chromaffin cells and neuroblasts via bridge and connecting progenitor cells and smFISH confirms neuroblasts, chromaffin cells, and SCPs to be localized close to each other within the adrenal gland. In addition to the SCP to neuroblast and SCP to chromaffin cell trajectories, a differentiation trajectory from sympathetic neuroblasts to chromaffin cells was determined by Kameneva et al. [5]. In contrast, no such connection between the two cell types was observed in studies by Jansky et al. and Kildisiute et al. [4, 6]. Future experiments will have to show if differentiation of neuroblasts to chromaffin cells (and probably vice versa) takes place in the human adrenal gland.

In contrast to the results obtained using human samples, pseudotime analyses by Furlan et al. in mice did not determine a trajectory from SCPs to sympathetic neuroblasts [3]. However, the authors claim in Kameneva et al. that the cells connecting SCPs and neuroblasts were overlooked due to the analysis of a limited number of cells by the plate-based smart-seq2 scRNA-seq protocol [5]. Re-analysis of the murine adrenal gland by scRNA-seq of more cells identified intermediate cells in the SCP to neuroblast transition. Lineage tracing confirmed SCPs as origin for sympathetic neuroblasts also in the developing mouse adrenal gland [5]. In contrast, sympathetic neuroblasts in suprarenal ganglia (SRG) and the sympathetic chain were identified to originate directly from migrating neural crest cells and not SCPs by lineage tracing [3].

Another recent study analyzed human adrenal gland development by scRNA-seq and identified SCPs to give rise to chromaffin cells and neuroblasts [7]. However, when analyzing data from Dong et al., together with published data on human adrenal glands in a combined analysis, cells identified as chromaffin cells by Dong et al. co-clustered with neuroblasts from the three other studies [4–6], whereas Dong et al. neuroblasts co-clustered with chromaffin cells (Fig. 7.1). The selection of marker genes by Dong et al. also suggested that chromaffin cells and neuroblasts were interchanged in this study [8, 9]. While classical neuronal marker genes like ISL1, PRPH, and NPY were used to identify chromaffin cells, chromaffin marker CHGB showed higher expression in cells identified as neuroblasts. Furthermore, cell type annotation performed here and in Kildisiute et al. is supported by expression of PNMT, encoding the enzyme that converts noradrenaline into adrenaline, in a subpopulation of cells identified as chromaffin cells. Secretion of adrenaline is a specific feature of a subset of mature chromaffin cells [1].

7.1.2 Sympathetic Neuroblasts in Adrenal Glands and in Sympathetic Ganglia Display Similar Transcriptomes

Sympathetic neurons are not only located in the adrenal gland but the majority of sympathetic neurons are located in paravertebral ganglia of the sympathetic chain and prevertebral ganglia in the abdomen [10]. To shed light on the development of neurons in sympathetic ganglia, paravertebral ganglia, and surrounding tissue from different developmental time points were profiled by snRNA-seq (Fig. 7.2a, unpublished data). Sympathetic ganglia comprised SCPs and sympathetic neuroblasts, but no chromaffin cells. In contrast to the adrenal gland, no cells connecting SCPs to neuroblasts were identified, indicating that neuroblasts in sympathetic ganglia do not originate from SCPs. This result is in line with a previous publication showing that SCPs do not give rise to sympathetic neurons in the suprarenal ganglion and sympathetic chain by

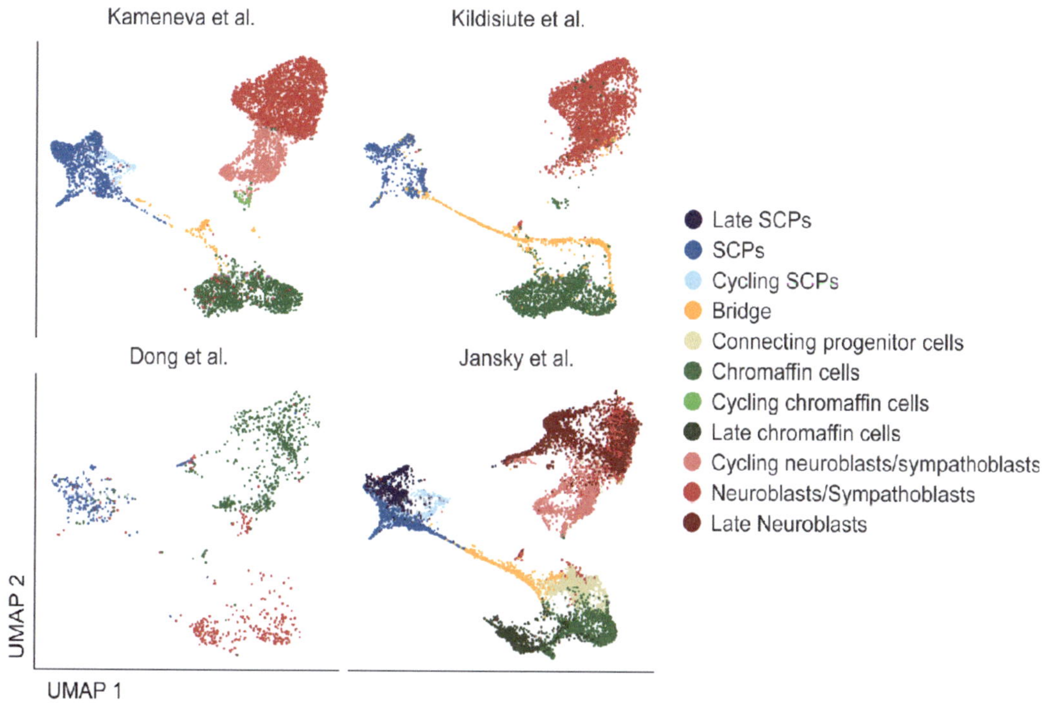

Fig. 7.1 Comparison of the adrenal medulla cell atlas to other published datasets, UMAP projections showing adrenal medullary cells from four publications, which were integrated into one combined UMAP, before the samples were split by publication. The cells are colored by adrenal medullary cell type. Number of cells: Kameneva et al.: n = 7487; Kildisiute et al.: n = 6451; Dong et al.: n = 1236; Jansky et al.: n = 10,739

lineage tracing in the mouse [3]. However, other explanations for the missing connection between SCPs and neuroblasts in human sympathetic ganglia remain. First, it is possible that too few cells were studied and the transitioning cells were missed. Second, the analyzed samples might cover developmental time points that are too late and the transition of SCPs to neuroblasts takes place before CS20. In the mouse, there is evidence that extra-adrenal neuroblasts arise earlier than intra-adrenal neuroblasts [11]. Future experiments, which cover earlier time points in the development of sympathetic ganglia, are necessary to clarify the yet imperfect picture. In order to explore how similar neuroblasts in the adrenal gland and neuroblasts in sympathetic ganglia are, transcriptional similarity between the two cell types was determined. Despite their potentially different origins, neuroblasts from the two locations display very comparable transcriptomes. This goes in line with another scRNA-seq study, which detected no marked differences between adrenal and ganglia sympathetic neuroblast transcriptomes in neither human nor murine data [11].

7.1.3 Migration and Specification of Neural Crest Cells Are Regulated by Activity of Distinct Transcription Factors

Sympathetic neurons and chromaffin cells arise directly or indirectly from the neural crest, a highly migratory multipotent cell population that, despite intensive study, remains largely enigmatic, especially in human embryos [12]. During development, trunk neural crest cells (NCCs) are specified at the neural plate border and migrate to sympathetic ganglia and the adrenal gland via a region close to the dorsal aorta and finally differentiate into the sympathetic or chromaffin lineages [12]. Recently, neural crest

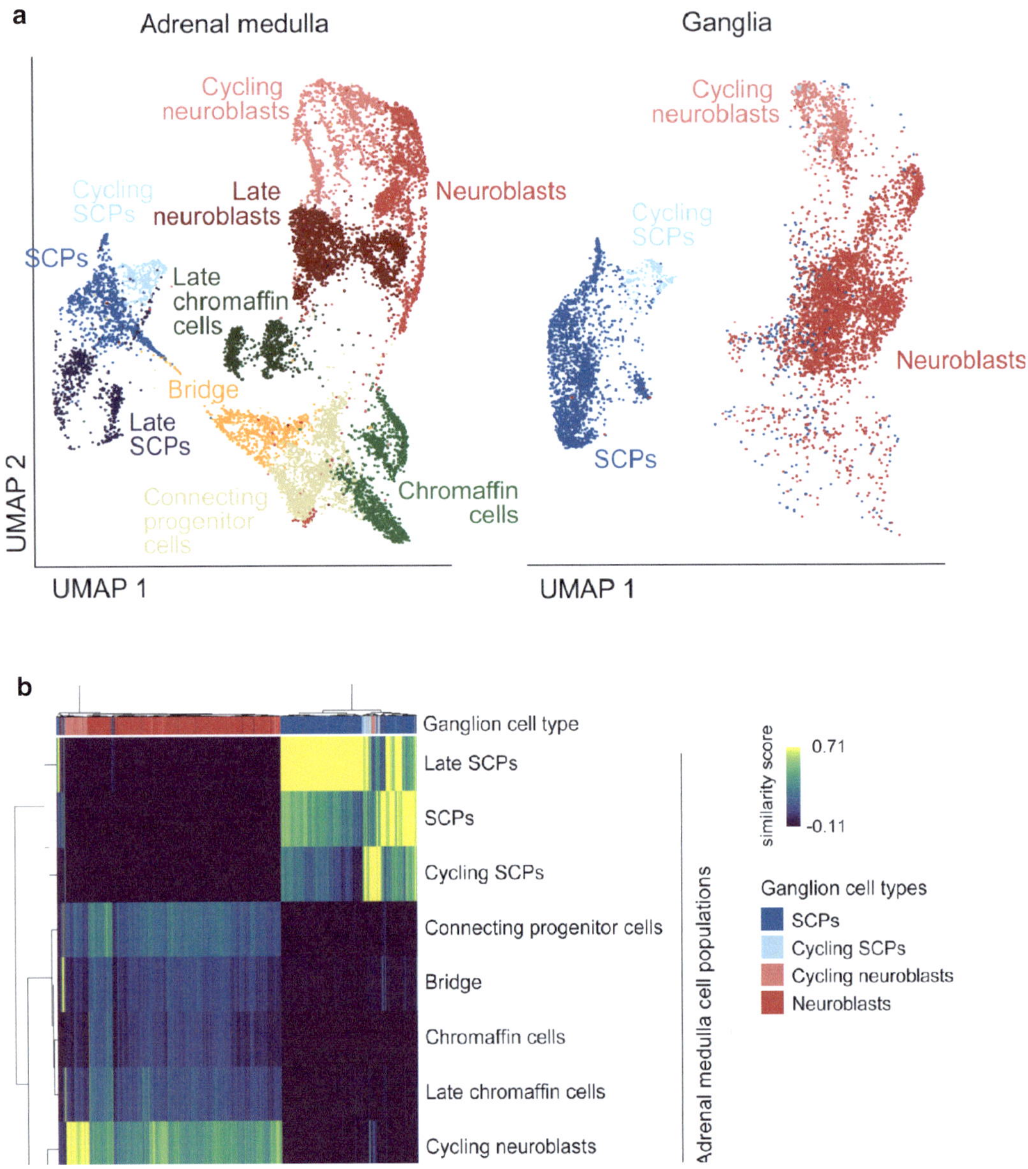

Fig. 7.2 (**a**) UMAP projections showing adrenal medullary cells and neuroblasts and SCPs from sympathetic ganglia, which were integrated into one combined UMAP, before the samples were split by localization. The cells are colored by cell type. (**b**) Heat map displaying similarity of single SCPs and neuroblasts derived from sympathetic ganglia to cell types in the adrenal medulla

cells and related cell types were studied by single-cell transcriptomics to expand the knowledge on their development. Three populations of NCCs were determined, including pre-EMT NCCs, EMT NCCs, and NCCs. Pre-EMT NCCs are early NCCs directly after specification from the neural tube, which still show some activity of neural tube-specific transcription factors like SOX9. Subsequently, the cells undergo epithelial-to-mesenchymal transition and migrate to target organs (EMT NCCs). Only after migration, NCCs showed high transcription factor activity of classical neural crest specifiers like SOX10 and FOXD3. These results are consistent with another single-cell study on early human embryo development [7]. In contrast, immunohistochemical stainings identified SOX10 protein expression in NCCs surrounding the dorsal aorta, but also in migrating NCCs [13]. Sensory neurons, which, like sympathetic neurons and chromaffin cells, arise from ventrally migrating trunk NCCs in dorsal root ganglia (DRG) were already detected as early as CS13. Migrating NCCs were primarily identified at CS13 and less at CS15, suggesting that neural crest migration is almost completed by CS15. Accordingly, IHC staining for neural crest markers identified no migrating trunk NCCs at CS18 anymore [13].

In addition to neural crest markers, NCCs showed activity of TFAP2B and MYCN, which were determined to be active in neuroblasts in sympathetic ganglia and the adrenal gland. This observation hints to the possibility that a subset of trunk neural crest cells might be primed for the sympathetic cell fate already at these early developmental stages. IHC in human embryos have shown that SOX10+, NGFR+ NCCs are located near the dorsal aorta at CS13, CS15, and CS18, where formation of primary ganglia is induced [13].

Together, these results indicate that neuroblasts in sympathetic ganglia might arise earlier than intra-adrenal neuroblasts and chromaffin cells. Also, it seems likely that they develop directly from NCCs instead of differentiation via SCPs. This hypothesis is further supported by the missing intermediate cells between SCPs and neuroblasts in sympathetic ganglia described here and lineage tracing experiments in mice [3]. Future snRNAseq experiments covering the developmental stages between CS15 and CS20 will provide more reliable insights into the developmental origins of sympathetic ganglia neurons. In addition, methods preserving spatial tissue organization like IHC or smFISH on human embryos are needed to validate localization of the analyzed cell types.

7.2 Developmental Programs in Neuroblastoma

7.2.1 Neuroblastomas Mirror Neuroblast Differentiation States

Neuroblastomas are thought to arise during the development of sympathetic neurons and chromaffin cells from the neural crest [14, 15, 16]. To define the specific cell type that neuroblastomas are likely to originate from, the transcriptomes of single neuroblastoma cells were studied and compared to transcriptomes of cell populations in the developing adrenal medulla [4]. Single neuroblastoma cells show closest similarity to developing sympathetic neuroblasts. Notably, different neuroblastoma subgroups vary in their differentiation state along the normal neuroblast differentiation trajectory. Low-risk tumors closely mirror the most differentiated late neuroblast population. In contrast, *MYCN*-amplified neuroblastomas show higher similarity to less differentiated early neuroblasts and also display features of bridge cells. *TERT*-rearranged and ALT tumors are intermediate between low-risk and *MYCN*-amplified tumors. A subgroup of tumors, termed neuroblastomas with mesenchymal features, are even less differentiated than *MYCN*-amplified tumors, resembling bridge and connecting progenitor cells in addition to chromaffin cells and early neuroblasts. Several other recent publications compared neuroblastoma cells to normal cells in the developing adrenal gland, but not all of them drew the same conclusions. Kildisiute et al. identified all neuroblastoma cells to have a sympathetic neuroblast (sympathoblast)-like phenotype [6]. Although this is generally consistent with results presented here, it seems that their tumor cohort does not contain any less differentiated tumors that show similarity to bridge cells, like it was seen for *MYCN*-amplified tumors and NBs with mesenchymal features in the study by Jansky et al. This observation illustrates the significance of a representative tumor panel, which, in Jansky et al., was accomplished through access to bulk RNA-seq and whole genome sequencing data for a large neuroblastoma cohort. Further, it highlights the advantages of snRNA-seq, which allows analysis of stored frozen samples, instead of using fresh tumor samples. Kildisiute et al. performed tumor-to-normal cell comparisons on clusters of cells instead of single-cell level, which might also explain the lack of bridge-like tumor cells. In the study conducted by Kameneva et al., the majority of tumor cells showed similarity to normal sympathetic neuroblasts (sympathoblasts), with some cells being assigned to normal chromaffin cells, which is in line with results presented in Jansky et al. [5]. In their study, no normal bridge cells were determined and therefore also not compared to neuroblastoma cells. Another study identified neuroblastomas to display a primarily chromaffin cell-like phenotype [7]. Considering that normal chromaffin cells and sympathetic neuroblasts were annotated incorrectly, as discussed above, their data also confirm the sympathetic neuroblast identity of neuroblastomas.

Taken together, the observed similarity of the neuroblastoma and the developing sympathetic neuroblast transcriptomes indicate that immature neuroblasts are the developmental origin of neuroblastoma. However, this approach is not able to unambiguously identify a tumor cell of origin, as tumor cells could further differentiate after acquisition of first alterations or dedifferentiate in response to oncogenic alterations (Fig. 7.3, dashed red arrows). Hence, immediate progenitors of sympathetic neuroblasts or more mature neuroblasts are also possible neuroblastoma origins. Another hint that sympathetic neuroblasts might indeed be the neuroblastoma cell of origin was identified by analysis of expression of cell identity genes harboring large super enhancers, which are occasionally involved in neuroblastoma-specific enhancer hijacking events. These highly active cell identity genes, whose enhancers drive expression of neuroblastoma oncogenes in a subset of tumors, were selectively expressed in the normal neuroblast trajectory [4]. These data suggest, that sympathetic neuroblasts are the cells in the developing adrenal medulla most susceptible to neuroblastoma oncogenic transformation. Expression of neuroblastoma oncogenic drivers in models of developing neuroblasts and related cell types may provide a better understanding of developmental origin and neuroblastoma initiation in the future.

Current transgenic neuroblastoma mouse models utilize ectopic expression of human *MYCN* under control of the Th promoter to target MYCN expression to neuroblastoma cells of origin [17]. However, the single-cell transcriptomic analyses of the developing human adrenal gland, presented in several recent publications, identified TH to be primarily expressed in chromaffin cells and only at lower levels in neuroblasts. Hence, MYCN expression is primarily targeted to the wrong cell type, which might explain why these models do not fully recapitulate human neuroblastomas.

Despite intensive research on new therapeutic targets for neuroblastoma therapy, effective options for high-risk tumors are lacking. Identification of neuroblasts as the transcriptionally most similar normal neuroblastoma counterpart will guide future studies on the functional evaluation of candidate genes as novel therapeutic targets. Careful comparison of sympathetic neuroblast and neuroblastoma expression profiles might give new insights into cancer drivers and enable identification of neuroblastoma identity genes with expression restricted to pre-natal tissues. Furthermore, these cancer to normal comparisons might facilitate determination of neuroblastoma-specific genes, which can be used to refine risk stratification.

Although few neuroblastoma cells displayed features of bridge cells or connecting progenitor cells, neuroblastomas generally showed very limited intra-tumoral heterogeneity. No distinct differentiation hierarchy as, for example, in medulloblastomas, which harbor cells with primitive progenitor properties and cells with

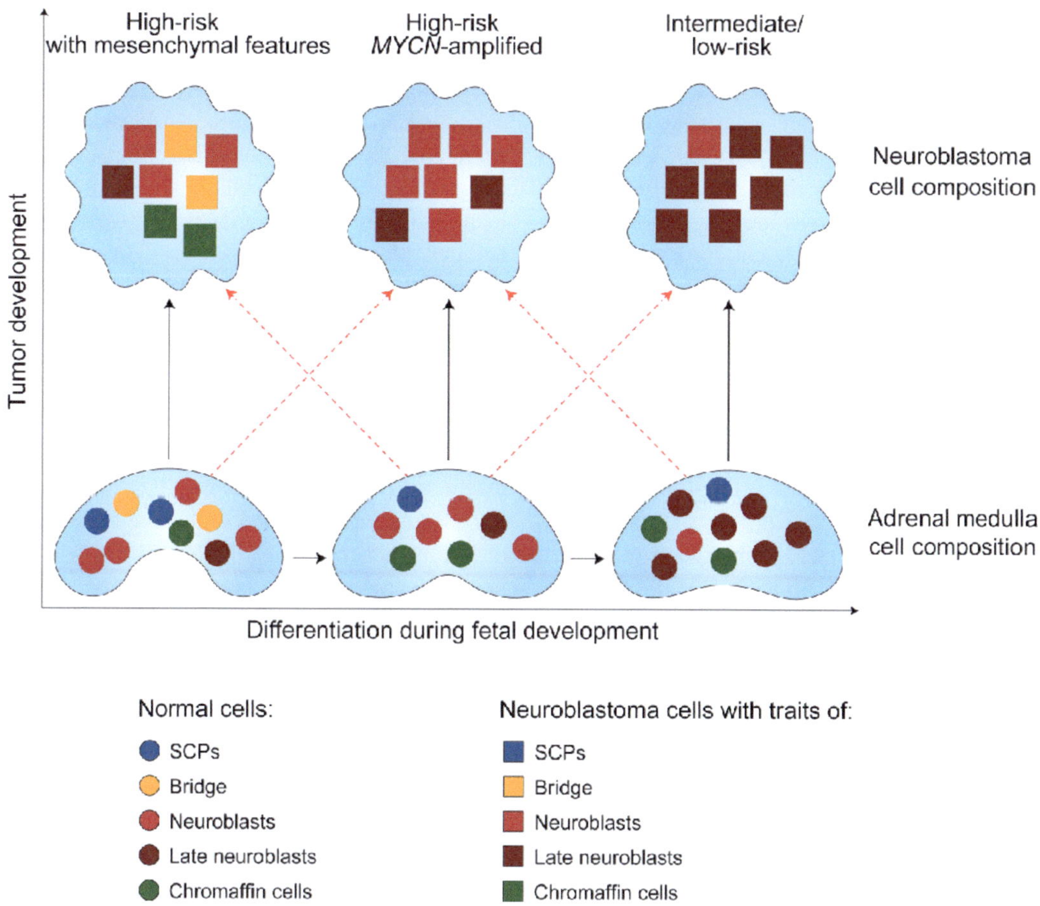

Fig. 7.3 Developmental phenotype of neuroblastoma subgroups. Schematic illustration of the composition of normal human adrenal glands during fetal development and the composition of neuroblastoma split by subgroups. Solid black arrows indicate the suggested origin of neuroblastoma subgroups at different developmental stages and dashed red arrows indicate alternative origins, involving differentiation or de-differentiation. Adapted from Rohrer et al. [31]

mature neuronal phenotype [18], was identified in neuroblastoma. These results suggest that neuroblastomas are more homogeneous than medulloblastomas. However, it is also possible that this is a limitation of 10x Genomics scRNA-seq, in which subtle changes in the differentiation state of the cells may not have been captured due to the limited number of genes detected per cell. A more in-depth analysis using for example smart-seq2, which captures a higher number of genes per cell and profiles the full-length transcript enabling detection of SNVs, could provide a better view on neuroblastoma intra-tumoral heterogeneity.

7.2.2 Neuroblastoma Differentiation along the Normal Neuroblast Trajectory Has Prognostic Impact

To further validate the developmental identity of neuroblastoma, bulk expression data from two large cohorts of neuroblastomas were deconvoluted using adrenal medullary cell population marker genes [4]. Developing neuroblasts were further validated as the likely neuroblastoma developmental origin. In these larger cohorts, differentiation state along the normal neuroblast trajectory was associated with patient risk and stage. Moreover, the fractions of more differentiated late neuroblast-like tumor cells and less differentiated cycling neuroblast-like tumor cells were predictive of patient survival. Contrary to this study, chromaffin cell, instead of neuroblast differentiation state, was identified to be predictive of neuroblastoma patient outcome by Dong et al. [7]. Considering their incorrect cell type annotation of chromaffin cells and neuroblasts, these results are in line with results presented here. Kameneva et al. also identified expression of the normal cycling sympathetic neuroblast signatures to be associated with poor patient survival, independent of *MYCN* amplification status and cell cycle genes [5]. In contrast, mature neuroblasts were associated with a good prognosis. Together this indicates that distinct developmental programs are expressed in different neuroblastoma subtypes and deconvolution of bulk expression data can be used to identify these programs.

7.2.3 Neuroblastoma Cell Lines Resemble the SCP to Neuroblast or Chromaffin Cell Differentiation Trajectory

To assess how well cell lines reflect neuroblastoma developmental identity, neuroblastoma cell lines were studied by scRNA-seq and compared to developing adrenal medullary cell populations [4]. Cell line SK-N-SH has previously been described to harbor neuroblastic, intermediate, and substrate-adherent cells [19, 20]. Super-enhancer profiling identified neuroblastic cells to show adrenergic identity and substrate-adherent cells to have mesenchymal identity [21]. Of note, the three cell populations were recovered by scRNA-seq analysis. Comparison to developing sympathoadrenal cells identified adrenergic cells to match to developing neuroblasts and mesenchymal cells to resemble primarily SCPs. Intermediate SK-N-SH cells showed similarity to a broad set of cell types, including bridge, connecting progenitor cells, chromaffin cells, and neuroblasts. Results for intermediate SK-N-SH cells are comparable to results for neuroblastomas with mesenchymal features, indicating that intermediate cells might represent NBs with mesenchymal features in culture. An in-depth comparison of the cells in the future might show if intermediate SK-N-SH cells truly resemble cells identified in neuroblastomas with mesenchymal features. Mesenchymal SK-N-SH cells with similarity to SCPs were even more undifferentiated along the normal SCP to neuroblast trajectory. Comparable malignant mesenchymal cells with features of SCPs were not identified in neuroblastoma tumors, which is consistent with Dong et al. and Kildisiute et al. [6, 7]. In contrast, a recent pre-print study, profiling neuroblastomas by scRNA-seq, identified malignant mesenchymal cells and malignant SCP-like cells in addition to malignant adrenergic cells within neuroblastoma tumors (Olsen et al., 2020, bioRxiv). Future single-cell transcriptomic studies on larger cohorts will have to show if malignant mesenchymal cells are rarely found in neuroblastomas or if cells identified as malignant cells by Olsen et al. are non-malignant normal mesenchymal and Schwann cells.

A possible explanation for the absence of mesenchymal neuroblastoma cells from patient tumors was proposed by another study. While neuroblastoma cells were identified to be plastic in vitro, the neuroblastoma phenotype was shown to be influenced by the tumor microenvironment, which strongly pushed cells towards an adrenergic phenotype in vivo [22]. Two out of three neuroblastomas with mesenchymal features, identified in the study presented by Jansky et al., were derived from metastatic sites, raising the question if the microenvironment in metastatic niches might, in contrast to primary neuroblastoma sites, influence neuroblastoma identity towards a more mesenchymal phenotype. Future studies will have to dissect how the microenvironment can influence neuroblastoma identity, which could come along with crucial implications for patients' individual prognosis and therapy. The finding that mutant RAS pathway genes can induce mesenchymal features in neuroblastoma published in Gartlgruber et al. indicates that specific mutations or rare combinations of mutations may promote a mesenchymal phenotype also in tumors [23]. The adrenergic neuroblastoma cell line Kelly showed a primarily chromaffin cell-like identity, which was not observed in adrenergic neuroblastoma tumors. Future studies will have to address if this is a cell culture artifact, or rare genetic alterations may transdifferentiate tumor cells towards the chromaffin cell lineage. Members of the JUN/FOS family of transcription factors were active in normal developing chromaffin cells and may therefore be interesting candidates for promoting a chromaffin cell-like identity.

7.2.4 Strategies to Release the Neuroblastoma Differentiation Block

Releasing blocked differentiation has been proposed as a promising therapeutic concept for neuroblastoma [24]. In Jansky et al., TFAP2B was identified as a key regulator during sympathetic neuroblast differentiation and transcription factor MYCN was active in developing neuroblasts and post-migrating neural crest cells. In neuroblastomas, MYCN was the main transcription factor active in *MYCN*-amplified tumors, whereas TFAP2B was primarily active in low-risk tumors. Due to their roles during normal neuroblast development and in neuroblastoma, both transcription factors were analyzed for their potential involvement in blocking neuroblastoma differentiation. Profiling *MYCN*-amplified neuroblastoma cells after knockdown of MYCN identified an increase in expression of signatures for normal neuroblasts and bridge cells, suggesting that oncogenic MYCN causes de-differentiation along the normal neuroblast lineage (Fig. 7.4). In addition, oncogenic MYCN was identified to promote proliferation, which is consistent with studies identifying MYCN to promote proliferation and to prevent differentiation of neuronal progenitor cells [25, 26]. Earlier, during development in neural crest cells, MYCN was described to promote neuronal differentiation [27]. Activity of TFAP2B in normal neuroblast development and low-risk neuroblastoma suggests loss of

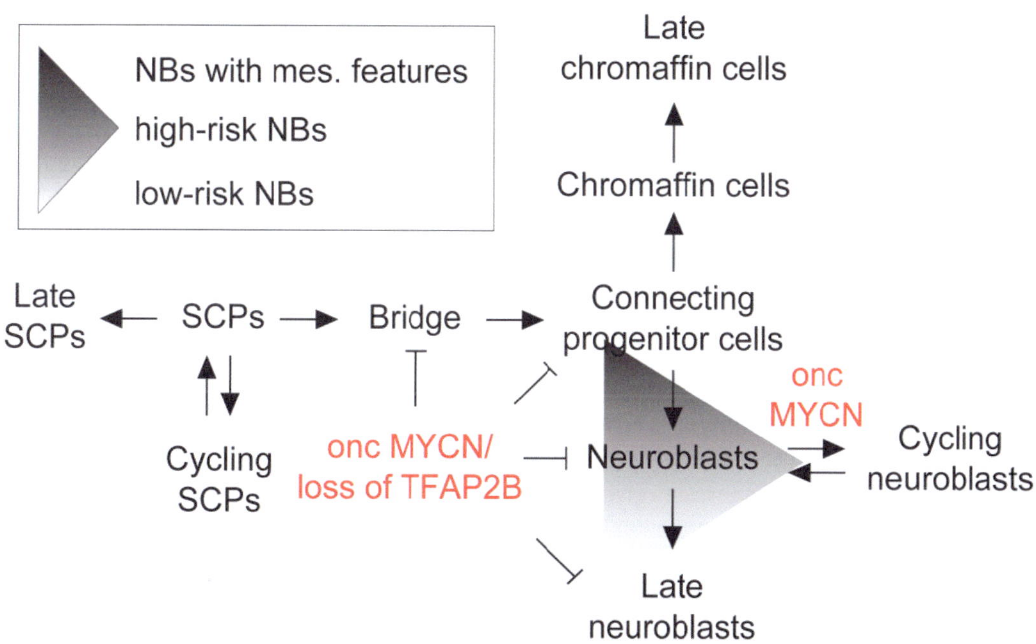

Fig. 7.4 Roles of TFAP2B and MYCN in blocking neuroblastoma differentiation. Schematic illustration depicting the influences of oncogenic MYCN and loss of TFAP2B on developmental programs in neuroblastoma. Adapted from Jansky et al. [4]

TFAP2B to block differentiation. Profiling of *MYCN*-amplified neuroblastoma cells after ectopic overexpression of TFAP2B identified increased expression of signatures for normal neuroblasts and chromaffin cells. These results indicate that normal differentiation can at least in part be restored by TFAP2B re-expression, which is in line with a study describing TFAP2B to mediate noradrenergic neuronal differentiation in neuroblastoma (Fig. 7.4) [28].

Retinoic acids are known to induce morphologic differentiation in neuroblastoma cell lines and are used in standard high-risk neuroblastoma therapy for the management of minimal residual disease after myeloablative therapy [29, 30]. To test whether differentiation along the normal neuroblast lineage is induced by ATRA treatment, expression profiles of neuroblastoma cells after ATRA treatment were analyzed. ATRA-treated cells showed morphological features of differentiation and increased expression of neuroblast differentiation markers, but also high fractions of less differentiated neuroblast-like cells. Presence of less differentiated neuroblasts suggests that normal differentiation cannot fully be restored by ATRA treatment. These results might explain why the therapeutic effect of retinoic acid therapy in the clinic is limited.

7.3 Conclusion and Perspectives

Using single-cell transcriptomics, several recent studies provided new insights into human development of sympathetic neurons and chromaffin cells. Especially in the developing adrenal gland, but also in sympathetic ganglia and the neural crest, the different cell populations and their lineage relationships and differentiation trajectories were resolved. In contrast to the previous view, late migrating SCPs were identified to give rise to chromaffin cells and sympathetic neuroblasts in the developing human adrenal gland. In addition, transient cell populations during this transition, bridge cells and connecting progenitor cells, were determined. The studies identified important transcription factors, which regulate fate decisions and characterized the expression profiles of the, to date largely inaccessible, human adrenal medullary cell types. In contrast to adrenal neuroblasts, there was no evidence for neuroblasts in sympathetic ganglia to arise from SCPs. However, the presented data indicate that sympathetic ganglia neuroblasts directly originate from neural crest cells. Additional snRNAseq experiments on more samples and earlier developmental time points are needed to further substantiate this hypothesis. Despite their potentially different origins, the transcriptomes of adrenal and ganglia sympathetic neuroblasts showed very high similarity. Additionally, the fate of neural crest cells was analyzed from their specification from the neural tube, followed by EMT and migration to the induction of differentiation programs. Moreover, the corresponding transcription factors regulating neural crest development were identified. Although new insights into the normal development of sympathoadrenal cells were gained, they were primarily studied to provide clues as to the origin of neuroblastoma. Hence, the central finding of these studies was that neuroblastomas transcriptionally resemble developing sympathetic neuroblasts. Notably, different neuroblastoma subgroups cover various differentiation states along the normal neuroblast differentiation trajectory. Neuroblastoma differentiation state along this normal neuroblast trajectory is associated with outcome. Although the present studies provided some evidence that neuroblasts are the cells that are at highest risk to acquire neuroblastoma-specific alterations, the neuroblastoma cell of origin could also differentiate or de-differentiate after acquisition of oncogenic alterations and hence be a more or less differentiated cell type. To unambiguously identify the cell of origin, neuroblastoma driver genes should be expressed in models covering all cell types during normal sympathetic neuron development in the future.

Heterogeneous neuroblastoma cell lines harboring mesenchymal subpopulations show similarity to normal SCPs, whereas no mesenchymal neuroblastoma cells with similarity to SCPs were detected in tumors. In tumors, neuroblastoma cells with some mesenchymal features showing similarity to bridge and connecting progenitor cells were identified. Future single-cell transcriptomic studies on a larger cohort of neuroblastomas are needed to clarify if mesenchymal neuroblastoma cells are a cell culture artifact or are present also in patient tumors. Thirant et al. describe an influence of the microenvironment on the mesenchymal or adrenergic neuroblastoma phenotype in vivo [22] and the neuroblastomas with mesenchymal features identified in this study were primarily derived from metastatic sites. Hence, the influence of the microenvironment, especially in the context of metastasis, on neuroblastoma identity should additionally be addressed in future experiments. Especially, identity of single neuroblastoma cells from different metastatic sites should be determined. Identification of strategies to overcome the differentiation block is an important therapeutic concept in neuroblastoma. Central regulators in normal neuroblast differentiation were identified. Targeting these regulators, for example, by inhibition of MYCN or re-expression of TFAP2B, was shown to at least partly restore normal neuroblast differentiation. Furthermore, by assessing retinoic acid differentiation therapy for the induction of normal neuroblast differentiation, the framework to evaluate future therapeutic concepts that are based on differentiation, is established. A future in depth comparison of normal neuroblast and neuroblastoma transcriptomes might enable identification and functional evaluation of novel candidate driver genes and improve risk stratification.

References

1. Anderson DJ, Michelsohn A. Role of glucocorticoids in the chromaffin-neuron developmental decision. Int J Dev Neurosci. 1989;7:475–87.
2. Unsicker K, Krisch B, Otten U, Thoenen H. Nerve growth factor-induced fiber outgrowth from isolated rat adrenal chromaffin cells: impairment by glucocorticoids. Proc Natl Acad Sci U S A. 1978;75:3498–502.
3. Furlan A, et al. Multipotent peripheral glial cells generate neuroendocrine cells of the adrenal medulla. Science. 2017;357:eaal3753.
4. Jansky S, et al. Single-cell transcriptomic analyses provide insights into the developmental origins of neuroblastoma. Nat Genet. 2021;53:683–93.
5. Kameneva P, et al. Single-cell transcriptomics of human embryos identifies multiple sympathoblast lineages with potential implications for neuroblastoma origin. Nat Genet. 2021;53:694–706.
6. Kildisiute G, et al. Tumor to normal single-cell mRNA comparisons reveal a pan-neuroblastoma cancer cell. Sci Adv. 2021;7:eabd3311.
7. Dong R, et al. Single-cell characterization of malignant phenotypes and developmental trajectories of adrenal neuroblastoma. Cancer Cell. 2020;38:716–33. e716.
8. Kildisiute G, Young MD, Behjati S. Pitfalls of applying mouse markers to human adrenal medullary cells. Cancer Cell. 2021;39:132–3.
9. Bedoya-Reina OC, Schlisio S. Chromaffin cells with Sympathoblast signature: too similar to keep apart? Cancer Cell. 2021;39:134–5.
10. Magro G, Grasso S. Immunohistochemical identification and comparison of glial cell lineage in foetal, neonatal, adult and neoplastic human adrenal medulla. Histochem J. 1997;29:293–9.
11. Kameneva P, et al. Evolutionary switch in expression of key markers between mouse and human leads to mis-assignment of cell types in developing adrenal medulla. Cancer Cell. 2021;39:590–1.
12. Duband JL, Monier F, Delannet M, Newgreen D. Epithelium-mesenchyme transition during neural crest development. Acta Anat (Basel). 1995;154:63–78.
13. Betters E, Liu Y, Kjaeldgaard A, Sundstrom E, Garcia-Castro MI. Analysis of early human neural crest development. Dev Biol. 2010;344:578–92.
14. Hoehner JC, et al. A developmental model of neuroblastoma: differentiating stroma-poor tumors' progress along an extra-adrenal chromaffin lineage. Lab Investig. 1996;75:659–75.
15. Maris JM, Hogarty MD, Bagatell R, Cohn SL. Neuroblastoma. Lancet. 2007;369:2106–20.
16. Ratner N, Brodeur GM, Dale RC, Schor NF. The "neuro" of neuroblastoma: neuroblastoma as a neurodevelopmental disorder. Ann Neurol. 2016;80:13–23.
17. Rasmuson A, et al. Tumor development, growth characteristics and spectrum of genetic aberrations in the TH-MYCN mouse model of neuroblastoma. PLoS One. 2012;7:e51297.
18. Hovestadt V, et al. Resolving medulloblastoma cellular architecture by single-cell genomics. Nature. 2019;572:74–9.
19. Biedler JL, Helson L, Spengler BA. Morphology and growth, tumorigenicity, and cytogenetics of human neuroblastoma cells in continuous culture. Cancer Res. 1973;33:2643–52.
20. Biedler JL, Roffler-Tarlov S, Schachner M, Freedman LS. Multiple neurotransmitter synthesis by human neuroblastoma cell lines and clones. Cancer Res. 1978;38:3751–7.
21. Boeva V, et al. Heterogeneity of neuroblastoma cell identity defined by transcriptional circuitries. Nat Genet. 2017;49:1408–13.

22. Thirant C, et al. Reversible transitions between noradrenergic and mesenchymal tumor identities define cell plasticity in neuroblastoma. Nat Commun. 2023;14:2575.
23. Gartlgruber M, et al. Super enhancers define regulatory subtypes and cell identity in neuroblastoma. Nat Cancer. 2021;2:114–28.
24. Matthay KK, et al. Successful treatment of stage III neuroblastoma based on prospective biologic staging: a Children's Cancer Group study. J Clin Oncol. 1998;16:1256–64.
25. Alam G, et al. MYCN promotes the expansion of Phox2B-positive neuronal progenitors to drive neuroblastoma development. Am J Pathol. 2009;175:856–66.
26. Ryl T, et al. Cell-cycle position of single MYC-driven cancer cells dictates their susceptibility to a chemotherapeutic drug. Cell Syst. 2017;5:237–50. e238.
27. Wakamatsu Y, Watanabe Y, Nakamura H, Kondoh H. Regulation of the neural crest cell fate by N-myc: promotion of ventral migration and neuronal differentiation. Development. 1997;124:1953–62.
28. Ikram F, et al. Transcription factor activating protein 2 beta (TFAP2B) mediates noradrenergic neuronal differentiation in neuroblastoma. Mol Oncol. 2016;10:344–59.
29. Matthay KK, et al. Long-term results for children with high-risk neuroblastoma treated on a randomized trial of myeloablative therapy followed by 13-cis-retinoic acid: a children's oncology group study. J Clin Oncol. 2009;27:1007–13.
30. Sidell N. Retinoic acid-induced growth inhibition and morphologic differentiation of human neuroblastoma cells in vitro. J Natl Cancer Inst. 1982;68:589–96.
31. Rohrer H. Linking human sympathoadrenal development and neuroblastoma. Nat Genet. 2021;53:593–4.

Neuroblastoma Tumor Microenvironment: Innate and Adaptive Immunity

8

Michael Zobel and Shahab Asgharzadeh

8.1 Introduction

For the majority of neuroblastoma patients who present with widely metastatic disease, long-term cure remains elusive despite multimodal therapy. The introduction of monoclonal antibody therapy targeting disialoganglioside (GD2) on the surface of neuroblastoma has led to improved outcomes for this population, along with that of patients with relapsed and/or refractory disease; however, long-term survival remains poor [1–4]. In contrast, there exists a subset of young patients (<18 months of age at diagnosis) with neuroblastoma who experience spontaneous tumor regression (stage MS) or have excellent long-term with modest chemotherapy survival despite metastatic disease (stage M with MYCN non-amplified tumors) [5, 6]. Recognition of the spontaneous regression phenomenon prompted investigation of tumor-associated antigens and tumor immune recognition by Hellstrom et al., with early in vitro investigations demonstrating that lymphocytes from children with neuroblastoma, and from their mothers, had anti-neuroblastoma activity [7–9]. While these findings did not consistently correlate with in vivo eradication, particularly for rapidly growing neuroblastoma, they did support a theory of immune recognition in neuroblastoma clearance. Since then, substantial investigation into the role of the tumor microenvironment (TME) in malignancies, including neuroblastoma, has elucidated some of the complex interactions between tumor and immune cells that mediate tumor establishment, persistence, and eradication. The persistently high relapse rate of neuroblastoma has shifted the focus of research toward elucidating both escape mechanisms intrinsic to neuroblastoma cells and mechanisms extrinsic to cells, yet within the TME, that limit the anti-tumor effects of innate and adaptive immune responses. Furthermore, the limited efficacy of chimeric antigen receptor (CAR) T cell therapies directed against neuroblastoma also suggests an immunosuppressive neuroblastoma TME [10–14]. Immune cells within the TME of many solid tumors are heterogeneous, which in neuroblastoma is affected by variable tumor biology and clinical features such as MYCN proto-oncogene amplification, the site of disease (e.g., bone marrow versus liver), and relapsed and/or refractory disease. Elucidating the identity of and frequency of immune cells, with improved understanding of their functional roles in the pathophysiology of the neuroblastoma TME, will help guide identification of novel immunotherapies.

M. Zobel
Cancer and Blood Disease Institute, Children's Hospital Los Angeles, Los Angeles, CA, USA

Division of Pediatric Surgery, Children's Hospital Los Angeles, Los Angeles, CA, USA

S. Asgharzadeh (✉)
Department of Pediatrics, Children's Hospital Los Angeles, Los Angeles, CA, USA
e-mail: sasgharzadeh@chla.usc.edu

S. Asgharzadeh, F. Westermann (eds.), *Neuroblastoma*, Pediatric Oncology,
https://doi.org/10.1007/978-3-031-51292-6_8

In this chapter, we aim to review the interaction of the innate immune system and neuroblastoma within the tumor microenvironment, followed by a review of the current understanding of the role played by the adaptive immune system. We will review the data available by cell type with a focus on human neuroblastoma, supplemented by supportive murine studies.

8.2 The Innate Immune System and Neuroblastoma

The innate immune system, comprising plasma proteins and cellular defenses, is involved in solid tumor recognition. However, immune-mediated destruction clearly fails given that many tumors persist despite these measurable innate defenses. Macrophages, dendritic cells (DCs), and neutrophils represent terminally differentiated myeloid cells that evolved as major protective effector cells against pathogens and are also crucial in tissue remodeling [15]. DCs and macrophages, the antigen presenting cells (APCs) of the innate immune system, play a key role in priming T cell responses of the adaptive immune system, and their function can be strongly influenced by the tumor microenvironment, as will be reviewed below. Natural killer (NK) cells, NKT cells, and γδ TCR-expressing T cells (γδT) have both positive and negative immune regulatory functions but can contribute to tumor control both through interactions with APCs and by affecting T cell cytokine production [16].

Tumor-associated macrophages (TAMs) and tumor-associated neutrophils (TANs) represent major components of the TME whose native immune functions have been repurposed to promote tumor growth, treatment resistance, and metastasis [17–19]. In addition, two major myeloid subgroups of MDSCs with distinct immunosuppressive functions also have been identified: monocytic (M-)MDSCs and polymorphonuclear cells (PMN-)MDSCs [20]. In various pathogenic conditions, including chronic inflammatory states, autoimmune diseases, and malignancies, excessive myelopoiesis can result in accumulation of immature myeloid cells that are distinct from their terminally differentiated counterparts (i.e., macrophages and neutrophils). Myelopoiesis is induced by GM-CSF, while G-CSF and M-CSF induce the differentiation of granulocytes and macrophages, respectively. This aberrant myelopoiesis is regulated by many factors, including GM-CSF, IL6, IL10, COX2, and VEGF, all of which contribute to the persistent expansion of the immature myeloid cells observed in these conditions. The broad term Myeloid-derived Suppressor Cells (MDSCs) was created to recognize their significant immunosuppressive capabilities in cancers [21]. Murine studies of inflammation demonstrated expansion of these heterogeneous immature myeloid cells with variable monocytic and neutrophil markers, including CD11b, Ly6C, Ly6G [22]. Given their potent immunosuppressive capabilities, the fundamental role of MDSCs in inflammation is likely to protect the host from tissue damage caused by uncontrolled immune responses in the setting of significant, chronic inflammation, and/or infection. Cancer cells likely coopt this activity to protect themselves from elimination by the immune system.

The specific markers that distinguish M-MDSCs and PMN-MDSCs, as well as those specific to immature early stage MDSCs (eMDSCs), have been evaluated systemically and described elsewhere [23, 24]. While markers that differentiate MDSCs have been described in mice, clear discernment of MDSCs in humans remains incomplete. Surface expression of CD14, CD33, CD11b, and HLA-DR has been used to characterize MDSCs in humans [20]. Irrespective, both M-MDSCs and PMN-MDSCs can inhibit immune activity of T cells and NK cells through secretion of reactive oxygen species (ROS), nitrogen oxide (NO), arginase-1, etc. and induction of regulatory T cells (Tregs) [25].

The identification of the various myeloid cells in tumors using standard immunohistochemistry techniques remains challenging. TAMs and M-MDSCs, and TANs and PMN-MDSCs, represent the continuum of differentiation in aberrant myelopoiesis in tumor development, but have been shown to have distinct biochemical and functional properties.

8.2.1 Tumor-Associated Macrophages (TAMs) and M-MDSC

Polarization of macrophages to either pro-tumorigenic or anti-tumorigenic phenotypes has been well-described with recent postulation that polarity exists along a continuum [26]. In vitro, macrophages that are activated via stimulation with IFN-γ, TNFα, and/or GM-CSF become M1 macrophages, and are thought to play a tumor-suppressive role via production of pro-inflammatory cytokines. Conversely, macrophages activated by immune complexes and/or specific interleukin cytokines become M2 macrophages that produce anti-inflammatory cytokines and are tumor-promoting, with direct effects on tumor angiogenesis, tumor growth, and suppression of other immune cells in the TME [27]. Macrophages found within tumors, TAMs, have been shown to suppress T cell proliferation and activation [28]. TAMs found in neuroblastoma possess the phenotype of M2 macrophages, express inflammatory cytokines (IL-1b, IL-6, IL-12, TNFα), and contribute to high IL-10 and TGF-β in the TME [29–32].

In patients with neuroblastoma, TAM infiltration into tumors has been studied to understand the implication in prognosis. Initial gene expression profiling study comparing children with metastatic disease lacking MYCN amplification revealed significant difference in genes and pathways related to immune cell and macrophage infiltration in those older than 18 months of age (high-risk by INPC criteria) compared to the younger cohort (intermediate-risk) [33]. IHC evaluation of MYCN non-amplified tumors of patients over 18 months of age revealed tumor infiltration of macrophages with a largely M2-like phenotype, and this was increased in metastatic tumors compared to locoregional tumors. A PCR-based 48-gene expression profiling of these tumor samples found that high expression of 14 tumor- and inflammation-related genes was predictive of progression-free survival (PFS), with significantly worsened PFS in tumors with higher expression profiles. Notably, the inflammation-related genes involved in polarization of TAMs (i.e., IL-6R, IL-10, CD16, CD14) were significant outcome predictors, supporting the association between TAM/MDSC polarization within the TME and poor prognosis [34].

Recent research has focused on better understanding the interaction of macrophages with other stromal cells, such as fibroblasts, within the TME. Hashimoto et al. suggest a relationship between macrophages and fibroblasts (also known as cancer-associated fibroblasts, or CAFs) that results in pro-tumor activation of both cell types and further promotes tumor proliferation [35]. They found that increased TAM infiltration in neuroblastoma samples, with a high density of co-localized macrophages and fibroblasts, was significantly correlated with higher clinical stage, MYCN amplification, an unfavorable histologic classification, and a higher COG risk classification. Furthermore, increased TAM infiltration was associated with the presence of bone marrow metastases, supporting the potential role of TAMs in the metastasis [35].

TAM recruitment to neuroblastoma tumors may also play a role in worsening prognosis via upregulation transcriptional expression of oncogenes. Hajidaniel et al. utilized a murine model of spontaneous MYCN non-amplified neuroblastoma and observed that macrophages recruited to the TME as TAMs enhanced local neuroblastoma proliferation in vivo, and also appeared to induce transcriptional upregulation of the MYC oncogene by these neuroblastoma cells in co-culture [36]. They further demonstrated that co-culture of human neuroblastoma cell lines with M2 macrophages resulted in increased MYC protein levels, providing evidence that macrophages may alter neuroblastoma cell MYCN amplification, worsening prognosis. Recent work by our group also show the cooperative nature of TAM with CAFs in culture with neuroblastoma leading to significant TGFβ1 levels required for suppression of NK and T-cell activities [37].

In neuroblastoma, there is evidence that presence or increase frequency of MDSC promotes development of tumors of TH-MYCN and NB-Tag transgenic mice as well as in syngeneic NSX2 models [38–40]. Most of these studies have used markers that are more consistent with current definition of M-MDSC, although in some cases, P-MDSC cannot be readily distinguished based on flow cytometry markers used. MDSCs in these pre-clinical models contributed to ROS, arginase-1 and TGFβ1 accumulation and in certain therapeutic models their inhibition reduced tumor growth kinetics and increased T-cell tumor infiltration [38–40]. MDSC inhibition via CSFR1 inhibition or Bruton's tyrosine kinase inhibition also potentiated effects of immune checkpoints in these murine models [41, 42]. There is very limited data on the frequency and type of MDSCs in human neuroblastoma tumors. Recent work by our group utilizing Imaging Mass Cytometry (IMC) shows evidence of M-MDSC and P-MDSC in tumors of children with refractory tumors (in preparation), and further studies utilizing high-parameter imaging or single-cell studies likely will further elucidate their prognostic significance.

8.2.2 Tumor-Associated Neutrophils (TANs) and PMN-MDSCs

Neutrophils are the most abundant immune cells in the peripheral blood and play a key role in innate defense against infection and are increasingly recognized for their role in tumor immunology. While their role in neuroblastoma is not well-understood, there is active investigation into the role of neutrophils in other solid tumors. While phenotypically similar to circulating neutrophils, TANs along with their immature versions (PMN-MDSCs) have near opposite functions and are immunosuppressive, inhibiting anti-tumor functions of T cells, NK cells, and other myeloid cells [43]. TANs have been identified within tumors with anti-tumor properties, like the TAMs previously described. Unfortunately, early studies exploring the role of neutrophils in cancer failed to differentiate TANs from PMN-MDSCs, contributing to confusion regarding their independent roles [44].

Traditionally, neutrophils were described as the first responders and mediators of target cell or pathogen death via a variety of mechanisms: phagocytosis, secretion of reactive oxygen species and/or hyperchlorous acid, TNFα and IFNγ production, degranulation and release of cytotoxic proteins and enzymes, TNF-related apoptosis-inducing ligand (TRAIL), or via antibody-dependent cell-mediated cytotoxicity. Their role in modulating adaptive immune responses along with their pro- and anti-tumorigenic properties are increasingly being explored [45]. Specifically, neutrophil polarization, similar to that of macrophages, has been described with separate identification of anti-tumor neutrophils (N1) and pro-tumorigenic neutrophils (N2). N1 neutrophils have cytotoxic potential and may play a role in antitumor immune memory, whereas N2 neutrophils may play a role in tumor growth, invasion, and metastasis [46, 47].

In neuroblastoma, neutrophils can mediate antibody-dependent cellular cytotoxicity (ADCC) via anti-GD2 antibody bound to GD2-expressing human neuroblastoma cell lines; however, conversely, they can also be growth promoting in the absence of antibody and/or GD2 expression [48]. Neutrophil-mediated lysis of human neuroblastoma cells requires neutrophil degranulation with the release of defensins, granular proteins that bind and permeabilize cells, and cathepsin-G, a protease directly involved in tumor lysis. Administration of granulocyte-macrophage colony stimulatory factor (GM-CSF) further enhances neutrophil ADCC via increased release of these lytic granular molecules [49]. Similar neutrophil ADCC findings have been shown in other solid tumor models in the presence of target-specific monoclonal antibodies, and this ADCC was also further enhanced by GM-CSF via increased expression of CD11/CD18 molecules [50, 51]. In a clinical trial, neuroblastoma patients treated with an anti-GD2 monoclonal antibody, 3F8, in combination with GM-CSF were found to have increased activation of granulocytes during therapy [52]. Furthermore, this increase in the frequency of activated granulocytes positively correlated with PFS, further supporting an anti-tumorigenic role of granulocytes in neuroblastoma eradication [52].

In contrast to these anti-tumor properties, pro-tumorigenic roles of TANs have been demonstrated in murine models of non-neuroblastoma solid tumors. Specifically, in an orthotopic small cell lung cancer murine model, TANs appeared to recruit immunosuppressive Tregs to the TME via increased secretion of the chemoattractant CCL17 relative to their splenic or circulating neutrophil counterparts [53]. N2-polarized TANs were able to attract significantly more Tregs than N1 TANs, an effect that was decreased in the presence of CCL17-neutralizing antibody and abrogated when neutrophils were depleted post-tumor inoculation. Additionally, neutrophil expression of CCL17 was only found in the tumor tissue, and not in adjacent, healthy lung. Given the immunosuppressive nature of Tregs, TAN-mediated recruitment of Tregs to the TME may represent a potential pro-tumorigenic role of neutrophils [53].

Though the current understanding of the pro-tumor function of neutrophils and neutrophil-derived cells in neuroblastoma is limited, there is evidence of a role. In human patients with refractory and relapsed neuroblastoma, PMN-MDSCs with immune inhibitory effects were enriched in the peripheral blood after treatment with GD2.CAR-T cells [54]. Furthermore, higher number of PMN-MDSCs relative to CAR-T cells were identified in patients that did not respond to therapy, whereas the opposite was observed in responders. When isolated, these PMN-MDSCs had strongly inhibitory effects on CAR-T cytotoxicity in vitro. Future research will hopefully elucidate clearer mechanisms of pro-tumor neutrophil and PMN-MDSC activity in neuroblastoma.

8.2.3 Dendritic Cells

Dendritic cells (DCs), upon activation and maturation, are potent antigen presenting cells that play a crucial role in connecting innate and adaptive immune responses via presentation of tumor-associated antigens (TAA), expression of co-stimulatory molecules key in T cell activation, and secretion of cytokines that supports NK cell activation. However, despite the anti-tumor potential of DCs, immune surveillance via antigen presentation is thought to be obstructed by downregulation within the neuroblastoma TME.

A macrophage/DC progenitor is the common origin for conventional DCs (cDCs), plasmacytoid DCs (pDCs), and monocytes which ultimately can differentiate into monocyte-derived dendritic cells (Mo-DCs) and inflammatory DCs. Conventional DCs are known to infiltrate tumor tissues, capture antigens released from tumor cells, and cross-present them to CD8 T cells, thus driving expansion of tumor-specific cytotoxic T-lymphocytes (CTLs) [55]. Plasmacytoid DCs specialize in secretion of type I interferons (IFNs) following stimulation of toll-like receptors (TLRs). Type I IFNs, particularly IFN-α, is a potent stimulator of NK cell tumor cytotoxicity and NK cells stimulated by TLR9-activated pDCs are cytotoxic against high-risk neuroblastoma cell lines (including GD2-negative cells) by antibody-dependent cellular cytotoxicity (ADCC) comparable to IL-2 stimulated NK cells in the presence of anti-GD2 antibody therapy [56].

Dendritic cell vaccine research has elucidated additional DC immune interactions in neuroblastoma. Tumor lysate-pulsed DCs administered to pediatric refractory solid tumor patients, including some with neuroblastoma, can elicit tumor-specific T cell expansion and, in some cases, mediate tumor regression [57]. However, separate work with vaccination of stage IV neuroblastoma patients with monocyte-derived DCs pulsed with autologous neuroblastoma tumor RNA failed to elicit a significant cell-mediated antitumor response (as measured by T cell proliferation assay), despite some patients having measurable increase in anti-tumor antibodies post-vaccination [58]. Profound chemotherapy-induced immunosuppression prior to vaccination is thought largely to blame for diminished vaccine-induced immune response. This is further supported by the fact that improved graft-versus-neuroblastoma effect can be seen when vaccination of neuroblastoma patients following allogenic transplant with DC vaccine is given in combination with donor lymphocyte infusion [59].

Tumor-associated DC dysfunction is unlikely attributable entirely to the lack of sufficient effector cells and in fact, in vitro human and murine neuroblastoma studies have shown neuroblastoma-associated gangliosides inhibit generation of functionally active DCs from monocytes [60]. Mo-DCs support NK cell effector functions and survival with a subsequent positive feedback loop with DCs in neuroblastoma [61]. In addition, DCs can promote NK cell activation, including IFN-γ secretion and cytolytic activation against tumor cells in other solid tumor models [62]. Given these anti-tumor functions supported by DCs, ganglioside-mediated DC suppression acts as a potential mechanism of neuroblastoma immune escape.

Neuroblastoma also expresses high amounts of galectin-1 (Gal-1), a glycan-binding protein with demonstrated role in cellular transformation, adhesion, migration, immunity, and angiogenesis, which all contribute to tumor progression. Gal-1 was shown in other solid tumors to control select T-helper-mediated effector functions and induce differentiation of tolerogenic DCs through IL-10 and IL-27 dependent pathways. Gal-1 blockade in neuroblastoma inhibited tumor growth via suppression of T cell cytotoxicity, IFN-γ production, and DC maturation in a murine model [63].

8.2.4 Natural Killer (NK) Cells

Natural killer (NK) cells play a key role in immune surveillance and tumor immunity and have been shown to have strong anti-neuroblastoma effector functions both in vitro and in vivo. In contrast to lack of research involving neutrophils and neuroblastoma, significant work has been done to elucidate NK cell functions within the neuroblastoma TME.

8.2.4.1 Activation and Anti-Neuroblastoma Activity

NK cell activation, and ultimately target/tumor cell cytotoxicity, is mediated by activating receptors on NK cells that recognize unique ligands on healthy and abnormal cells; these include NKp46, NKp30, NKp44, NKG2D, and DNAM-1. These non-major histocompatibility class (MHC) I ligands expressed on healthy cells are often upregulated and over-expressed following malignant transformation. Following ligand binding at activating receptors, activated NK cells become potent mediators of anti-tumor immunity. However, NK activation is counterbalanced by inhibitory receptors and ligands, with deference to NK inhibition when both receptor types are engaged on a target cell. Additionally, the presence of HLA class I molecules on healthy cells that bind NK-inhibitory receptors act as a second layer of protection against normal autologous cell destruction. While NK-inhibitory dominance and protection of autologous cells is crucial, this represents a potential area of exploitation by neuroblastoma cells to avoid immune detection. In vitro models have shown neuroblastoma cells upregulate NK-inhibitory HLA class I expression in response to IFN-γ, which effectively decreases their susceptibility to autologous NK-mediated cytotoxicity [64]. It is possible that this upregulation occurs in neuroblastoma cells in vivo, particularly following anti-GD2 therapy that engages NK cells through FcγR interactions, leading to NK cell activation and increased release of IFN-γ [65].

Neuroblastoma may also downregulate expression of NK-activating ligands such as PVR (CD155). Neuroblasts isolated from the bone marrow of stage IV neuroblastoma patients, while overall low in HLA class I expression, exhibited varied expression of PVR, with expression present in samples at disease onset, yet absent in relapse samples [66].

When activation signals predominate and NK-cell activating receptors bind their respective ligands on tumor cells (NKG2D receptor to MICA/B, or ULBPs and DNAM-1 receptor to PVR and Nectin-2), cytolytic granules are released inducing tumor cell lysis. Separately, NK cells can upregulate expression of death receptor ligands, Fas ligand, and tumor necrosis factor-related apoptosis-inducing ligand (TRAIL), which can bind tumor cells and directly trigger death-receptor pathways leading to tumor cell death. Both NK lytic functions are further enhanced through interaction with activated dendritic cells (DC) and the type I interferons (IFNs) they produce. In neuroblastoma, TLR-9-activated plasmacytoid DCs have been shown to increase NK cell lytic activity against NBL cells in vitro and this increase was independent of tumor cell GD2 expression, occurred with or without anti-GD2 antibody, was mediated via cytolytic granule release and TRAIL-mediated apoptosis, and was dependent on pDC produced IFNα [56].

While potent on their own, NK cells can also mediate neuroblastoma cytotoxicity through tumor-directed antibody via Fc recognition. In the presence of GD2-directed antibody, both murine-derived anti-GD2 and/or human-murine chimeric anti-GD2 antibody, NK cells have been shown to be potent effectors of anti-neuroblastoma ADCC in addition to their antibody-independent cytotoxic potential [67]. Sensitized NK cells also play a role in priming tumor cells for recognition by cytotoxic T-lymphocytes (CTLs) by driving increased surface expression of MHC-I on neuroblastoma cells, a process thought to be secondary to contact-dependent IFNγ secretion [68].

8.2.4.2 Inhibition

Through interaction at inhibitory immunoreceptors (killer immunoglobulin-like receptors (KIR) or NKG2A/CD94 heterodimers) differentially expressed on the surface of NK cells, NK cell activation is counterbalanced with inhibitory signals following binding of various HLA molecules on target cells [56, 69]. While tumor cells lacking HLA class-I molecules and expressing non-MHC-I molecules bind and activate NK cells triggering tumor cell lysis, other tumor cells can exploit this delicate balance by expressing HLA class I molecules that bind inhibitory receptors and escape NK cell directed lysis.

Analysis of KIR, HLA, and FcR allele genotypes in a cohort of 38 relapsed/refractory neuroblastoma patients treated with anti-GD2-IL2 immunoconjugate therapy found KIR/KIR-ligand mismatch in 24 of 38. Of those patients, seven experienced either a complete response or partial response, whereas no response to therapy was seen in KIR-matched patients, indicating KIR-mediated NK cell inhibition can play a significant role in therapy resistance [70, 71]. Separate immunotherapy studies in neuroblastoma have elucidated TGF-β within the TME as another negative regulator of NK-mediated ADCC of neuroblastoma cells [37, 65, 72, 73]. Via activation of the STAT3 and SMAD2/3 pathways in NK cells, IL-6 and TGF-β1 suppress IL-2 induction of cytotoxicity, granzyme A and B release, perforin expression, and IFN-γ secretion by NK cells [74].

MYCN expression in human neuroblastoma cell lines is also inversely correlated with expression of ligands recognized by NK activating receptors NKG2D and DNAM1. In a MYCN-inducible cell line, downregulation of MYCN resulted in enhanced expression of the activating ligands MICA, ULBPs, and PVR, which resulted in tumor cells being more susceptible to NK-mediated recognition and cell lysis [75]. Given the significantly worsened prognosis for patients with MYCN-amplified neuroblastoma, this diminished expression of NK-activating receptors may have clinically significant effects on anti-tumor NK cell activity.

8.2.5 Natural Killer T (NKT) Cells

Natural killer T cells (NKT) are a subset of T lymphocytes but possess many innate-like properties and as such are generally considered a bridge between innate and adaptive immune responses. There are two main groups of NKTs: Type I invariant NKT (iNKT) cells and Type II NKT cells. iNKT cells are characterized by expression of an invariant T cell receptor (TCR) α-chain, Vα24-Jα18, in combination with limited beta-chain repertoire, whereas Type II NKT cells express a broad range of TCR chain combinations. These cells recognize lipid antigens presented by CD1d, an MHC-like molecule, and their tissue localization is largely chemokine driven [76, 77].

Most research involving NKT cells in neuroblastoma has focused on iNKT cells. Consistent with their innate classification, iNKT cells traffic to neuroblastoma where they can be activated and rapidly produce cytokines that further drive an adaptive response. iNKT trafficking to neuroblastoma is mediated by CCL2 via CCR2 receptors expressed on the surface of iNKT cells [78]. In a study of 98 untreated primary stage IV neuroblastoma tumor samples, a combination of RT-PCR, microarray gene expression profiling, and immunofluorescent microscopy was used to quantify iNKT cell infiltration; infiltration was identified in 53% of samples with iNKT-positive tumors demonstrating greater expression of CCL2 [78]. Furthermore, TCR-stimulated iNKT cells produce IL-2 and IFN-gamma that has been shown to activate and induce NK cell cytotoxicity of neuroblastoma in vitro [79]. While the ability of iNKT cells to directly kill neuroblastoma is low given that most neuroblastomas are CD1d-negative, iNKTs can still impede CD1d-negative neuroblastoma growth and survival through direct cytotoxicity of CD1d + TAMs and monocytes within the TME; this results in effective reduction of pro-tumorigenic IL-6 otherwise produced by these cells [31].

Invariant NKT infiltration is associated with favorable clinical outcome in neuroblastoma and other cancers. iNKT infiltration also has been found to be inversely correlated with MYCN amplification, with little if any iNKT infiltration found in MYCN-amplified tumors. To explain this, previous studies have identified an inverse correlation between MYCN amplification and expression of the chemokine instrumental in iNKT trafficking to the TME, CCL2 [78]. In MYCN-overexpressing neuroblastoma xenografts, there was an impaired ability to attract human NKT cells, along with T cells and monocytes, with the mechanism thought to be MYCN-induced repression of CCL2 expression, in a STAT3-independent manner [32]. The repression of CCL2 expression by MYCN, with subsequent decreased iNKT trafficking, serves as a potential mechanism of immune evasion by neuroblastoma. Mechanisms involved in iNKT cell expansion in the TME have not yet been fully elucidated, but the therapeutic potential of iNKT-mediated immunotherapy is being explored, including iNKT stimulation, adoptive transfer, and CAR-iNKTs [76, 79–88].

8.2.6 Cytokines and Chemokines in the Neuroblastoma Tumor Microenvironment

Chemokines and cytokines released by cells of the innate immune system provide critical interactions between immune cells and drive cell migration, activation (or inhibition), expansion, and persistence (or quiescence). While the immune cell-specific cytokine production will be discussed elsewhere, we will review the known chemokine production by neuroblastoma cells which serves an important role in immune modulation within the TME.

Chemokines produced by neuroblastoma cells contribute to varied leukocyte chemoattraction to the TME, resulting in both pro- or anti-tumor effects. These chemokines can also have direct effects on surrounding stromal cells, inducing additional cytokine and chemokine production that may impact angiogenesis, tumor metastases, leukocyte migration, and immunoregulation [89].

CCL2 is secreted by neuroblastoma cell lines and is expressed in stage IV neuroblastoma tumors along with CXCL12, CCL5, and CCL21. Interestingly, CCL2 expression was found to be inversely correlated with MYCN amplification with correspondingly decreased NKT cell infiltration [78]. CX3CL1 (fractalkine), a chemokine involved in leukocyte adhesion and migration, has been found in greater than 90% of human neuroblastoma samples and is also thought to contribute to chemoattraction of NK cells, γδT cells, and CD8 CTLs to the TME, all of which express its receptor, CX3CR1 [90]. Both CCL2 expression and CX3CL1 gene expression are inversely correlated with MYCN amplification, supporting the "cold" TME in MYCN-amplified tumors [78, 90]. However, higher expression of these cytokines does not equate to greater anti-tumor effects, as infiltrating T cells are dysfunctional due to low levels of IL2 [90], and attraction of monocytes by CCL2 leads to their conversion to TAMs and enhanced TGFβ1 production [37].

Xenograft models in neuroblastoma have allowed for identification of the chemokine receptors CXCR4 and CXCR7 along with their ligand, CXCL12. These are believed to be mediators of primary and secondary neuroblastoma growth with distinct correlation between expression and growth patterns. CXCR4 expression is more often found in highly aggressive, undifferentiated tumors which readily disseminate to liver and lungs in xenografts, while CXCR7 expression is associated with differentiated, mature neuroblastoma tumors and is associated with metastases to the adrenal glands and liver in murine models; co-expression of both CXCR4 and CXCR7 seems to induce bone marrow metastases [91]. Interestingly, neuroblastoma derived TGFβ1 has been shown to play an immunomodulatory role by upregulating expression of CXCR4 and CXCR3 in NK cells, with a dose-dependent correlation seen between TGFβ1 levels and chemokine receptor expression [72].

Transcriptomic data from primary, MYCN-amplified neuroblastoma tumors have demonstrated low IFN-pathway activity and chemokine expression with poor T-cell infiltration. Conversely, small molecule IFN-pathway activation was significantly increased with MYCN-depletion, leading to increased chemokine expression, including CXCL10, and thus increased T-cell recruitment in vitro [92]. IFN-gamma treatment pre-clinical models of neuroblastoma have been shown to induce upregulation of MHC class I expression on neuroblastoma tumor cells, with enhanced infiltration of T cells into the tumor. Interestingly, 5-day subcutaneous injection of INF-gamma to five children with relapsed neuroblastoma demonstrated upregulation of MHC class 1 and infiltration of T cells in 2 out of 5 patients [93].

Neuroblastoma has also been noted to induce cytokine expression, particularly IL-6, by immune and stromal cells within the TME. Neuroblastoma induces increased IL-6 production by TAMs in vitro and by bone marrow stromal cells in vivo, and a combination of TAMs and stromal cells leads to enhanced expression of cytokines in all these cells [37, 94]. Recombinant human IL-6 in vitro leads to increased proliferation in neuroblastoma cells that express IL-6R, and even had a protective effect against etoposide-induced apoptosis [94].

8.3 The Adaptive Immune System and Neuroblastoma

The introduction of immunotherapy-based treatments for neuroblastoma represented a revolutionary change that highlights the importance of the adaptive immune system in understanding this disease. For most childhood cancers, it has historically been held that the anti-tumor properties of the adaptive immune system are limited because self-reactive T cells are eliminated during thymopoeisis to prevent autoimmunity [95]. In neuroblastoma, this seemed consistent given an overall absence of T cells within neuroblastoma tumors and no perceived clinical benefit to immune-stimulating interventions, namely, vaccination. However, there may be no better example of the efficacy of antibody-based tumor-directed therapy than dinutuximab, the monoclonal antibody therapy that binds a surface GD2 glycolipid expressed nearly ubiquitously on neuroblastoma cell surfaces. The cells of the adaptive immune system are thus deserving of important consideration in this context.

8.3.1 T Lymphocytes

A complete understanding of the role of T lymphocytes in the natural response to neuroblastoma remains evasive. The types of T cells most worthy of discussion within the context of neuroblastoma are CD4+ "helper" cells, cytotoxic CD8+ cells, and regulatory T cells (Tregs). Though grouped together in name, studies have demonstrated unique functions of each cell type in neuroblastoma. As with other cancers, the degree of T cell infiltration into neuroblastoma tumors is a key prognostic indicator. In low-risk neuroblastoma, locoregional tumors demonstrated greater infiltration of all T cell types and this correlated with improved survival, which contrasted with worsened T cell organization in tumors with poorer prognosis [96]. CD4+ T cells appear to be major participants in the protumorigenic effect of the adaptive immune system in neuroblastoma [97]. In a highly penetrant MYCN amplified neuroblastoma mouse model, depletion of CD4+ T cells prevented tumor formation, suggesting that helper T cells are pathogenic in the neuroblastoma tumor microenvironment. Interestingly, in this model, depletion of CD8+ T cells did not curtail tumor development.

A key mediator of T cell infiltration in tumors is downregulation of major histocompatibility complex (MHC) class I antigens. Most neuroblastoma cell lines exhibit low MHC class I expression; however, there is no clear, direct relationship between of MHC class I expression and disease severity. Furthermore, downregulation of classical MHC class I results in upregulation of nonclassical complexes, including HLA-G, which worsens prognosis [98]. While downregulation of MHC class I antigens may limit interaction with cytotoxic T cells, it increases susceptibility to KIR-matched natural killer cells [64]. This "double-edged sword" phenomenon exemplifies the challenges of immune-based neuroblastoma therapies. As it is, interferon gamma treatment, as well as NF-kb and IRF1, can restore MHC class I presentation, but the benefit remains unclear and impractical given that IFN-gamma treatment induces negative feedback loops that limit long-term effects [93, 96].

In addition to the T cell types of primary interest, γδT cells have innate and adaptive immune system characteristics and are capable of cytotoxicity without the help of APCs and do not require MHC class I or II peptide presentation. Enriched γδT cells isolated from the peripheral blood of neuroblastoma patients were found to have significant antibody-dependent and innate cytotoxicity against neuroblastoma [99]. These cells, and others yet to be studied in this context, provide targets for future therapeutic research, and could be utilized as cell sources for engineered cells expressing chimeric antigen receptors [100].

Regulatory T cells (Tregs) are immunosuppressive cells that mediate tolerance and maintain immunologic homeostasis by suppressing aberrant immune responses. In tumor immunology, however, Treg immune suppressive functions can be exploited by tumor cells as they can inhibit effective antitumor immune responses. Limited knowledge of Treg-specific immunophenotypic markers limited the ability to study this population until identification of the Treg lineage transcriptional factor FOXP3. In other cancers, Tregs within the TME portend a poor prognosis. While not directly reported in neuroblastoma, MYCN amplification corresponds with a higher number of Tregs in the peripheral blood and bone marrow [101]. In murine neuroblastoma model Neuro2a, Treg depletion with anti-CD25 monoclonal antibody (mAb) resulted in tumor rejection and increased survival of treated mice. This in conjunction with in vitro work showing no direct effects of mAb therapy on immune cell function supports the role of Tregs in suppression of immune responses to tumor [102]. In this model, delivery of a cell-based anti-neuroblastoma vaccine resulted in increased survival when an anti-CD25 mAb preceded vaccination. Additional work using an anti-CD4 mAb to induce Treg depletion showed similar improved vaccine response and neuroblastoma rejection [103]. Furthermore, ex vivo depletion of CD25+ Treg cells, followed by sensitization and adoptive transfer of the remaining T cells, resulted in enhanced anti-tumor vaccine efficacy, similar to the observed effects of in vivo CD4 depletion, but with the added benefits of elevated tumor-reactive CD4+ and CD8+ T cells and improved T-cell memory [104].

Human studies of Tregs in neuroblastoma patients have demonstrated limited and contradictory results. One study without healthy control patients was unable to measure significant Treg frequency in peripheral blood of patients with either high- or low-risk neuroblastoma [105]. A separate single-center, prospective study of 14 patients identified higher Treg frequency in patients with neuroblastoma as compared to healthy patients, and a significantly higher frequency in patients with tumors greater than 10 cm in size as compared to smaller tumors [106]. Unfortunately, this study did not identify differences in Treg frequency between patients with metastatic and local disease. Conversely, a more recent study of 27 patients with neuroblastoma identified a lower Treg frequency in the peripheral blood and bone marrow as compared to healthy controls, questioning the significance of Treg frequency and demonstrating that there may be unrecognized reasons for this variation [101].

8.3.2 B-Lymphocytes

Though a vast majority of the research of the adaptive immune system in patients with neuroblastoma has centered on T cells, there is increasing interest in the role of B lymphocytes and plasma cells. B cells pose a particularly exciting prospect given the incomplete current understanding of T cell involvement and the limited efficacy of T cell centered therapies, as discussed above. Collectively termed tumor-infiltrating B lymphocytes, or TIL-Bs, these frequently exist in close association with other T cells, particularly in tumors containing a high density of immune cells [107]. In one study of a large number of independent gene expression datasets, the presence of B cells in neuroblastoma tumors was associated with greater overall survival and longer recurrence-free survival [108]. B cells are not frequently seen on biopsies of neuroblastoma tumors, but this may reflect sampling error as B cells have been described to congregate in organized lymphoid structures on the periphery of tumors [109].

While the exact role of B cells in neuroblastoma remains unclear, T cells interact with plasma cell to induce production of antibodies necessary for an antibody-mediated immune response to tumor cells. In one study, 74 human patients with neuroblastoma, increased γδT cells were isolated in patients with neuroblastoma with increased serum IgG levels. The source of the IgG was found to be mature B cells, which interestingly were present in significantly lower frequency in neuroblastoma patients, but which exhibited significant upregulation of CD23 [110]. The clinical relevance of increased circulating antibody will be reviewed below.

8.3.3 Antibodies in the Neuroblastoma Tumor Microenvironment

Antibodies have been the focus of research in neuroblastoma for 50 years. In 1978, Brandeis et al. described the presence of circulating immune complexes in the serums of children with neuroblastoma, and noted a relationship: a greater concentration of immune complexes correlated with a higher stage of disease [111]. More recent observations also suggest the significance of antibody-mediated processes with the disease. The observation that a subset of very young patients with neuroblastoma, specifically those with stage 4S disease, will experience spontaneous regression of their disease supports the role of immune surveillance in tumor eradication. Anti-neuroblastoma IgM antibodies have been described in the serum of healthy adults and has been shown to mediate complement-dependent anti-neuroblastoma cytotoxic activity in vitro via the classical pathway of activation [112]. Furthermore, anti-tumor IgM antibody recognized an antigen unique to human neuroblastoma cell lines, had anti-neuroblastoma activity in xenografts, and was largely absent from the serums of sampled patients with active disease, providing support for possible antibody-mediated tumor cytotoxicity [113]. Interestingly, these antibodies were only present in a small percentage of healthy donors and the clinical implications remain unclear [114]. Opsoclonus-myoclonus in the young neuroblastoma patients, thought to be mediated by cross-reactivity of an anti-neuroblastoma antibody to an antigen also expressed on nervous system components, provides another potential clue for the immunogenicity of neuroblastoma and potential innate humoral response.

Despite the evidence that neuroblastoma-directed antibodies exist in some patients, patients with advanced disease are likely have overcome their antibody-mediated immune surveillance due to yet unknown reasons. This may be in part because, in comparison to other solid tumors, neuroblastoma is relatively devoid of neo-antigens. Regardless of this limitation, one of the most significant therapeutic breakthroughs in pediatric oncologic history was targeting GD2, with the monoclonal antibody dinutuximab. Introduction of dinutuximab after induction chemotherapy in newly diagnosed patients with high-risk neuroblastoma resulted in improved outcome [1]. For children with refractory/relapse disease, combining chemotherapy with dinutuximab (chemoimmunotherapy) resulted in an impressive clinical response [3, 4]. The success of anti-GD2 therapy served as the validation for a novel treatment approach using this approach and chimeric antigen receptor (CAR) T cells. However, the mechanisms of response or resistance, especially in chemoimmunotherapy, are currently unknown and likely attributable to patient's immune response and their tumors' microenvironment [4].

8.3.4 Mechanisms of Immune Evasion by Neuroblastoma

The progression of neuroblastoma despite the presence of the aforementioned immune cells within the tumor microenvironment implies strongly that neuroblastoma employs techniques that suppress and evade immune function. The most relevant mechanisms of evasion are a low baseline immunogenicity, deactivation of innate immune cells, and indirect and direct immunosuppression.

Through downregulation of MHC class I antigens (see "T cells" above), neuroblastoma can significantly limit the effect of cytotoxic T cells. Cytotoxic T cells recognizing Survivin, a widely expressed tumor-associated antigen, can be consistently detected in blood of patients with high-risk neuroblastoma. Increase in cytotoxic T cells are also observed in tumors with higher levels of neoantigens [115]. Despite this evidence of robust immune anti-tumor recognition, tumoral T cell infiltration in these patients was strikingly low, suggesting an intact cellular response at some point during pathogenesis, but an overall failure of cellular immunosurveillance [109]. The low classic MHC class I expression observed in undifferentiated neuroblastomas may thus represent an early immune escape event, limiting the efficacy of programmed effectors of anti-tumor function. MHC class I expression is also dependent on MYCN amplification status, with lower expression in amplified tumors, which may explain the observed prognostic implications [115]. There are likely numerous additional undiscovered factors that further contribute to the T cell exclusion observed in COG-designated high-risk tumors compared to low-risk tumors [96].

NK cells are known effective killers of neuroblastoma cells in vitro; however, they are significantly less effective in vivo, suggesting an escape mechanism of tumor cells. It is known that neuroblastoma cells exhibit low expression of multiple ligands responsible for NK cell activation which may in large part explain the relative ineffectiveness of innate cell function in vivo [116]. Another mechanism of NK cell evasion is via production of TGF-β and by the overexpression of B7-H3 molecules, which directly inhibit NK cell cytotoxicity [37, 66, 117, 118]. In opposition of these effects, the efficacy of NK cell killing is significantly increased in the setting of dinutuximab bound to GD2 on the surface of neuroblastoma cells. Furthermore, delivery of ex vivo-activated NK cells and dinutuximab in a mouse model of a neuroblastoma results in significantly improved survival, particularly when treated prior to surgical resection of the primary tumor [119, 120].

Direct and indirect immunosuppressive mechanisms by neuroblastoma cells are the final technique for immune evasion. One such mechanism relies on interruption of the interaction between cytotoxic T cells and antigen presentation by inducing dendritic cell dysfunction. When in direct contact with DCs, neuroblastoma cells inhibit DC maturation, interfere with T cell activation, and induce DC apoptosis [121]. Apoptosis occurs due to Fas binding and FasL expression correlates with MYCN amplification [122]. Another mechanism of immune evasion is via direct release of suppressors of lymphocyte function including TGFβ, arginase-2, and MIF [123]. TGF-β has been shown to directly impair NK cell function with increased TGF-β expression in tumors correlating with poor prognosis [31, 37]. Arginase, which breaks down arginine that is essential for lymphocytes, suppresses immune cell functions in the TME. In neuroblastoma, high levels of arginase correlated with higher tumor burden and reduced survival [124].

8.4 Conclusion

The relationship between neuroblastoma tumor cells and immune cells within the tumor microenvironment is critical to the pathogenesis of disease. A thorough understanding of the immune system provides the necessary context for identifying potential immune-modulating therapies. Identifying the repertoire of immune cell infiltrates and circulating immune cells post-therapy and at time of relapse remains a challenge. The single-cell resolution technologies will inevitably provide further insights into TME composition and alteration in cytokine milieu and understanding these new found interactions could identify novel therapeutic opportunities. The next therapeutic breakthrough in neuroblastoma treatment will very likely arise from novel techniques for altering the neuroblastoma tumor microenvironment.

References

1. Yu AL, Gilman AL, Ozkaynak MF, London WB, Kreissman SG, Chen HX, et al. Anti-GD2 Antibody with GM-CSF, Interleukin-2, and Isotretinoin for Neuroblastoma. New England Journal of Medicine. 2010;363(14):1324–34. https://doi.org/10.1056/NEJMoa0911123.
2. Zhou MJ, Doral MY, DuBois SG, Villablanca JG, Yanik GA, Matthay KK. Different outcomes for relapsed versus refractory neuroblastoma after therapy with (131)I-metaiodobenzylguanidine ((131)I-MIBG). Eur J Cancer. 2015;51(16):2465–72. https://doi.org/10.1016/j.ejca.2015.07.023.
3. Mody R, Naranjo A, Van Ryn C, Yu AL, London WB, Shulkin BL, et al. Irinotecan-temozolomide with temsirolimus or dinutuximab in children with refractory or relapsed neuroblastoma (COG ANBL1221): an open-label, randomised, phase 2 trial. Lancet Oncol. 2017; https://doi.org/10.1016/S1470-2045(17)30355-8.
4. Mody R, Yu AL, Naranjo A, Zhang FF, London WB, Shulkin BL, et al. Irinotecan, temozolomide, and dinutuximab with GM-CSF in children with refractory or relapsed neuroblastoma: a report from the Children's Oncology Group. J Clin Oncol. 2020;38(19):2160–9. https://doi.org/10.1200/JCO.20.00203.
5. Irwin MS, Naranjo A, Zhang FF, Cohn SL, London WB, Gastier-Foster JM, et al. Revised neuroblastoma risk classification system: a report from the Children's oncology group. J Clin Oncol. 2021;39(29):3229–41. https://doi.org/10.1200/JCO.21.00278.
6. Schmidt ML, Lukens JN, Seeger RC, Brodeur GM, Shimada H, Gerbing RB, et al. Biologic factors determine prognosis in infants with stage IV neuroblastoma: a prospective Children's Cancer Group study. J Clin Oncol. 2000;18(6):1260–8. https://doi.org/10.1200/JCO.2000.18.6.1260.
7. Hellstrom I, Hellstrom KE, Bill AH, Pierce GE, Yang JP. Studies on cellular immunity to human neuroblastoma cells. Int J Cancer. 1970;6(2):172–88.
8. Hellstrom IE, Hellstrom KE, Pierce GE, Bill AH. Demonstration of cell-bound and humoral immunity against neuroblastoma cells. Proc Natl Acad Sci U S A. 1968;60(4):1231–8.
9. Hellstrom KE, Hellstrom I. Immunity to neuroblastomas and melanomas. Annu Rev Med. 1972;23:19–38. https://doi.org/10.1146/annurev.me.23.020172.000315.
10. Heczey A, Louis CU, Savoldo B, Dakhova O, Durett A, Grilley B, et al. CAR T cells administered in combination with lymphodepletion and PD-1 inhibition to patients with neuroblastoma. Mol Ther. 2017;25(9):2214–24. https://doi.org/10.1016/j.ymthe.2017.05.012.
11. Louis CU, Savoldo B, Dotti G, Pule M, Yvon E, Myers GD, et al. Antitumor activity and long-term fate of chimeric antigen receptor-positive T cells in patients with neuroblastoma. Blood. 2011;118(23):6050–6. https://doi.org/10.1182/blood-2011-05-354449.
12. Pule MA, Savoldo B, Myers GD, Rossig C, Russell HV, Dotti G, et al. Virus-specific T cells engineered to coexpress tumor-specific receptors: persistence and antitumor activity in individuals with neuroblastoma. Nat Med. 2008;14(11):1264–70. https://doi.org/10.1038/nm.1882.
13. Straathof K, Flutter B, Wallace R, Jain N, Loka T, Depani S, et al. Antitumor activity without on-target off-tumor toxicity of GD2-chimeric antigen receptor T cells in patients with neuroblastoma. Sci Transl Med. 2020;12(571) https://doi.org/10.1126/scitranslmed.abd6169.
14. Park JR, Digiusto DL, Slovak M, Wright C, Naranjo A, Wagner J, et al. Adoptive transfer of chimeric antigen receptor re-directed cytolytic T lymphocyte clones in patients with neuroblastoma. Mol Ther. 2007;15(4):825–33. https://doi.org/10.1038/sj.mt.6300104.

15. Wynn TA, Chawla A, Pollard JW. Macrophage biology in development, homeostasis and disease. Nature. 2013;496(7446):445–55. https://doi.org/10.1038/nature12034.
16. Hagerling C, Casbon AJ, Werb Z. Balancing the innate immune system in tumor development. Trends Cell Biol. 2015;25(4):214–20. https://doi.org/10.1016/j.tcb.2014.11.001.
17. Ojalvo LS, Whittaker CA, Condeelis JS, Pollard JW. Gene expression analysis of macrophages that facilitate tumor invasion supports a role for Wnt-signaling in mediating their activity in primary mammary tumors. J Immunol. 2010;184(2):702–12. https://doi.org/10.4049/jimmunol.0902360.
18. Sidibe A, Ropraz P, Jemelin S, Emre Y, Poittevin M, Pocard M, et al. Angiogenic factor-driven inflammation promotes extravasation of human proangiogenic monocytes to tumours. Nat Commun. 2018;9(1):355. https://doi.org/10.1038/s41467-017-02610-0.
19. Hughes R, Qian BZ, Rowan C, Muthana M, Keklikoglou I, Olson OC, et al. Perivascular M2 macrophages stimulate tumor relapse after chemotherapy. Cancer Res. 2015;75(17):3479–91. https://doi.org/10.1158/0008-5472.Can-14-3587.
20. Gabrilovich DI. Myeloid-derived suppressor cells. Cancer Immunol Res. 2017;5(1):3–8. https://doi.org/10.1158/2326-6066.Cir-16-0297.
21. Gabrilovich DI, Bronte V, Chen SH, Colombo MP, Ochoa A, Ostrand-Rosenberg S, et al. The terminology issue for myeloid-derived suppressor cells. Cancer Res. 2007;67(1):425.; author reply 6. https://doi.org/10.1158/0008-5472.CAN-06-3037.
22. Bronte V, Chappell DB, Apolloni E, Cabrelle A, Wang M, Hwu P, et al. Unopposed production of granulocyte-macrophage colony-stimulating factor by tumors inhibits CD8+ T cell responses by dysregulating antigen-presenting cell maturation. J Immunol. 1999;162(10):5728–37.
23. Bronte V, Brandau S, Chen SH, Colombo MP, Frey AB, Greten TF, et al. Recommendations for myeloid-derived suppressor cell nomenclature and characterization standards. Nat Commun. 2016;7:12150. https://doi.org/10.1038/ncomms12150.
24. Mandruzzato S, Brandau S, Britten CM, Bronte V, Damuzzo V, Gouttefangeas C, et al. Toward harmonized phenotyping of human myeloid-derived suppressor cells by flow cytometry: results from an interim study. Cancer Immunol Immunother. 2016;65(2):161–9. https://doi.org/10.1007/s00262-015-1782-5.
25. Gabrilovich DI, Ostrand-Rosenberg S, Bronte V. Coordinated regulation of myeloid cells by tumours. Nat Rev Immunol. 2012;12(4):253–68. https://doi.org/10.1038/nri3175.
26. Biswas SK, Mantovani A. Macrophage plasticity and interaction with lymphocyte subsets: cancer as a paradigm. Nat Immunol. 2010;11(10):889–96. https://doi.org/10.1038/ni.1937.
27. Afik R, Zigmond E, Vugman M, Klepfish M, Shimshoni E, Pasmanik-Chor M, et al. Tumor macrophages are pivotal constructors of tumor collagenous matrix. J Exp Med. 2016;213(11):2315–31. https://doi.org/10.1084/jem.20151193.
28. DeNardo DG, Ruffell B. Macrophages as regulators of tumour immunity and immunotherapy. Nat Rev Immunol. 2019;19(6):369–82. https://doi.org/10.1038/s41577-019-0127-6.
29. Sohara Y, Shimada H, Minkin C, Erdreich-Epstein A, Nolta JA, DeClerck YA. Bone marrow mesenchymal stem cells provide an alternate pathway of osteoclast activation and bone destruction by cancer cells. Cancer Res. 2005;65(4):1129–35. https://doi.org/10.1158/0008-5472.CAN-04-2853.
30. Kim J, Bae JS. Tumor-associated macrophages and neutrophils in tumor microenvironment. Mediat Inflamm. 2016;2016:6058147. https://doi.org/10.1155/2016/6058147.
31. Song L, Asgharzadeh S, Salo J, Engell K, Wu HW, Sposto R, et al. Valpha24-invariant NKT cells mediate antitumor activity via killing of tumor-associated macrophages. J Clin Invest. 2009;119(6):1524–36. https://doi.org/10.1172/jci37869.
32. Song L, Ara T, Wu HW, Woo CW, Reynolds CP, Seeger RC, et al. Oncogene MYCN regulates localization of NKT cells to the site of disease in neuroblastoma. J Clin Invest. 2007;117(9):2702–12. https://doi.org/10.1172/jci30751.
33. Asgharzadeh S, Pique-Regi R, Sposto R, Wang H, Yang Y, Shimada H, et al. Prognostic significance of gene expression profiles of metastatic neuroblastomas lacking MYCN gene amplification. J Natl Cancer Inst. 2006;98(17):1193–203. https://doi.org/10.1093/jnci/djj330.
34. Asgharzadeh S, Salo JA, Ji L, Oberthuer A, Fischer M, Berthold F, et al. Clinical significance of tumor-associated inflammatory cells in metastatic neuroblastoma. J Clin Oncol. 2012;30(28):3525–32. https://doi.org/10.1200/jco.2011.40.9169.
35. Hashimoto O, Yoshida M, Koma Y, Yanai T, Hasegawa D, Kosaka Y, et al. Collaboration of cancer-associated fibroblasts and tumour-associated macrophages for neuroblastoma development. J Pathol. 2016;240(2):211–23. https://doi.org/10.1002/path.4769.
36. Hadjidaniel MD, Muthugounder S, Hung LT, Sheard MA, Shirinbak S, Chan RY, et al. Tumor-associated macrophages promote neuroblastoma via STAT3 phosphorylation and up-regulation of c-MYC. Oncotarget. 2017;8(53):91516–29. https://doi.org/10.18632/oncotarget.21066.
37. Louault K, Porras T, Lee MH, Muthugounder S, Kennedy RJ, Blavier L, et al. Fibroblasts and macrophages cooperate to create a pro-tumorigenic and immune resistant environment via activation of TGF-beta/IL-6 pathway in neuroblastoma. Onco Targets Ther. 2022;11(1):2146860. https://doi.org/10.1080/2162402X.2022.2146860.
38. Santilli G, Piotrowska I, Cantilena S, Chayka O, D'Alicarnasso M, Morgenstern DA, et al. Polyphenon [corrected] E enhances the antitumor

immune response in neuroblastoma by inactivating myeloid suppressor cells. Clin Cancer Res. 2013;19(5):1116–25. https://doi.org/10.1158/1078-0432.CCR-12-2528.
39. Shirinbak S, Chan RY, Shahani S, Muthugounder S, Kennedy R, Hung LT, et al. Combined immune checkpoint blockade increases CD8+CD28+PD-1+ effector T cells and provides a therapeutic strategy for patients with neuroblastoma. Onco Targets Ther. 2021;10(1):1838140. https://doi.org/10.1080/2162402X.2020.1838140.
40. Bianchi G, Vuerich M, Pellegatti P, Marimpietri D, Emionite L, Marigo I, et al. ATP/P2X7 axis modulates myeloid-derived suppressor cell functions in neuroblastoma microenvironment. Cell Death Dis. 2014;5:e1135. https://doi.org/10.1038/cddis.2014.109.
41. Ishfaq M, Pham T, Beaman C, Tamayo P, Yu AL, Joshi S. BTK inhibition reverses MDSC mediated immunosuppression and enhances response to anti-PDL1 therapy in neuroblastoma. Cancers (Basel). 2021;13(4) https://doi.org/10.3390/cancers13040817.
42. Mao Y, Eissler N, Blanc KL, Johnsen JI, Kogner P, Kiessling R. Targeting suppressive myeloid cells potentiates checkpoint inhibitors to control spontaneous neuroblastoma. Clin Cancer Res. 2016;22(15):3849–59. https://doi.org/10.1158/1078-0432.CCR-15-1912.
43. Ostrand-Rosenberg S, Sinha P, Beury DW, Clements VK. Cross-talk between myeloid-derived suppressor cells (MDSC), macrophages, and dendritic cells enhances tumor-induced immune suppression. Semin Cancer Biol. 2012;22(4):275–81. https://doi.org/10.1016/j.semcancer.2012.01.011.
44. Zhou J, Nefedova Y, Lei A, Gabrilovich D. Neutrophils and PMN-MDSC: their biological role and interaction with stromal cells. Semin Immunol. 2018;35:19–28. https://doi.org/10.1016/j.smim.2017.12.004.
45. Zilio S, Serafini P. Neutrophils and granulocytic MDSC: the Janus god of cancer immunotherapy. Vaccine. 2016;4(3) https://doi.org/10.3390/vaccines4030031.
46. Piccard H, Muschel RJ, Opdenakker G. On the dual roles and polarized phenotypes of neutrophils in tumor development and progression. Crit Rev Oncol Hematol. 2012;82(3):296–309. https://doi.org/10.1016/j.critrevonc.2011.06.004.
47. Sionov RV, Fridlender ZG, Granot Z. The multifaceted roles neutrophils play in the tumor microenvironment. Cancer Microenviron. 2015;8(3):125–58. https://doi.org/10.1007/s12307-014-0147-5.
48. Chen RL, Reynolds CP, Seeger RC. Neutrophils are cytotoxic and growth-inhibiting for neuroblastoma cells with an anti-GD2 antibody but, without cytotoxicity, can be growth-stimulating. Cancer Immunol Immunother. 2000;48(11):603–12.
49. Barker E, Reisfeld RA. A mechanism for neutrophil–mediated lysis of human neuroblastoma cells. Cancer Res. 1993;53(2):362–7.
50. Kushner BH, Cheung NK. Absolute requirement of CD11/CD18 adhesion molecules, FcRII and the phosphatidylinositol-linked FcRIII for monoclonal antibody-mediated neutrophil antihuman tumor cytotoxicity. Blood. 1992;79(6):1484–90.
51. van Egmond M, Bakema JE. Neutrophils as effector cells for antibody-based immunotherapy of cancer. Semin Cancer Biol. 2013;23(3):190–9. https://doi.org/10.1016/j.semcancer.2012.12.002.
52. Cheung IY, Hsu K, Cheung NK. Activation of peripheral-blood granulocytes is strongly correlated with patient outcome after immunotherapy with anti-GD2 monoclonal antibody and granulocyte-macrophage colony-stimulating factor. J Clin Oncol. 2012;30(4):426–32. https://doi.org/10.1200/jco.2011.37.6236.
53. Mishalian I, Bayuh R, Eruslanov E, Michaeli J, Levy L, Zolotarov L, et al. Neutrophils recruit regulatory T-cells into tumors via secretion of CCL17—a new mechanism of impaired antitumor immunity. Int J Cancer. 2014;135(5):1178–86. https://doi.org/10.1002/ijc.28770.
54. Tumino N, Besi F, Martini S, Di Pace AL, Munari E, Quatrini L, et al. Polymorphonuclear myeloid-derived suppressor cells are abundant in peripheral blood of cancer patients and suppress natural killer cell anti-tumor activity. Front Immunol. 2021;12:803014. https://doi.org/10.3389/fimmu.2021.803014.
55. Woo SR, Corrales L, Gajewski TF. Innate immune recognition of cancer. Annu Rev Immunol. 2015;33:445–74. https://doi.org/10.1146/annurev-immunol-032414-112043.
56. Cordeau M, Belounis A, Lelaidier M, Cordeiro P, Sartelet H, Herblot S, et al. Efficient killing of high risk neuroblastoma using natural killer cells activated by plasmacytoid dendritic cells. PLoS One. 2016;11(10):e0164401. https://doi.org/10.1371/journal.pone.0164401.
57. Geiger JD, Hutchinson RJ, Hohenkirk LF, McKenna EA, Yanik GA, Levine JE, et al. Vaccination of pediatric solid tumor patients with tumor lysate-pulsed dendritic cells can expand specific T cells and mediate tumor regression. Cancer Res. 2001;61(23):8513–9.
58. Caruso DA, Orme LM, Amor GM, Neale AM, Radcliff FJ, Downie P, et al. Results of a phase I study utilizing monocyte-derived dendritic cells pulsed with tumor RNA in children with stage 4 neuroblastoma. Cancer. 2005;103(6):1280–91. https://doi.org/10.1002/cncr.20911.
59. Ash S, Stein J, Askenasy N, Yaniv I. Immunomodulation with dendritic cells and donor lymphocyte infusion converge to induce graft vs neuroblastoma reactions without GVHD after allogeneic bone marrow transplantation. Br J Cancer.

2010;103(10):1597–605. https://doi.org/10.1038/sj.bjc.6605924.
60. Shurin GV, Shurin MR, Bykovskaia S, Shogan J, Lotze MT, Barksdale EM Jr. Neuroblastoma-derived gangliosides inhibit dendritic cell generation and function. Cancer Res. 2001;61(1):363–9.
61. Valteau-Couanet D, Leboulaire C, Maincent K, Tournier M, Hartmann O, Benard J, et al. Dendritic cells for NK/LAK activation: rationale for multicellular immunotherapy in neuroblastoma patients. Blood. 2002;100(7):2554–61. https://doi.org/10.1182/blood.V100.7.2554.
62. Fernandez NC, Lozier A, Flament C, Ricciardi-castagnoli P, Bellet D, Suter M, et al. Dendritic cells directly trigger NK cell functions: cross-talk relevant in innate anti-tumor immune responses in vivo. Nat Med. 1999;5(4):405–11.
63. Soldati R, Berger E, Zenclussen AC, Jorch G, Lode HN, Salatino M, et al. Neuroblastoma triggers an immunoevasive program involving galectin-1-dependent modulation of T cell and dendritic cell compartments. Int J Cancer. 2012;131(5):1131–41. https://doi.org/10.1002/ijc.26498.
64. Raffaghello L, Prigione I, Bocca P, Morandi F, Camoriano M, Gambini C, et al. Multiple defects of the antigen-processing machinery components in human neuroblastoma: immunotherapeutic implications. Oncogene. 2005;24(29):4634–44. https://doi.org/10.1038/sj.onc.1208594.
65. Bottino C, Dondero A, Bellora F, Moretta L, Locatelli F, Pistoia V, et al. Natural killer cells and neuroblastoma: tumor recognition, escape mechanisms, and possible novel immunotherapeutic approaches. Front Immunol. 2014;5:56. https://doi.org/10.3389/fimmu.2014.00056.
66. Castriconi R, Dondero A, Augugliaro R, Cantoni C, Carnemolla B, Sementa AR, et al. Identification of 4Ig-B7-H3 as a neuroblastoma-associated molecule that exerts a protective role from an NK cell-mediated lysis. Proc Natl Acad Sci U S A. 2004;101(34):12640–5. https://doi.org/10.1073/pnas.0405025101.
67. Zeng Y, Fest S, Kunert R, Katinger H, Pistoia V, Michon J, et al. Anti-neuroblastoma effect of ch14.18 antibody produced in CHO cells is mediated by NK-cells in mice. Mol Immunol. 2005;42(11):1311–9. https://doi.org/10.1016/j.molimm.2004.12.018.
68. Spel L, Boelens JJ, van der Steen DM, Blokland NJ, van Noesel MM, Molenaar JJ, et al. Natural killer cells facilitate PRAME-specific T-cell reactivity against neuroblastoma. Oncotarget. 2015;6(34):35770–81. https://doi.org/10.18632/oncotarget.5657.
69. Campoli M, Ferrone S. Tumor escape mechanisms: potential role of soluble HLA antigens and NK cells activating ligands. Tissue Antigens. 2008;72(4):321–34. https://doi.org/10.1111/j.1399-0039.2008.01106.x.
70. Delgado DC, Hank JA, Kolesar J, Lorentzen D, Gan J, Seo S, et al. Genotypes of NK cell KIR receptors, their ligands, and Fcgamma receptors in the response of neuroblastoma patients to Hu14.18-IL2 immunotherapy. Cancer Res. 2010;70(23):9554–61. https://doi.org/10.1158/0008-5472.can-10-2211.
71. Tarek N, Le Luduec JB, Gallagher MM, Zheng J, Venstrom JM, Chamberlain E, et al. Unlicensed NK cells target neuroblastoma following anti-GD2 antibody treatment. J Clin Invest. 2012;122(9):3260–70. https://doi.org/10.1172/jci62749.
72. Castriconi R, Dondero A, Bellora F, Moretta L, Castellano A, Locatelli F, et al. Neuroblastoma-derived TGF-beta1 modulates the chemokine receptor repertoire of human resting NK cells. J Immunol. 2013;190(10):5321–8. https://doi.org/10.4049/jimmunol.1202693.
73. Zenarruzabeitia O, Vitalle J, Astigarraga I, Borrego F. Natural killer cells to the attack: combination therapy against neuroblastoma. Clin Cancer Res. 2017;23(3):615–7. https://doi.org/10.1158/1078-0432.Ccr-16-2478.
74. Xu Y, Sun J, Sheard MA, Tran HC, Wan Z, Liu WY, et al. Lenalidomide overcomes suppression of human natural killer cell anti-tumor functions by neuroblastoma microenvironment-associated IL-6 and TGFβ1. Cancer Immunol Immunother. 2013;62(10):1637–48. https://doi.org/10.1007/s00262-013-1466-y.
75. Brandetti E, Veneziani I, Melaiu O, Pezzolo A, Castellano A, Boldrini R, et al. MYCN is an immunosuppressive oncogene dampening the expression of ligands for NK-cell-activating receptors in human high-risk neuroblastoma. Onco Targets Ther. 2017;6(6):e1316439. https://doi.org/10.1080/2162402x.2017.1316439.
76. Tian G, Courtney AN, Jena B, Heczey A, Liu D, Marinova E, et al. CD62L+ NKT cells have prolonged persistence and antitumor activity in vivo. J Clin Invest. 2016;126(6):2341–55. https://doi.org/10.1172/jci83476.
77. Bennstein SB. Unraveling natural killer T-cells development. Front Immunol. 2017;8:1950. https://doi.org/10.3389/fimmu.2017.01950.
78. Metelitsa LS, Wu HW, Wang H, Yang Y, Warsi Z, Asgharzadeh S, et al. Natural killer T cells infiltrate neuroblastomas expressing the chemokine CCL2. J Exp Med. 2004;199(9):1213–21. https://doi.org/10.1084/jem.20031462.
79. Metelitsa LS, Naidenko OV, Kant A, Wu HW, Loza MJ, Perussia B, et al. Human NKT cells mediate antitumor cytotoxicity directly by recognizing target cell CD1d with bound ligand or indirectly by producing IL-2 to activate NK cells. J Immunol. 2001;167(6):3114–22.
80. Giaccone G, Punt CJ, Ando Y, Ruijter R, Nishi N, Peters M, et al. A phase I study of the natural killer T-cell ligand alpha-galactosylceramide (KRN7000) in patients with solid tumors. Clin Cancer Res. 2002;8(12):3702–9.
81. Ishikawa A, Motohashi S, Ishikawa E, Fuchida H, Higashino K, Otsuji M, et al. A phase I study of

alpha-galactosylceramide (KRN7000)-pulsed dendritic cells in patients with advanced and recurrent non-small cell lung cancer. Clin Cancer Res. 2005;11(5):1910–7. https://doi.org/10.1158/1078-0432.CCR-04-1453.
82. Nagato K, Motohashi S, Ishibashi F, Okita K, Yamasaki K, Moriya Y, et al. Accumulation of activated invariant natural killer T cells in the tumor microenvironment after alpha-galactosylceramide-pulsed antigen presenting cells. J Clin Immunol. 2012;32(5):1071–81. https://doi.org/10.1007/s10875-012-9697-9.
83. Nieda M, Okai M, Tazbirkova A, Lin H, Yamaura A, Ide K, et al. Therapeutic activation of Valpha24+Vbeta11+ NKT cells in human subjects results in highly coordinated secondary activation of acquired and innate immunity. Blood. 2004;103(2):383–9. https://doi.org/10.1182/blood-2003-04-1155.
84. Mise N, Takami M, Suzuki A, Kamata T, Harada K, Hishiki T, et al. Antibody-dependent cellular cytotoxicity toward neuroblastoma enhanced by activated invariant natural killer T cells. Cancer Sci. 2016;107(3):233–41. https://doi.org/10.1111/cas.12882.
85. Bae EA, Seo H, Kim BS, Choi J, Jeon I, Shin KS, et al. Activation of NKT cells in an anti-PD-1-resistant tumor model enhances antitumor immunity by reinvigorating exhausted CD8 T cells. Cancer Res. 2018;78(18):5315–26. https://doi.org/10.1158/0008-5472.CAN-18-0734.
86. Kunii N, Horiguchi S, Motohashi S, Yamamoto H, Ueno N, Yamamoto S, et al. Combination therapy of in vitro-expanded natural killer T cells and alpha-galactosylceramide-pulsed antigen-presenting cells in patients with recurrent head and neck carcinoma. Cancer Sci. 2009;100(6):1092–8. https://doi.org/10.1111/j.1349-7006.2009.01135.x.
87. Shin T, Nakayama T, Akutsu Y, Motohashi S, Shibata Y, Harada M, et al. Inhibition of tumor metastasis by adoptive transfer of IL-12-activated Valpha14 NKT cells. Int J Cancer. 2001;91(4):523–8. https://doi.org/10.1002/1097-0215(20010215)91:4<523::aid--ijc1087>3.0.co;2-l.
88. Heczey A, Liu D, Tian G, Courtney AN, Wei J, Marinova E, et al. Invariant NKT cells with chimeric antigen receptor provide a novel platform for safe and effective cancer immunotherapy. Blood. 2014;124(18):2824–33. https://doi.org/10.1182/blood-2013-11-541235.
89. Somasundaram R, Herlyn D. Chemokines and the microenvironment in neuroectodermal tumor-host interaction. Semin Cancer Biol. 2009;19(2):92–6. https://doi.org/10.1016/j.semcancer.2008.11.002.
90. Zeng Y, Huebener N, Fest S, Weixler S, Schroeder U, Gaedicke G, et al. Fractalkine (CX3CL1)- and interleukin-2-enriched neuroblastoma microenvironment induces eradication of metastases mediated by T cells and natural killer cells. Cancer Res. 2007;67(5):2331–8. https://doi.org/10.1158/0008-5472.CAN-06-3041.
91. Muhlethaler-Mottet A, Liberman J, Ascencao K, Flahaut M, Balmas Bourloud K, Yan P, et al. The CXCR4/CXCR7/CXCL12 Axis is involved in a secondary but complex control of neuroblastoma metastatic cell homing. PLoS One. 2015;10(5):e0125616. https://doi.org/10.1371/journal.pone.0125616.
92. Layer JP, Kronmuller MT, Quast T, van den Boorn-Konijnenberg D, Effern M, Hinze D, et al. Amplification of N-Myc is associated with a T-cell-poor microenvironment in metastatic neuroblastoma restraining interferon pathway activity and chemokine expression. Onco Targets Ther. 2017;6(6):e1320626. https://doi.org/10.1080/2162402x.2017.1320626.
93. Reid GS, Shan X, Coughlin CM, Lassoued W, Pawel BR, Wexler LH, et al. Interferon-gamma-dependent infiltration of human T cells into neuroblastoma tumors in vivo. Clin Cancer Res. 2009;15(21):6602–8. https://doi.org/10.1158/1078-0432.CCR-09-0829.
94. Ara T, Song L, Shimada H, Keshelava N, Russell HV, Metelitsa LS, et al. Interleukin-6 in the bone marrow microenvironment promotes the growth and survival of neuroblastoma cells. Cancer Res. 2009;69(1):329–37. https://doi.org/10.1158/0008-5472.CAN-08-0613.
95. Anderson J, Majzner RG, Sondel PM. Immunotherapy of neuroblastoma: facts and hopes. Clin Cancer Res. 2022;28(15):3196–206. https://doi.org/10.1158/1078-0432.CCR-21-1356.
96. Mina M, Boldrini R, Citti A, Romania P, D'Alicandro V, De Ioris M, et al. Tumor-infiltrating T lymphocytes improve clinical outcome of therapy-resistant neuroblastoma. Onco Targets Ther. 2015;4(9):14. https://doi.org/10.1080/2162402x.2015.1019981.
97. Van de Velde LA, Allen EK, Crawford JC, Wilson TL, Guy CS, Russier M, et al. Neuroblastoma formation requires unconventional CD4 T cells and Arginase-1-dependent myeloid cells. Cancer Res. 2021;81(19):5047–59. https://doi.org/10.1158/0008-5472.CAN-21-0691.
98. Morandi F, Cangemi G, Barco S, Amoroso L, Giuliano M, Gigliotti AR, et al. Plasma levels of soluble HLA-E and HLA-F at diagnosis may predict overall survival of neuroblastoma patients. Biomed Res Int. 2013;2013:956878. https://doi.org/10.1155/2013/956878.
99. Fisher JP, Yan M, Heuijerjans J, Carter L, Abolhassani A, Frosch J, et al. Neuroblastoma killing properties of Vdelta2 and Vdelta2-negative gammadeltaT cells following expansion by artificial antigen-presenting cells. Clin Cancer Res. 2014;20(22):5720–32. https://doi.org/10.1158/1078-0432.ccr-13-3464.
100. Saura-Esteller J, de Jong M, King LA, Ensing E, Winograd B, de Gruijl TD, et al. Gamma Delta T-cell based cancer immunotherapy: past-present-future. Front Immunol. 2022;13:915837. https://doi.org/10.3389/fimmu.2022.915837.

101. Morandi F, Pozzi S, Barco S, Cangemi G, Amoroso L, Carlini B, et al. CD4(+)CD25(hi)CD127(−) Treg and CD4(+)CD45R0(+)CD49b(+)LAG3(+) Tr1 cells in bone marrow and peripheral blood samples from children with neuroblastoma. Onco Targets Ther. 2016;5(12):e1249553. https://doi.org/10.1080/2162402x.2016.1249553.
102. Johnson BD, Jing W, Orentas RJ. CD25+ regulatory T cell inhibition enhances vaccine-induced immunity to neuroblastoma. J Immunother (Hagerstown, Md : 1997). 2007;30(2):203–14. https://doi.org/10.1097/01.cji.0000211336.91513.dd.
103. Croce M, Corrias MV, Orengo AM, Brizzolara A, Carlini B, Borghi M, et al. Transient depletion of CD4(+) T cells augments IL-21-based immunotherapy of disseminated neuroblastoma in syngeneic mice. Int J Cancer. 2010;127(5):1141–50. https://doi.org/10.1002/ijc.25140.
104. Jing W, Yan X, Hallett WH, Gershan JA, Johnson BD. Depletion of CD25(+) T cells from hematopoietic stem cell grafts increases posttransplantation vaccine-induced immunity to neuroblastoma. Blood. 2011;117(25):6952–62. https://doi.org/10.1182/blood-2010-12-326108.
105. Gowda M, Godder K, Kmieciak M, Worschech A, Ascierto M-L, Wang E, et al. Distinct signatures of the immune responses in low risk versus high risk neuroblastoma. J Transl Med. 2011;9(1):170. https://doi.org/10.1186/1479-5876-9-170.
106. Tilak T, Sherawat S, Agarwala S, Gupta R, Vishnubhatla S, Bakhshi S. Circulating T-regulatory cells in neuroblastoma: a pilot prospective study. Pediatr Hematol Oncol. 2014;31(8):717–22. https://doi.org/10.3109/08880018.2014.886002.
107. Laumont CM, Banville AC, Gilardi M, Hollern DP, Nelson BH. Tumour-infiltrating B cells: immunological mechanisms, clinical impact and therapeutic opportunities. Nat Rev Cancer. 2022;22(7):414–30. https://doi.org/10.1038/s41568-022-00466-1.
108. Schaafsma E, Jiang C, Cheng C. B cell infiltration is highly associated with prognosis and an immune-infiltrated tumor microenvironment in neuroblastoma. J Cancer Metastasis Treat. 2021;7(34) https://doi.org/10.20517/2394-4722.2021.72.
109. Coughlin CM, Fleming MD, Carroll RG, Pawel BR, Hogarty MD, Shan X, et al. Immunosurveillance and survivin-specific T-cell immunity in children with high-risk neuroblastoma. J Clin Oncol. 2006;24(36):5725–34. https://doi.org/10.1200/jco.2005.05.3314.
110. Mou W, Han W, Ma X, Wang X, Qin H, Zhao W, et al. gammadeltaTFH cells promote B cell maturation and antibody production in neuroblastoma. BMC Immunol. 2017;18(1):36. https://doi.org/10.1186/s12865-017-0216-x.
111. Brandeis WE, Helson L, Wang Y, Good RA, Day NK. Circulating immune complexes in sera of children with neuroblastoma: correlation with stage of disease. J Clin Invest. 1978;62(6):1201–9. https://doi.org/10.1172/JCI109240.
112. Ollert MW, David K, Schmitt C, Hauenschild A, Bredehorst R, Erttmann R, et al. Normal human serum contains a natural IgM antibody cytotoxic for human neuroblastoma cells. Proc Natl Acad Sci U S A. 1996;93(9):4498–503.
113. David K, Ollert MW, Juhl H, Vollmert C, Erttmann R, Vogel CW, et al. Growth arrest of solid human neuroblastoma xenografts in nude rats by natural IgM from healthy humans. Nat Med. 1996;2(6):686–9.
114. Devarapu SK, Mamidi S, Ploger F, Dill O, Blixt O, Kirschfink M, et al. Cytotoxic activity against human neuroblastoma and melanoma cells mediated by IgM antibodies derived from peripheral blood of healthy donors. Int J Cancer. 2016;138(12):2963–73. https://doi.org/10.1002/ijc.30025.
115. Wei JS, Kuznetsov IB, Zhang S, Song YK, Asgharzadeh S, Sindiri S, et al. Clinically relevant cytotoxic immune cell signatures and clonal expansion of T-cell receptors in high-risk MYCN-not-amplified human neuroblastoma. Clin Cancer Res. 2018;24(22):5673–84. https://doi.org/10.1158/1078-0432.CCR-18-0599.
116. Veneziani I, Fruci D, Compagnone M, Pistoia V, Rossi P, Cifaldi L. The BET-bromodomain inhibitor JQ1 renders neuroblastoma cells more resistant to NK cell-mediated recognition and killing by downregulating ligands for NKG2D and DNAM-1 receptors. Oncotarget. 2019;10(22):2151–60. https://doi.org/10.18632/oncotarget.26736.
117. Cohen PS, Letterio JJ, Gaetano C, Chan J, Matsumoto K, Sporn MB, et al. Induction of transforming growth factor beta 1 and its receptors during all-trans-retinoic acid (RA) treatment of RA-responsive human neuroblastoma cell lines. Cancer Res. 1995;55(11):2380–6.
118. Seaman S, Stevens J, Yang MY, Logsdon D, Graff-Cherry C, St CB. Genes that distinguish physiological and pathological angiogenesis. Cancer Cell. 2007;11(6):539–54. https://doi.org/10.1016/j.ccr.2007.04.017.
119. Barry WE, Jackson JR, Asuelime GE, Wu HW, Sun J, Wan Z, et al. Activated natural killer cells in combination with anti-GD2 antibody Dinutuximab improve survival of mice after surgical resection of primary neuroblastoma. Clin Cancer Res. 2019;25(1):325–33. https://doi.org/10.1158/1078-0432.CCR-18-1317.
120. Zobel MJ, Zamora AK, Wu HW, Sun J, Lascano D, Malvar J, et al. Initiation of immunotherapy with activated natural killer cells and anti-GD2 antibody dinutuximab prior to resection of primary neuroblastoma prolongs survival in mice. J Immunother Cancer. 2020;8(2) https://doi.org/10.1136/jitc-2020-001560.
121. Chen X, Doffek K, Sugg SL, Shilyansky J. Neuroblastoma cells inhibit the immunostimulatory function of dendritic cells. J Pediatr Surg. 2003;38(6):901–5. https://doi.org/10.1016/s0022-3468(03)00119-2.

122. Gross N, Balmas K, Beretta Brognara C, Tschopp J. Expression of Fas (APO-1/CD95) and Fas ligand (FasL) in human neuroblastoma. Med Pediatr Oncol. 2001;36(1):111–4. https://doi.org/10.1002/1096-911x(20010101)36:1<111::Aid--mpo1026>3.0.Co;2-3.
123. Wienke J, Dierselhuis MP, Tytgat GAM, Kunkele A, Nierkens S, Molenaar JJ. The immune landscape of neuroblastoma: challenges and opportunities for novel therapeutic strategies in pediatric oncology. Eur J Cancer. 2021;144:123–50. https://doi.org/10.1016/j.ejca.2020.11.014.
124. Mussai F, Egan S, Hunter S, Webber H, Fisher J, Wheat R, et al. Neuroblastoma arginase activity creates an immunosuppressive microenvironment that impairs autologous and engineered immunity. Cancer Res. 2015;75(15):3043–53. https://doi.org/10.1158/0008-5472.CAN-14-3443.

9 Neuroblastoma Tumor Microenvironment: Non-Immune Cells and Exosomes

Lucia Borriello, Laurence Blavier, and Yves A. DeClerck

9.1 Introduction

It is clear that non-malignant cells in the tumor microenvironment (TME) are not innocent bystanders but can positively or negatively affect the growth, survival, and metastatic potential of tumor cells [1]. Innate and adaptive immune cells like neutrophils, macrophages, NK cells, T and B lymphocytes, whose function in the TME of neuroblastoma (NB) is described in another chapter, have been the focus of much attention recently with new developments in immunotherapy. However, non-immune cells such as endothelial cells (EC), pericytes, Schwann cells (SC), and cancer-associated fibroblasts (CAF) are also present in the stroma of NB tumors. The presence of SC in NB tumors was recognized in the early 1980s [2] as a marker of favorable outcome [3], and the contribution of EC and tumor-derived vascular endothelial cell growth factor (VEGF) to NB progression was recognized in the late 1990s [4]. The presence of alpha smooth muscle actin (α-SMA) positive cancer-associated fibroblasts has been more recently reported [5, 6]. Over the last two decades, we have gained a significantly better understanding of the mechanisms by which non-immune stromal cells affect the behavior of tumor cells, and of the mechanism of communication between these cells and NB cells and immune cells in the TME. Some of this knowledge has begun to translate into clinical trials, targeting non-immune cells or pathways they activate in NB (Fig. 9.1).

L. Borriello
Department of Cancer and Cellular Biology, Lewis Katz School of Medicine, Temple University, Philadelphia, USA

Fox Chase Cancer Center, Cancer Signaling and Tumor Microenvironment Program, Philadelphia, USA

L. Blavier
The Saban Research Institute, Children's Hospital Los Angeles, Los Angeles, CA, USA

Division of Hematology, Oncology and Blood and Bone Marrow Transplantation, Department of Pediatrics, Keck School of Medicine, University of Southern California, Los Angeles, CA, USA

Y. A. DeClerck (✉)
The Saban Research Institute, Children's Hospital Los Angeles, Los Angeles, CA, USA

Division of Hematology, Oncology and Blood and Bone Marrow Transplantation, Department of Pediatrics, Keck School of Medicine, University of Southern California, Los Angeles, CA, USA

Department of Biochemistry and Molecular Medicine, Keck School of Medicine, University of Southern California, Los Angeles, CA, USA
e-mail: declerck@usc.edu

S. Asgharzadeh, F. Westermann (eds.), *Neuroblastoma*, Pediatric Oncology,
https://doi.org/10.1007/978-3-031-51292-6_9

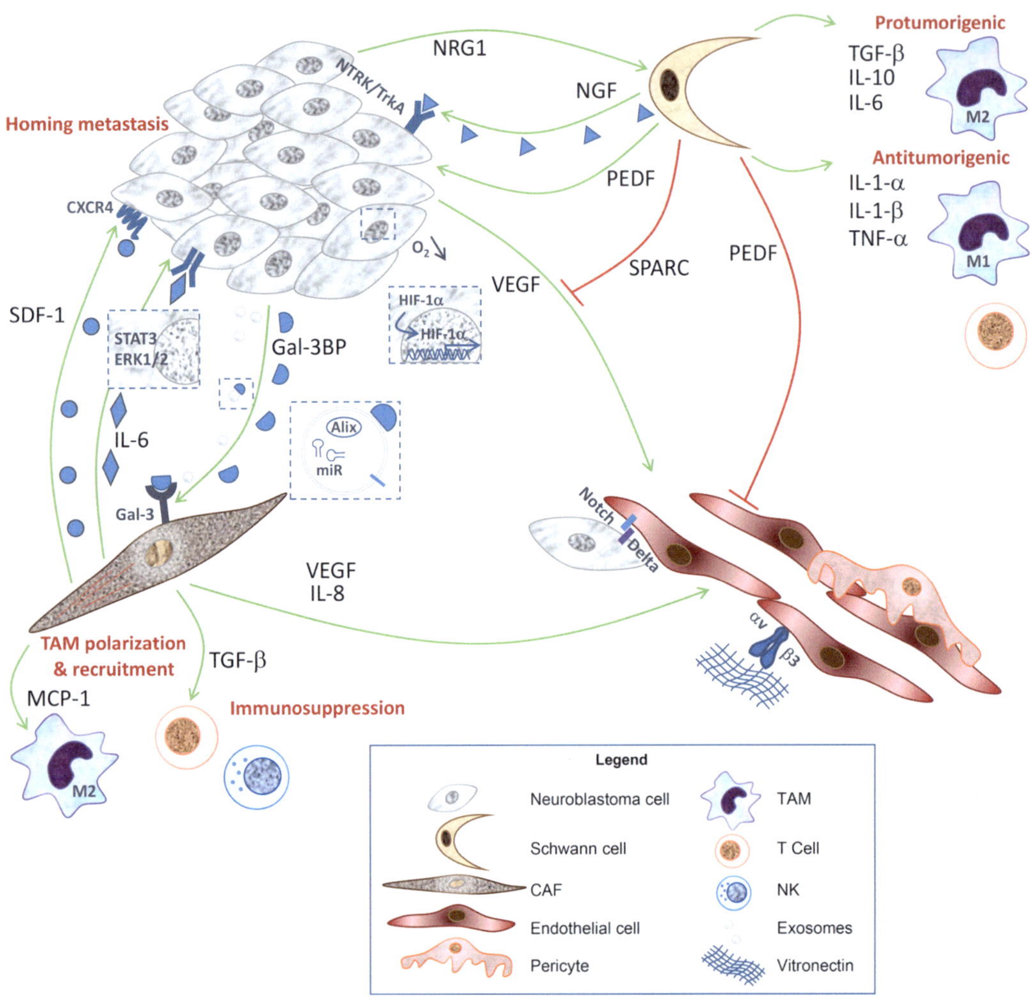

Fig. 9.1 Schematic representation of neuroblastoma tumor microenvironment where Schwann cells, endothelial cells, and cancer-associated fibroblasts, communicate with tumor cells and modulate immune response

9.2 Schwann Cells Contribute to an Unfavorable Soil

The presence of SC is a well-recognized hallmark of more benign NB tumors and their absence (Schwannian stroma-poor) is a key feature characterizing aggressive stroma-poor tumors associated with an unfavorable outcome [3]. The origin of SC in NB is the subject of controversy. Whereas some studies have suggested a neoplastic origin by demonstrating that they share chromosomal abnormalities such as loss of heterozygosity at 1p36 or 11q23, microsatellite mutations and even MYCN amplification seen in NB cells [7], other studies have shown that SC do not share genetic alterations commonly seen in NB and ganglia cells in NB [8]. The interaction between SC and NB cells is reciprocal [9]. When stimulated by neuregulin (NRG1), a cell adhesion molecule produced by NTRK1/TrkA expressing NB cells, SC secrete nerve growth factor (NGF), the ligand for NTRK/TrkA cells, that inhibits NB cell growth and stimulates differentiation [9]. SC are attracted to NB tumors by the production of neuregulin-1 (NRG1) [9] and produce the secreted acid protein rich in cysteine (SPARC), an anti-angiogenic molecule that reduces VEGF-A expression in NB cells [10–14], therefore reducing tumor vascularization. SC are also a source of pigmented epithelium-derived factor (PEDF), an inhibitor of angiogenesis that also promotes NB cell differentiation [15]. Whether the presence of SC in the stroma of NB tumors could affect immune response is not known. Their function and survival are affected by inflammation in NB tumors. For example, high motility group box 1 (HMGB1), a master regulator of inflammation, induces autophagy in SC and suppresses their anti-tumor activity promoting NB cell growth [16]. There is also evidence in models of nerve injury and repair that SC affect the immune response. Responsible for myelination of peripheral nerve and conductivity, SC actively contribute to inflammation during nerve injury and repair [17] by acting as antigen-presenting cells expressing MCHII molecules and being a source of cytokines and chemokines that contribute to an inflammatory reaction. They produce interleukin (IL)-1α and IL-1β, tumor necrosis factor (TNF)-α, and IL-6 that promote T cell proliferation and activation, and stimulate the immune system, a role that would be consistent with their well-known anti-tumoral function. Much more should be learned on the immune modulatory function of SC in NB.

9.3 Endothelial Cells and Pericytes in NB Vascularization

EC in the vasculature of NB tumors originate from three sources, neighboring vessels, EC precursor cells (EPC) recruited from the bone marrow, and tumor cells through vascular mimicry [18, 19]. The general observation that a disrupted vasculature with leaky EC and disrupted pericytes is a feature of aggressive tumors is also true in NB. Blood vessels are larger, more abundant and more irregularly shaped in high-risk tumors with poor prognostic factors than in tumors associated with a more favorable outcome [20]. NB tumors typically develop their vasculature through the production of VEGF by tumor cells under hypoxic conditions. MYCN plays a particularly important role in angiogenesis. The expression of hypoxia-inducible factor-1α (HIF-1α) is higher in *MYCN*-amplified tumors and MYCN can override HIF-1α inhibition. HIF-1α and MYCN are also essential for the Warburg effect (aerobic glycolysis) by activating the transcription of multiple glycolytic genes [21]. HIF-1α expression is enhanced by factors that increase the expression of *MYCN* or regulate its nuclear translocation, like Aurora kinases [22]. VEGF is not the only pathway driving angiogenesis in NB. For example, activation of NOTCH in EC by the ligand Delta expressed by NB cells increases EC proliferation and survival [23, 24]. However, inhibition of NOTCH causes a paradoxical activation of liver cells promoting angiogenesis and liver metastasis in mice [25]. *MYCN*-amplified tumors have higher expression of αvβ3 integrin in EC, which stimulates EC attachment to vitronectin and migration, and increases PI3K signaling, EC proliferation and survival [26]. Tumor cells are not the only source of angiogenic factors in NB, macrophages and CAF (see below) are also a source on pro-angiogenic molecules like VEGF and IL-8 [6, 27].

Pericytes, which originate from mesenchymal stromal cells (MSC) present in adjacent tissues or recruited from the bone marrow in a PDGFB and PDGFR-β dependent mechanism, also contribute to the tumor vasculature in NB [28]. Their presence around EC is regulated by the matrix metalloproteinase (MMP)-9, as NB tumor-bearing MMP-9 null mice show a disrupted vasculature with increased leakiness and fewer pericytes [29].

9.4 Cancer-Associated Fibroblasts; Newly Recognized Contributors to the Soil in NB Tumors

The presence of CAF in tumors has been recognized for many years, in particular in pancreatic and breast cancers where they contribute to a desmoplastic reaction, increase tissue stiffness, and promote the proliferation and invasion of cancer cells. CAF represent a heterogeneous population of mesenchymal cells expressing a variety of markers such as fibroblast specific protein (FSP) 1 (aka S100A4), fibroblast activation protein α (FAP-α, aka dipeptidyl peptidase IV), α-SMA, PDGFR-β, β1 integrin (CD29), in addition to other proteins such as thrombospondin-1, tenascin-C and stromelysin, desmin-1 and VEGF-A [30, 31]. In contrast to normal resting fibroblasts, CAF rapidly proliferate, secrete an abundance of extracellular matrix (ECM) proteins, including collagen and fibronectin, and are migratory. When activated by the presence of tumor cells, these fibroblasts become "educated" and secrete inflammatory molecules [32–35]. There is strong evidence that a major source of CAF are bone marrow-derived MSC, multipotent cells that have the ability to differentiate into adipocytes, chondrocytes, pericytes, EC, and induced pluripotent stem cells (iPSC) [32–36].

The presence of CAF in NB tumors was first identified by L. Cohn's group, who reported the presence of α-SMA positive non-pericyte cells in NB tumors and demonstrated that the presence of these cells is associated with an increase in microvascular proliferation and a decrease in SC in tumors from patients with overall poorer clinical outcome [5], thus suggesting that CAF contribute to an environment that is favorable to NB cells. The mechanisms by which these CAF contribute to a pro-tumorigenic TME have been recently reported. CAF that share phenotypic and functional characteristics of MSC have been isolated from NB tumors and shown to express several markers of activated CAF-like FAP-α and α-SMA as well as markers of MSC like CD105, CD90, and CD73. These CAF-MSC promote NB cell growth and survival, and enhance resistance to chemotherapy [6] by secreting multiple cytokines and chemokines such as IL-6, IL-8, VEGF-A, monocyte chemoattractant protein (MCP) 1 (aka CCL2), and stromal-derived factor (SDF) 1 (aka CXCL-12) that have broad pro-tumorigenic effects on NB cells and stromal cells in the TME [37, 38]. These cytokines and chemokines activate STAT3 and ERK1/2-mediated signaling in NB cells that stimulate NB cell proliferation, survival, and drug resistance [39]. MSC also protect NB cells from H_2O_2-induced oxidative stress by their capacity to produce and activate antioxidant enzymes and to downregulate superoxide dismutase [40]. CAF-derived cytokines not only target NB cells but also non-malignant cells in the TME of NB tumors. IL-6 activates osteoclasts in the bone marrow that promote the formation of osteolytic metastasis [41]. VEGF and IL-8 stimulate angiogenesis and MCP-1 is a chemoattractant for monocytes and macrophages. SDF-1 promotes the recruitment of CXCR4 expressing tumor cells to the metastatic niche [42, 43]. CAF and MSC are a source of TGF-β, which has a potent immunosuppressive activity on NK and T cells and promotes immune escape [44].

In NB tumors, CAF are often present at sites of tumor infiltration with tumor-associated macrophages (TAM), and there is a direct correlation between the expression of CD163 (a marker of M2 polarized macrophages) and FAP-α expression in data set analysis of NB tumors [6]. CAF expressing prostaglandin synthase are present with M2 macrophages in an inflammatory subtype of NB tumors [45, 46]. The number of TAM and CAF significantly correlates with clinical stage, *MYCN* amplification, bone marrow metastasis, histological type, and risk classification [46]. Once activated, CAF enhance the invasive ability of peripheral blood mononuclear cell (PBMC)-derived macrophages, polarizing them toward an M2-like phenotype [46]. Vice versa, TAM enhance not only the invasive abilities of CAF but also their proliferation. TAM enhance CAF-induced STAT3 activation in NB cells by being a source of the soluble agonistic receptor for IL-6, sIL-6R [39].

MSC present in NB tumors are not only precursors of CAF but also adipocytes, which raises the question whether adipocytes could contribute to the TME of NB. The presence of adipocytes in NB and NB metastatic lesions has not been carefully examined but NB cells express the receptor for leptin, the main cytokine produced by adipocytes, and stimulation of this receptor has been reported to activate STAT3 and promote NB cell survival [47, 48].

9.5 Tumor Cell–Stromal Cell Communication in the TME of NB: A Role for Extracellular Vesicles?

Communication between tumor cells and stromal cells occurs through contact-dependent and contact-independent mechanisms. In the case of NB, most of the mechanisms of communication reported are contact-independent and mediated by soluble proteins such as growth factors (NGF, VEGF, TGF-β, PEDF), cytokines (IL-6, IL-8, IL-10), chemokines (CXCL-12) or other factors (SPARC, Gal-3BP). There has, however, been more recent evidence that extracellular vesicles (EV) released by tumor cells in the extracellular milieu and captured by stromal cells in the TME could play a role. EV represent a large family of vesicles ranging from 20 nm to 5 μm in diameter that can be classified in three main groups based on their size, their subcellular origin, and their composition: (1) exosomes originating from late endosomes (aka multivesicular bodies—MVB); (2) microvesicles issued from the budding of the plasma membrane during cell stress; and (3) apoptotic bodies released by dying cells [38, 49].

Exosomes are cup-shaped vesicles of 30 to 120 nm in size that contain a large variety of proteins, lipids, metabolites, and nucleic acids, including regulatory miR that act as shuttles mediating the communication between tumor cells and stromal cells in both directions [49]. Our laboratory has recently shown that exosomes derived from NB cells induce in MSC the production of cytokines and chemokines such as IL-6, IL-8, VEGF, and MCP-1 [38]. Exosomes differentiate from other EV by the presence of specific proteins such as tetraspanins (CD9, CD63, and CD81), heat shock proteins (HSP70, HSP90), major histocompatibility complex (MHC) class I and class II, proteins of the endosomal sorting complex required for transport (ESCRT) components (TSG101 and Alix). They have a unique biogenesis as they derive from intra-luminal vesicles (ILV) formed by inward budding in late endosomes (MVB) [50, 51]. When MVB fuse with lysosomes, their cargo is degraded, but when they fuse with the plasma membrane, ILV are released into the extracellular space as exosomes [52, 53].

The protein content of the cargo of exosomes from several NB cells includes, in addition to the exosomal markers (CD63, CD9, CD81, Hsp70, Hsp90, and Alix), disialoganglioside (GD)-2 and proteins involved in tumor progression such as CD147 (basigin), a multifunctional protein involved in invasion and metastasis, and CD276/B7-H3, an immune checkpoint protein that protects NB cells from attack by NK cells [54]. A more recent comparative analysis of the proteomic cargo of exosomes isolated from NB cell lines derived from primary tumors (IMR32 and IGR-NB8) vs. cell lines derived from bone marrow metastasis (SK-N-SH, SH-SY5Y, IGR-N91, SK-N-BE(2)-C, and LAN-1) [55] revealed that primary tumor exosomes contain a higher level of proteins involved in ECM assembly and adhesion, as well as in neuronal development, whereas exosomes isolated from bone-marrow metastasis exhibit proteins involved in ameboidal cell migration and mitochondrial activity. These observations suggest that proteomic profiling of NB-derived exosomes reflects the biology of the tumor, raising the possibility that the analysis of exosomes from the peripheral blood may be a liquid biopsy biomarker for clinical outcome. This possibility, however, requires further investigation.

EV also contain regulatory non-coding RNA. The profile of miR content of EV from two *MYCN*-amplified NB cell lines revealed the presence of several oncogenic miRNAs associated with a range of cellular and molecular functions related to cell growth, cancer progression, and drug resistance [56]. Exosomal miRNAs are also involved in a reciprocal interaction between NB cells and monocytes where NB cells release exosomes containing miR-21, which, when captured by monocytes, binds to toll-like receptor 8 (TLR8) triggering an NF-κB-mediated pro-inflammatory response in monocytes. This response includes the upregulation of miR-155 that is shuttled by macrophage-derived exosomes to NB cells where it targets the inhibitor of telomerase, telomeric repeat binding factor 1 (TERF1), promoting increased resistance to cisplatin of NB cells [57]. There is thus much experimental evidence suggesting that NB-derived exosomes could play an important role in the communication between NB cells and stromal cells in the TME. However, presently, most if not all of this evidence is from experiments performed in co-cultures in vitro. The demonstration that exosomes play a critical role in the TME of NB is awaiting experimental evidence in vivo [55].

9.6 Therapeutic Implications

Evidence that several non-immune stromal cells in the TME of NB have a pro-tumorigenic role is supporting the development of strategies to target these cells or their effects. These strategies can be classified in three main approaches: (1) Approaches that target the production or activity of cytokines/chemokines released by stromal cells upon exposure to NB cells or released by NB cells to educate stromal cells; (2) Approaches that target pathways that are specifically activated in NB cells by non-immune stromal cells; and (3) Approaches directly targeting non-immune cells.

9.6.1 Targeting Cytokines

Anti VEGF therapy was among the first strategies targeting cytokines in the TME. Avastin (bevacizumab), in combination with chemotherapy, radiotherapy, or IMBG-based therapy, has been the subject of several clinical trials in patients with NB (Table 9.1). The New Advances in Neuroblastoma Therapy (NANT) consortium completed a trial combining bevacizumab with zoledronic acid and cyclophosphamide in patients with refractory/recurrent high-risk neuroblastoma, demonstrating the safety of bevacizumab in young patients, an observation which was confirmed in children with other malignancies [58].

Table 9.1 Open clinical trials using agents that target the tumor microenvironment in neuroblastoma with sponsor institution, NCT number, and status as of May 2018 indicated

Trial	Sponsor	Number	Status
Cyclophosphamide, Topotecan, and bevacizumab (CTB) in patients with relapsed/refractory Ewing's sarcoma and neuroblastoma	Memorial Sloan Kettering Cancer Center	NCT01492673	Active, not recruiting
Bevacizumab, irinotecan and Temozolomide for relapsed or refractory neuroblastoma	Memorial Sloan Kettering Cancer Center	NCT01114555	Active, not recruiting
Anti-angiogenic therapy with radiotherapy for pediatric neuroblastoma	Xinhua Hospital, Shanghai Jiao Tong University School of Medicine	NCT02615106	Recruiting
N2007–02: Bevacizumab, cyclophosphamide and Zoledronic acid in patients with recurrent or refractory high-risk neuroblastoma	New Approaches to Neuroblastoma Therapy Consortium	NCT00885326	Active, not recruiting
Iodine I 131 monoclonal antibody 3F8 and bevacizumab in treating patients with relapsed or refractory neuroblastoma	Memorial Sloan Kettering Cancer Center	NCT00450827	Completed
Activity study of bevacizumab with Temozolomide ± irinotecan for neuroblastoma in children (BEACON)	University of Birmingham	NCT02308527	Recruiting
Sorafenib and cyclophosphamide/Topotecan in patients with relapsed and refractory neuroblastoma	New Approaches to Neuroblastoma Therapy Consortium	NCT02298348	Recruiting
Ruxolitinib in treating young patients with relapsed or refractory solid tumor, leukemia, or myeloproliferative disease	Children's Oncology Group	NCT01164163	Completed
Next generation personalized neuroblastoma therapy (NEPENTHE)	Children's Hospital of Philadelphia	NCT02780128	Recruiting

A recently completed Phase II trial on bevacizumab with irinotecan and temozolomide in patients with refractory/relapsed NB demonstrated that the combination is well tolerated, but the addition of bevacizumab does not improve response rates in resistant NB compared to historical data for chemotherapy alone [59]. Recent preclinical observations in animal models suggest that normalization of the tumor vasculature with bevacizumab may promote the infiltration of NB tumors with anti-GD2 CAR-T cells and result in high production of interferon gamma and antitumor effect of CAR-T cells, suggesting that bevacizumab could be used in combination with CAR-T cell therapy to circumvent the low recruitment of these cells in solid tumors [60].

The use of SPARC as a therapeutic tool has been considered, but because of the complexity of the protein, its multiple domain, lack of small active peptide, and elevated levels in more metastatic cancer, its therapeutic use has not been tested in phase I clinical trials [61].

Targeting other cytokines such as IL-6, IL-8, or CCL2/MCP-1 has not been tested in clinical trials in patients with NB tumors. Considering the broad spectrum of cytokines and chemokines secreted by stromal cells in the TME of NB cells, it is unlikely that targeting a single cytokine will result in a substantial anti-tumor effect in patients as numerous alternate pathways of communication between stromal cells and NB cells are involved. For example, we have recently shown in genetically engineered mice developing *MYC*-non amplified NB tumors, that the ablation of IL-6 does not prevent tumor growth and STAT3 activation in NB cells [62].

9.6.2 Targeting Pathways

The use of small molecule inhibitors of pathways that are not constitutively activated in NB cells but activated upon interaction with stromal cells in the TME deserves further consideration. Among them are in particular STAT3, which is specifically activated by interaction with MSC, CAF, and TAM and ERK1/2 [1]. Sorafenib, a broad-spectrum kinase inhibitor with pre-clinical activity in NB [63–65], is presently tested in combination with cyclophosphamide and topotecan in a phase I trial in patients with relapsed and refractory NB by NANT [66]. The Children's Oncology Group completed a phase I study on ruxolitinib, a JAK2/STAT3 inhibitor in children with refractory/relapsed solid tumors including NB, and in leukemia and myeloproliferative neoplasms [67]. It was well tolerated and is now in several phase II clinical trials in children with leukemia and graft versus host disease. Trametinib, a small molecule inhibitor of MEK [68], is tested in a phase I/II study in children with plexiform neurofibroma in combination with dabrafenib and in patients with glioma harboring the BRAF mutation. It is included in the arsenal of drugs in the next generation personalized NB therapy trials (NEPENTHE) for patients with recurrent/relapsed NB tumors harboring mutations in the RAS-MAPK pathway.

9.6.3 Targeting Stromal Cells

Metronomic chemotherapy that uses low doses of continuously applied chemotherapeutic agents represents such an attempt to target EC. In a recently published study of 23 patients with recurrent or refractory high-risk NB treated with celecoxib and metronomics cyclophosphamide, vinblastine, and etoposide for up to 24 months, the metronomic approach although similarly effective as standard intensive therapy had lower toxicity and was applicable in an outpatient setting [69]. Targeting osteoclasts with the bisphosphonate zoledronic acid with metronomic cyclophosphamide was also shown to be well tolerated with clinical and biologic responses in patients with recurrent/refractory metastatic NB [70].

Specifically targeting CAF is challenging considering the heterogeneous nature of these cells and the need for specific markers to target pro-tumorigenic CAF, but it is an attractive approach considering the well demonstrated pro-tumorigenic activity of these cells and their role in immune escape. So far, preclinical experiments have focused on targeting FAP-α. A humanized monoclonal antibody (sibrotuzumab) against FAP-α has been developed and tested in the clinic, but it showed little efficacy due to lack of a strong antibody-dependent cellular toxicity and significant side effects [71, 72]. CAR-T cells engineered with a chimeric anti-FAP-α receptor have been tested in pre-clinical tumor models with some effect [73, 74].

SC are difficult to grow and amplify in vitro, and we still know little of their anti-tumor activity and potential use in cell therapy approaches. However, there is recent evidence that SC can be expanded from human pluripotent stem cells in chemically defined conditions [75] and could be used to treat demyelination disorders and injuries to the peripheral nervous system. Whether these cells could be part of cell therapy approaches to NB has not been considered and explored so far.

9.7 Conclusion

It is clear that non-immune cells play an active role in the TME of NB tumors, communicating not only with tumor cells but also with immune cells. Whereas our knowledge of the contribution of immune cells in NB is well advanced, our knowledge of the contribution of non-immune cells, and in particular fibroblasts, lags behind and represents a new area of exploration in the field that should lead to novel therapeutic intervention. How these cells control the immune system and allow NB cells to escape is of particular interest.

References

1. Borriello L, Seeger RC, Asgharzadeh S, DeClerck YA. More than the genes, the tumor microenvironment in neuroblastoma. Cancer Lett. 2016;380(1):304–14. https://doi.org/10.1016/j.canlet.2015.11.017.
2. Taxy JB. Electron microscopy in the diagnosis of neuroblastoma. Arch Pathol Lab Med. 1980;104(7):355–60.
3. Burgues O, Navarro S, Noguera R, Pellin A, Ruiz A, Castel V, et al. Prognostic value of the international neuroblastoma pathology classification in neuroblastoma (Schwannian stroma-poor) and comparison with other prognostic factors: a study of 182 cases from the Spanish neuroblastoma registry. Virchows Arch. 2006;449(4):410–20. https://doi.org/10.1007/s00428-006-0253-y.
4. Rossler J, Breit S, Havers W, Schweigerer L. Vascular endothelial growth factor expression in human neuroblastoma: up-regulation by hypoxia. Int J Cancer. 1999;81(1):113–7.
5. Zeine R, Salwen HR, Peddinti R, Tian Y, Guerrero L, Yang Q, et al. Presence of cancer-associated fibroblasts inversely correlates with Schwannian stroma in neuroblastoma tumors. Mod Pathol. 2009;22(7):950–8. https://doi.org/10.1038/modpathol.2009.52.
6. Borriello L, Nakata R, Sheard MA, Fernandez GE, Sposto R, Malvar J, et al. Cancer-associated fibroblasts share characteristics and protumorigenic activity with mesenchymal stromal cells. Cancer Res. 2017;77(18):5142–57. https://doi.org/10.1158/0008-5472.can-16-2586.
7. Mora J, Akram M, Cheung NK, Chen L, Gerald WL. Laser-capture microdissected Schwannian and neuroblastic cells in stage 4 neuroblastomas have the same genetic alterations. Med Pediatr Oncol. 2000;35(6):534–7.
8. Angelini P, Baruchel S, Marrano P, Irwin MS, Thorner PS. The neuroblastoma and ganglion components of nodular ganglioneuroblastoma are genetically similar: evidence against separate clonal origins. Mod Pathol. 2015;28(2):166–76. https://doi.org/10.1038/modpathol.2014.90.
9. Pajtler KW, Mahlow E, Odersky A, Lindner S, Stephan H, Bendix I, et al. Neuroblastoma in dialog with its stroma: NTRK1 is a regulator of cellular cross-talk with Schwann cells. Oncotarget. 2014;5(22):11180–92.
10. Huang D, Rutkowski JL, Brodeur GM, Chou PM, Kwiatkowski JL, Babbo A, et al. Schwann cell-conditioned medium inhibits angiogenesis. Cancer Res. 2000;60(21):5966–71.
11. Boyineni J, Tanpure S, Gnanamony M, Antony R, Fernandez KS, Lin J, et al. SPARC overexpression combined with radiation retards angiogenesis by suppressing VEGF-A via miR410 in human neuroblastoma cells. Int J Oncol. 2016;49(4):1394–406. https://doi.org/10.3892/ijo.2016.3646.
12. Chlenski A, Liu S, Guerrero LJ, Yang Q, Tian Y, Salwen HR, et al. SPARC expression is associated with impaired tumor growth, inhibited angiogenesis and changes in the extracellular matrix. Int J Cancer. 2006;118(2):310–6.
13. Chlenski A, Guerrero LJ, Peddinti R, Spitz JA, Leonhardt PT, Yang Q, et al. Anti-angiogenic SPARC peptides inhibit progression of neuroblastoma tumors. Mol Cancer. 2010;9:138. https://doi.org/10.1186/1476-4598-9-138.
14. Chlenski A, Liu S, Crawford SE, Volpert OV, DeVries GH, Evangelista A, et al. SPARC is a key Schwannian-derived inhibitor controlling neuroblastoma tumor angiogenesis. Cancer Res. 2002;62(24):7357–63.
15. Crawford SE, Stellmach V, Ranalli M, Huang X, Huang L, Volpert O, et al. Pigment epithelium-derived

factor (PEDF) in neuroblastoma: a multifunctional mediator of Schwann cell antitumor activity. J Cell Sci. 2001;114(Pt 24):4421–8.
16. Liu Y, Song L. HMGB1-induced autophagy in Schwann cells promotes neuroblastoma proliferation. Int J Clin Exp Pathol. 2015;8(1):504–10.
17. Tzekova N, Heinen A, Kury P. Molecules involved in the crosstalk between immune- and peripheral nerve Schwann cells. J Clin Immunol. 2014;34(Suppl 1):S86–104. https://doi.org/10.1007/s10875-014-0015-6.
18. Pezzolo A, Parodi F, Corrias MV, Cinti R, Gambini C, Pistoia V. Tumor origin of endothelial cells in human neuroblastoma. J Clin Oncol Off J Am Soc Clin Oncol. 2007;25(4):376–83. https://doi.org/10.1200/jco.2006.09.0696.
19. Jodele S, Chantrain CF, Blavier L, Lutzko C, Crooks GM, Shimada H, et al. The contribution of bone marrow derived cells to the tumor vasculature in neuroblastoma is matrix metalloproteinase-9 dependent. Cancer Res. 2005;65(8):3200–8.
20. Tadeo I, Bueno G, Berbegall AP, Fernandez-Carrobles MM, Castel V, Garcia-Rojo M, et al. Vascular patterns provide therapeutic targets in aggressive neuroblastic tumors. Oncotarget. 2016;7(15):19935–47. https://doi.org/10.18632/oncotarget.7661.
21. Qing G, Skuli N, Mayes PA, Pawel B, Martinez D, Maris JM, et al. Combinatorial regulation of neuroblastoma tumor progression by N-Myc and hypoxia inducible factor HIF-1alpha. Cancer Res. 2010;70(24):10351–61. https://doi.org/10.1158/0008-5472.can-10-0740.
22. Romain C, Paul P, Kim KW, Lee S, Qiao J, Chung DH. Targeting Aurora kinase-a downregulates cell proliferation and angiogenesis in neuroblastoma. J Pediatr Surg. 2014;49(1):159–65. https://doi.org/10.1016/j.jpedsurg.2013.09.051.
23. Gorantla B, Bhoopathi P, Chetty C, Gogineni VR, Sailaja GS, Gondi CS, et al. Notch signaling regulates tumor-induced angiogenesis in SPARC-overexpressed neuroblastoma. Angiogenesis. 2013;16(1):85–100. https://doi.org/10.1007/s10456-012-9301-1.
24. Hernandez SL, Banerjee D, Garcia A, Kangsamaksin T, Cheng WY, Anastassiou D, et al. Notch and VEGF pathways play distinct but complementary roles in tumor angiogenesis. Vasc Cell. 2013;5(1):17. https://doi.org/10.1186/2045-824x-5-17.
25. Banerjee D, Hernandez SL, Garcia A, Kangsamaksin T, Sbiroli E, Andrews J, et al. Notch suppresses angiogenesis and progression of hepatic metastases. Cancer Res. 2015;75(8):1592–602. https://doi.org/10.1158/0008-5472.can-14-1493.
26. Erdreich-Epstein A, Singh AR, Joshi S, Vega FM, Guo P, Xu J, et al. Association of high microvessel alphavbeta3 and low PTEN with poor outcome in stage 3 neuroblastoma: rationale for using first in class dual PI3K/BRD4 inhibitor, SF1126. Oncotarget. 2017;8(32):52193–210. https://doi.org/10.18632/oncotarget.13386.
27. Asgharzadeh S, Salo JA, Ji L, Oberthuer A, Fischer M, Berthold F, et al. Clinical significance of tumor-associated inflammatory cells in metastatic neuroblastoma. J Clin Oncol. 2012;30(28):3525–32. https://doi.org/10.1200/JCO.2011.40.9169.
28. Abramsson A, Lindblom P, Betsholtz C. Endothelial and nonendothelial sources of PDGF-B regulate pericyte recruitment and influence vascular pattern formation in tumors. J Clin Invest. 2003;112(8):1142–51.
29. Chantrain CF, Shimada H, Jodele S, Groshen S, Ye W, Shalinsky DR, et al. Stromal matrix metalloproteinase-9 regulates the vascular architecture in neuroblastoma by promoting pericyte recruitment. Cancer Res. 2004;64(5):1675–86.
30. Spaeth EL, Dembinski JL, Sasser AK, Watson K, Klopp A, Hall B, et al. Mesenchymal stem cell transition to tumor-associated fibroblasts contributes to fibrovascular network expansion and tumor progression. PLoS One. 2009;4(4):e4992.
31. Costa A, Kieffer Y, Scholer-Dahirel A, Pelon F, Bourachot B, Cardon M, et al. Fibroblast heterogeneity and immunosuppressive environment in human breast cancer. Cancer Cell. 2018;33:463. https://doi.org/10.1016/j.ccell.2018.01.011.
32. Von Luttichau I, Notohamiprodjo M, Wechselberger A, Peters C, Henger A, Seliger C, et al. Human adult CD34- progenitor cells functionally express the chemokine receptors CCR1, CCR4, CCR7, CXCR5, and CCR10 but not CXCR4. Stem Cells Dev. 2005;14(3):329–36. https://doi.org/10.1089/scd.2005.14.329.
33. Honczarenko M, Le Y, Swierkowski M, Ghiran I, Glodek AM, Silberstein LE. Human bone marrow stromal cells express a distinct set of biologically functional chemokine receptors. Stem Cells. 2006;24(4):1030–41. https://doi.org/10.1634/stemcells.2005-0319.
34. Ringe J, Strassburg S, Neumann K, Endres M, Notter M, Burmester GR, et al. Towards in situ tissue repair: human mesenchymal stem cells express chemokine receptors CXCR1, CXCR2 and CCR2, and migrate upon stimulation with CXCL8 but not CCL2. J Cell Biochem. 2007;101(1):135–46. https://doi.org/10.1002/jcb.21172.
35. Spaeth E, Klopp A, Dembinski J, Andreeff M, Marini F. Inflammation and tumor microenvironments: defining the migratory itinerary of mesenchymal stem cells. Gene Ther. 2008;15(10):730–8.
36. Yagi H, Soto-Gutierrez A, Parekkadan B, Kitagawa Y, Tompkins RG, Kobayashi N, et al. Mesenchymal stem cells: mechanisms of immunomodulation and homing. Cell Transplant. 2010;19(6):667–79. https://doi.org/10.3727/096368910X508762.
37. Silverman AM, Nakata R, Shimada H, Sposto R, DeClerck YA. A galectin-3-dependent pathway upregulates interleukin-6 in the microenvironment of human neuroblastoma. Cancer Res. 2012;72(9):2228–38.
38. Nakata R, Shimada H, Fernandez GE, Fanter R, Fabbri M, Malvar J, et al. Contribution of neuroblastoma-

derived exosomes to the production of pro-tumorigenic signals by bone marrow mesenchymal stromal cells. J Extracell Vesicles. 2017;6(1):1332941. https://doi.org/10.1080/20013078.2017.1332941.
39. Ara T, Nakata R, Sheard MA, Shimada H, Buettner R, Groshen SG, et al. Critical role of STAT3 in IL-6-mediated drug resistance in human neuroblastoma. Cancer Res. 2013;73(13):3852–64. https://doi.org/10.1158/0008-5472.CAN-12-2353.
40. Lanza C, Morando S, Voci A, Canesi L, Principato MC, Serpero LD, et al. Neuroprotective mesenchymal stem cells are endowed with a potent antioxidant effect in vivo. J Neurochem. 2009;110(5):1674–84.
41. Sohara Y, Shimada H, Minkin C, Erdreich-Epstein A, Nolta JA, DeClerck YA. Bone marrow mesenchymal stem cells provide an alternate pathway of osteoclast activation and bone destruction by cancer cells. Cancer Res. 2005;65(4):1129–35.
42. Ma M, Ye JY, Deng R, Dee CM, Chan GC. Mesenchymal stromal cells may enhance metastasis of neuroblastoma via SDF-1/CXCR4 and SDF-1/CXCR7 signaling. Cancer Lett. 2011;312(1):1–10. https://doi.org/10.1016/j.canlet.2011.06.028.
43. Muhlethaler-Mottet A, Liberman J, Ascencao K, Flahaut M, Balmas Bourloud K, Yan P, et al. The CXCR4/CXCR7/CXCL12 axis is involved in a secondary but complex control of neuroblastoma metastatic cell homing. PLoS One. 2015;10(5):e0125616. https://doi.org/10.1371/journal.pone.0125616.
44. Bianchi G, Morandi F, Cilli M, Daga A, Bocelli-Tyndall C, Gambini C, et al. Close interactions between mesenchymal stem cells and neuroblastoma cell lines lead to tumor growth inhibition. PLoS One. 2012;7(10):e48654. https://doi.org/10.1371/journal.pone.0048654.
45. Larsson K, Kock A, Idborg H, Arsenian Henriksson M, Martinsson T, Johnsen JI, et al. COX/mPGES-1/PGE2 pathway depicts an inflammatory-dependent high-risk neuroblastoma subset. Proc Natl Acad Sci U S A. 2015;112(26):8070–5. https://doi.org/10.1073/pnas.1424355112.
46. Hashimoto O, Yoshida M, Koma YI, Yanai T, Hasegawa D, Kosaka Y, et al. Collaboration of cancer-associated fibroblasts and tumour-associated macrophages for neuroblastoma development. J Pathol. 2016;240:211. https://doi.org/10.1002/path.4769.
47. Wang R, Swick AG. Identification and characterization of a leptin-responsive neuroblastoma cell line. Biochem Biophys Res Commun. 2009;379(4):835–9. https://doi.org/10.1016/j.bbrc.2008.12.157.
48. Russo VC, Metaxas S, Kobayashi K, Harris M, Werther GA. Antiapoptotic effects of leptin in human neuroblastoma cells. Endocrinology. 2004;145(9):4103–12. https://doi.org/10.1210/en.2003-1767.
49. Antonyak MA, Cerione RA. Microvesicles as mediators of intercellular communication in cancer. Methods Mol Biol. 2014;1165:147–73. https://doi.org/10.1007/978-1-4939-0856-1_11.
50. Thery C, Zitvogel L, Amigorena S. Exosomes: composition, biogenesis and function. Nat Rev Immunol. 2002;2(8):569–79.
51. Lotvall J, Hill AF, Hochberg F, Buzas EI, Di Vizio D, Gardiner C, et al. Minimal experimental requirements for definition of extracellular vesicles and their functions: a position statement from the International Society for Extracellular Vesicles. J Extracell Vesicles. 2014;3:26913. https://doi.org/10.3402/jev.v3.26913.
52. Kowal J, Tkach M, Thery C. Biogenesis and secretion of exosomes. Curr Opin Cell Biol. 2014;29:116–25. https://doi.org/10.1016/j.ceb.2014.05.004.
53. Colombo M, Raposo G, Thery C. Biogenesis, secretion, and intercellular interactions of exosomes and other extracellular vesicles. Annu Rev Cell Dev Biol. 2014;30:255–89. https://doi.org/10.1146/annurev-cellbio-101512-122326.
54. Marimpietri D, Petretto A, Raffaghello L, Pezzolo A, Gagliani C, Tacchetti C, et al. Proteome profiling of neuroblastoma-derived exosomes reveal the expression of proteins potentially involved in tumor progression. PLoS One. 2013;8(9):e75054. https://doi.org/10.1371/journal.pone.0075054.
55. Colletti M, Petretto A, Galardi A, Di Paolo V, Tomao L, Lavarello C, et al. Proteomic analysis of neuroblastoma-derived exosomes: new insights into a metastatic signature. Proteomics. 2017;17:23–4. https://doi.org/10.1002/pmic.201600430.
56. Haug BH, Hald OH, Utnes P, Roth SA, Lokke C, Flaegstad T, et al. Exosome-like extracellular vesicles from MYCN-amplified neuroblastoma cells contain oncogenic miRNAs. Anticancer Res. 2015;35(5):2521–30.
57. Challagundla KB, Wise PM, Neviani P, Chava H, Murtadha M, Xu T, et al. Exosome-mediated transfer of microRNAs within the tumor microenvironment and neuroblastoma resistance to chemotherapy. J Natl Cancer Inst. 2015;107(7):djv135. https://doi.org/10.1093/jnci/djv135.
58. Millan NC, Poveda MJ, Cruz O, Mora J. Safety of bevacizumab in patients younger than 4 years of age. Clin Transl Oncol. 2016;18(5):464–8. https://doi.org/10.1007/s12094-015-1389-5.
59. Modak S, Kushner BH, Basu E, Roberts SS, Cheung NK. Combination of bevacizumab, irinotecan, and temozolomide for refractory or relapsed neuroblastoma: results of a phase II study. Pediatr Blood Cancer. 2017;64(8):1. https://doi.org/10.1002/pbc.26448.
60. Bocca P, Carlo ED, Caruana I, Emionite L, Cilli M, De Angelis B, et al. Bevacizumab-mediated tumor vasculature remodelling improves tumor infiltration and antitumor efficacy of GD2-CAR T cells in a human neuroblastoma preclinical model. Onco Targets Ther. 2017;7(1):e1378843. https://doi.org/10.1080/2162402x.2017.1378843.
61. Feng J, Tang L. SPARC in tumor pathophysiology and as a potential therapeutic target. Curr Pharm Des. 2014;20(39):6182–90.
62. Hadjidaniel MD, Muthugounder S, Hung LT, Sheard MA, Shirinbak S, Chan RY, et al. Tumor-

associated macrophages promote neuroblastoma via STAT3 phosphorylation and up-regulation of c-MYC. Oncotarget. 2017;8(53):91516–29. https://doi.org/10.18632/oncotarget.21066.
63. Yang F, Jove V, Buettner R, Xin H, Wu J, Wang Y, et al. Sorafenib inhibits endogenous and IL-6/S1P induced JAK2-STAT3 signaling in human neuroblastoma, associated with growth suppression and apoptosis. Cancer Biol Ther. 2012;13(7):534.
64. Chai H, Luo AZ, Weerasinghe P, Brown RE. Sorafenib downregulates ERK/Akt and STAT3 survival pathways and induces apoptosis in a human neuroblastoma cell line. Int J Clin Exp Pathol. 2010;3(4):408–15.
65. Kakodkar NC, Peddinti RR, Tian Y, Guerrero LJ, Chlenski A, Yang Q, et al. Sorafenib inhibits neuroblastoma cell proliferation and signaling, blocks angiogenesis, and impairs tumor growth. Pediatr Blood Cancer. 2012;59(4):642–7. https://doi.org/10.1002/pbc.24004.
66. Okada K, Nakano Y, Yamasaki K, Nitani C, Fujisaki H, Hara J. Sorafenib treatment in children with relapsed and refractory neuroblastoma: an experience of four cases. Cancer Med. 2016;5(8):1947–9. https://doi.org/10.1002/cam4.784.
67. Loh ML, Tasian SK, Rabin KR, Brown P, Magoon D, Reid JM, et al. A phase 1 dosing study of ruxolitinib in children with relapsed or refractory solid tumors, leukemias, or myeloproliferative neoplasms: a children's oncology group phase 1 consortium study (ADVL1011). Pediatr Blood Cancer. 2015;62(10):1717–24. https://doi.org/10.1002/pbc.25575.
68. Vennepureddy A, Thumallapally N, Motilal Nehru V, Atallah JP, Terjanian T. Novel drugs and combination therapies for the treatment of metastatic melanoma. J Clin Med Res. 2016;8(2):63–75. https://doi.org/10.14740/jocmr2424w.
69. Berthold F, Homberg M, Proleskovskaya I, Mazanek P, Belogurova M, Ernst A, et al. Metronomic therapy has low toxicity and is as effective as current standard treatment for recurrent high-risk neuroblastoma. Pediatr Hematol Oncol. 2017;34(5):308–19. https://doi.org/10.1080/08880018.2017.1373314.
70. Russell HV, Groshen SG, Ara T, DeClerck YA, Hawkins R, Jackson HA, et al. A phase I study of zoledronic acid and low-dose cyclophosphamide in recurrent/refractory neuroblastoma: a new approaches to neuroblastoma therapy (NANT) study. Pediatr Blood Cancer. 2011;57(2):275–82. https://doi.org/10.1002/pbc.22821.
71. Scott AM, Wiseman G, Welt S, Adjei A, Lee FT, Hopkins W, et al. A phase I dose-escalation study of sibrotuzumab in patients with advanced or metastatic fibroblast activation protein-positive cancer. Clin Cancer Res. 2003;9(5):1639–47.
72. Lee J, Fassnacht M, Nair S, Boczkowski D, Gilboa E. Tumor immunotherapy targeting fibroblast activation protein, a product expressed in tumor-associated fibroblasts. Cancer Res. 2005;65(23):11156–63. https://doi.org/10.1158/0008-5472.can-05-2805.
73. Wang LC, Lo A, Scholler J, Sun J, Majumdar RS, Kapoor V, et al. Targeting fibroblast activation protein in tumor stroma with chimeric antigen receptor T cells can inhibit tumor growth and augment host immunity without severe toxicity. Cancer Immunol Res. 2014;2(2):154–66. https://doi.org/10.1158/2326-6066.cir-13-0027.
74. Kakarla S, Chow KK, Mata M, Shaffer DR, Song XT, Wu MF, et al. Antitumor effects of chimeric receptor engineered human T cells directed to tumor stroma. Mol Ther. 2013;21(8):1611–20. https://doi.org/10.1038/mt.2013.110.
75. Kim HS, Lee J, Lee DY, Kim YD, Kim JY, Lim HJ, et al. Schwann cell precursors from human pluripotent stem cells as a potential therapeutic target for myelin repair. Stem Cell Reports. 2017;8(6):1714–26. https://doi.org/10.1016/j.stemcr.2017.04.011.

Metastatic Disease Burden

10

Araz Marachelian and Meredith S. Irwin

10.1 Introduction

10.1.1 Metastatic Disease Predicts Outcome

At diagnosis more than half of neuroblastoma patients present with evidence of distant metastatic disease [1, 2]. The presence of metastases is defined similarly across different staging systems and is classified as Stage 4 in the INSS (International Neuroblastoma Staging system) [3] and Stage M in the INRG (International Neuroblastoma Risk Group) staging system. The presence of distant metastases is a robust independent risk factor for outcome. In the largest analysis to date using the International Neuroblastoma Risk Group (INRG) database of 8800 patients treated in North America, Europe, Australia, and Japan between 1990–2002, patients with INSS 4 had significantly inferior outcomes (5-year EFS, 42%) compared to those with INSS 1,2,3 and 4S (5-year EFS, 91%) [4]. In addition to stage, the majority of neuroblastoma risk classification systems incorporates additional robust, statistically validated prognostic factors, including all or some of the following – age, *MYCN* amplification status, presence of segmental chromosome aberrations (SCAs), and histology [4, 5] (see also Chap. 1). In most classification systems, including the INRG, all patients >18 months with metastatic disease, as well as patients of any age with metastatic disease with *MYCN* amplification, are classified as high-risk. Current therapy for most high-risk neuroblastoma patients includes three phases—induction chemotherapy, consolidation with one or two autologous stem cell transplants, followed by anti-GD2 containing immunotherapy regimens (Fig. 10.1). With this aggressive therapy, approximately half of patients are now cured [5, 6]. In contrast, infants (<12mo) and subsets of toddlers (12–18mo) with biologically favorable metastatic disease characterized by the absence of *MYCN* amplification are classified as intermediate risk neuroblastoma and recent trials demonstrate more favorable outcomes (5-year EFS >80% [7] with only 4–8 cycles of chemotherapy).

The most common sites of distant metastases at diagnosis are the bone, bone marrow, lymph nodes, and liver. The involvement of metastatic sites at diagnosis was recently characterized for the INRG cohort of patients diagnosed between 1974 and 2015, which included 6508 patients with specific data on metastatic sites. Metastases were documented in bone marrow (56%), bone

A. Marachelian
USC Keck School of Medicine and Children's Hospital Los Angeles, Los Angeles, CA, USA
e-mail: amarachelian@chla.usc.edu

M. S. Irwin (✉)
Hospital for Sick Children, University of Toronto, Toronto, ON, Canada
e-mail: meredith.irwin@sickkids.ca

S. Asgharzadeh, F. Westermann (eds.), *Neuroblastoma*, Pediatric Oncology,
https://doi.org/10.1007/978-3-031-51292-6_10

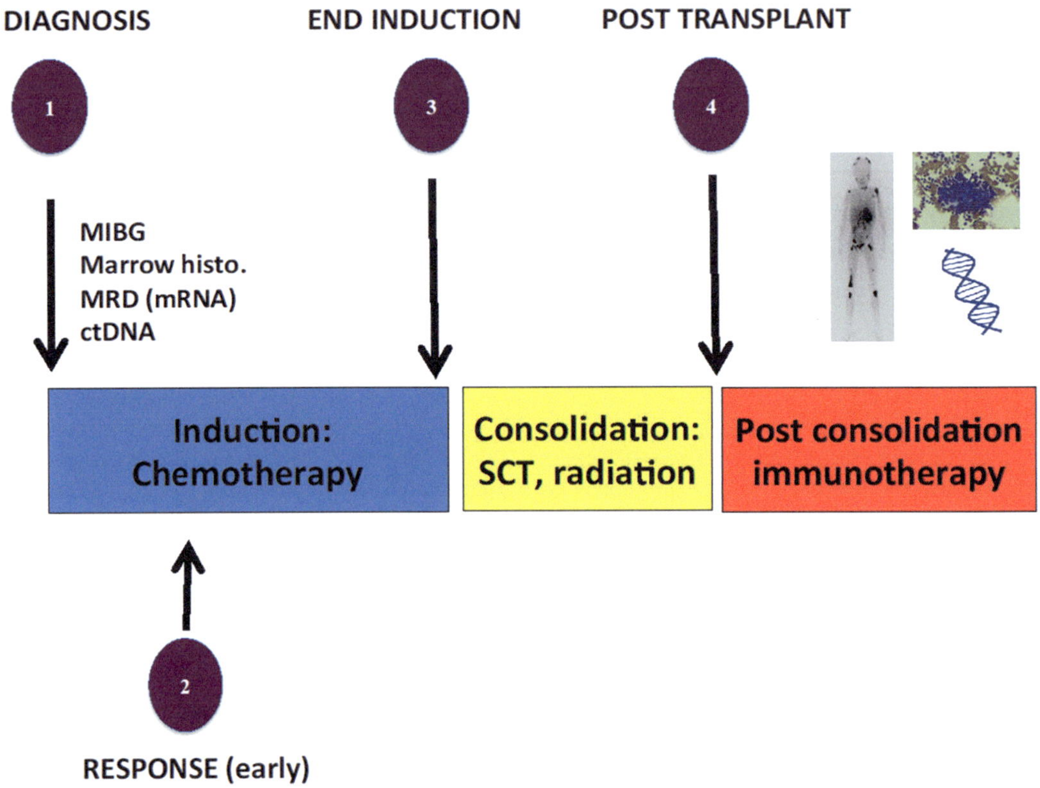

Fig. 10.1 Treatment regimen for high-risk neuroblastoma assessments for metastatic burden. Shown are the three phases of therapy for patients with high-risk neuroblastoma used in most International clinical trials. Patients receive 5–6 cycles of induction chemotherapy. During induction, most patients undergo resection of the primary tumor (often after 4–5 cycles of chemotherapy). The second phase is one or more cycles of high dose chemotherapy followed by autologous stem cell rescue (also referred to as stem cell transplant, SCT) and radiation to the local tumor bed +/− residual metastatic bony sites. Following SCT, patients are treated with immunotherapy with anti-GD2 antibody and cytokines. Assessment for metastatic burden takes place at multiple time points, including (1) diagnosis, (2) during induction/early response, (3) end of induction, and (4) post- SCT. The standard-of-care assessments for metastatic disease at these time points include imaging with MIBG scans (PET for MIBG-non avid patients), and bone marrow histology. Newer techniques to monitor metastatic burden and response to therapy include RT-PCR to assess tumor-specific transcripts in the bone marrow or peripheral blood or circulating tumor DNA (ctDNA)isolated from the serum

(47%), lymph nodes (24%), liver (21%), lung (3%), skin (4%), and CNS (1%) [2]. At recurrence, metastatic disease is even more common [8] and involves similar sites to those at diagnosis; however, in comparison to diagnosis, there is an increase in the incidence of CNS (parenchymal and leptomeningeal) disease at the time of relapse [9, 10]. The pattern and burden of metastatic disease at diagnosis is not incorporated into current risk stratification systems; however, evidence suggests that in certain cases, these factors may influence prognosis. For example, analyses of the INRG database of 8800 patients treated between 1990–2002 have shown that patients with distinct sites of metastases have differing outcomes. Rare patients with metastases that are limited to only distant lymph nodes ('stage 4 N') have more favorable outcomes (5-year EFS 77± 4% and OS 85 ± 3%) than those with other sites (35 ± 1% and OS 42 ± 1%) [11]. In contrast, those with involvement of the bone, bone marrow, lungs, or liver have inferior outcomes when compared to those without involvement of each of those sites [12]. Whether these sites are associated with adverse outcome due to challenges with local control at those anatomic locations or differing biology that makes them more therapy-resistant is unclear.

The impact of the burden of disease at diagnosis or during therapy is less well-studied, but increasingly quantitative imaging and laboratory assays to detect disease burden are being incorporated into prospective clinical trials. In retrospective studies, there has been some evidence to support the role for metastatic burden as a prognostic risk factor. In an INRG analysis, we developed a metastatic site index (MSI) to quantitatively score the number of systems or compartments with metastatic disease ranging from 1 to 8 based on the presence or absence of involvement of the bone, bone marrow, liver, lung, lymph nodes, skin, distant lymph node, and CNS. Limited metastatic disease associated with an MSI of 1 was associated with more favorable outcomes than those with MSI >1 (54 ± 2% versus 31 ± 1%) [12]. In patients >18 months of age, the survival was progressively worse with increasing MSI detected in patients with MSI of 1, 2–3, and 4–6. Higher MSI also correlated with increased levels of ferritin and LDH, two statistically robust markers of disease burden often used in centers with limited resources in which to perform MIBG scans or biomarkers [13]. This suggests that the involvement of more compartments or MSI may reflect a higher level of disseminated disease. Interestingly, this adverse outcome was less prominent in patients treated with autologous stem cell transplants, which may support the concept that a higher burden of disease at diagnosis may require higher intensity of therapy. Additional prospective studies are required to determine whether detecting metastatic disease at diagnosis and additional time-points during therapy, such as the end of induction, predicts outcome using newer, more sensitive methods (summarized in Fig. 10.1). Further data supporting the prognostic importance of detecting burden of metastatic disease by specific imaging and laboratory methods is discussed below in sections on Imaging and MRD.

10.2 Current Methods for Detection and Staging of Metastatic Disease

10.2.1 INRC

Given the significance of metastatic disease in prognosis and risk classification systems used to tailor therapy, accurate detection of metastatic disease at diagnosis and during therapy is important. In order to compare outcomes across clinical trials and different consortium groups, there have been significant international efforts to standardize these criteria, which resulted in the International Neuroblastoma Response Criteria (INRC). The INRC was recently revised in 2017 [2] and applies to both newly diagnosed and relapsed/refractory patients. The criteria integrate the response of the primary tumor and metastatic sites to determine an overall disease response. The revised INRC is described in several recent consensus publications, which specifically outline criteria for metastatic disease detection of bone marrow, bone, and soft tissue sites, including bone marrow histologic-based assays [14] and imaging methods [2].

10.2.2 Imaging Metastatic Response Criteria

There have been minor changes to the revised INRC in terms of assessing primary tumor response, which now relies on RECIST criteria [15]. Imaging to detect metastases at diagnosis and to determine metastatic response include a combination of anatomic/cross-sectional methods and functional or radionucleotide-based scans. These scans are used to detect soft tissue, including both lymph nodes and non-lymph node soft tissues and bone involvement. Most imaging-based metastatic assessments rely on nuclear medicine-based techniques, most commonly I-^{123} or -^{131} MIBG (meta-iodobenzylguanidine), which is now considered the standard detection method in the revised 2017 INRC. MIBG detects neuroblastoma within the bone marrow, cortical bone, and soft tissue. Uptake is dependent on the expression of the norepinephrine receptor and is detected in approximately 90% of neuroblastoma tumors. Many different systems have been developed to use MIBG scans to semi-quantitatively score metastatic involvement, and international consensus guidelines were developed in 2010 [16]. Several retrospective studies have demonstrated that the relative score of metastatic involvement on MIBG scan at diagnosis and/or end of induction chemotherapy predicts overall outcome [17–24]. The two most common—Curie and SIOPEN-scores—have been shown to have comparable ability to predict outcome [25]. The Curie score evaluates 10 sites, including 9 skeletal and a tenth site for soft tissue lesions, using a score of 0–3. The SIOPEN score evaluates skeletal MIBG uptake on a 0–6 scale in 12 anatomical body segments with a maximal score of 72.

The largest and most recent studies have focused on determining whether a particular absolute score or relative score cut-off at different time points during treatment, most commonly at the end of induction, can be used to predict relapse and thus identify a cohort of patients with high-risk neuroblastoma with a high likelihood to recur. A COG study of 280 patients included MIBG scans that were centrally reviewed and represented disease assessments at multiple time points during treatment on the COG A3973 Phase III trial. Patients with a Curie score > 2 at the end of induction had an inferior outcome when compared to those with a Curie score of ≤2, and this effect was independent of other known prognostic factors such as *MYCN* status (3-y EFS: 15.4% ± 5.3% vs. 44.9% ± 3.9%) [26]. Although absolute Curie scores at diagnosis were not prognostic, any MIBG-avid disease post-autologous stem cell transplant (Curie score > 0) predicted patients with a significantly worse outcome (3-y EFS: 28.9% ± 6.8% vs. 49.3% ± 4.9%). The SIOPEN scoring system was also evaluated using centrally reviewed scans from 341 patients treated on the SIOPEN/HR-NBL-1 study. In this study, a cut-off score of >3 was predictive of inferior outcome. The 5-year EFS for patients with SIOPEN score ≤ 3 were 47 ± 7% and 26 ± 3% for >3 at diagnosis. At the end of induction, the differences were 36 ± 4% vs. 14 ± 4% [23].

These findings suggest that metastatic response using semi-quantitative scores has strong predictive value in identifying patients who will go on to recurrence. Thus, there are active discussions in several large clinical trial consortium groups to potentially incorporate semi-quantitative scores into risk stratification systems, and future clinical trials may use this response to identify patients to treat with different therapies, including those that include high dose MIBG. Whether a relative score of 2 or 3 for Curie and SIOPEN scores, respectively, will remain prognostic in patients treated with current era therapies remains unknown since many of the studies demonstrating prognostic significance included only a minority of patients who received anti-GD2 containing immunotherapies.

In addition to MIBG scans, there has been increasing interest in using CT-PET (positron emission tomography) and increasingly MRI–PET to assess metastatic disease. For the subset of neuroblastoma patients with MIBG-non avid disease, PET scans have largely replaced technetium bone scans as the preferred method to detect metastatic disease at diagnosis and during treatment [2]. For the majority of patients with MIBG-avid disease, it is not clear that PET provides any additional benefit in characterizing metastatic burden at diagnosis or during treatment [27, 28]. However, there are small case reports and series that suggest that PET may be beneficial at later time points (e.g., post completion of therapy) to distinguish active poorly differentiated neuroblastoma from more differentiated, mature neuroblastoma [29, 30]. Additional studies will be required to determine the situations for which PET scans provide additional value in the assessment of metastatic disease or predicting outcome for patients with MIBG-avid disease, especially with PET scanning limitations for bony disease.

10.2.3 Bone Marrow Metastatic Staging and INRC Criteria

Aspirates and trephine biopsies of the bone marrow (usually sampled bilaterally) have been used for decades to detect metastatic involvement of the bone marrow. Standardized assessment has been hampered by the nature of bone marrow disease, which is patchy or heterogeneous, operator/sample variability, and reliance on morphology assessment by hematoxylin and eosin (H and E) staining. The revised INRC recommends the use of immunostaining using immunohistology and/or immunocytology in biopsies and aspirates, respectively, to distinguish neuroblastoma cells from other bone marrow cellular populations and to more accurately quantitate disease burden [14]. The scoring for percent involvement is defined by the number of neuroblastoma cells divided by hematopoietic or mononuclear cells on aspirate and quantifying tumor infiltration by calculating the percentage of the surface area involved by neuroblastic tumor in biopsies. In addition, the new guidelines include clarification that the site with the highest burden or percentage of neuroblastoma cells should be used in determining response. Furthermore, rather than categorizing involvement as binary (positive or negative), the revised INRC includes a new category of 'minimal disease', which is defined as more than 0% and ≤ 5% infiltration. Whether this relatively lower burden of disease is associated with different clinical feature or outcomes will be important to study prospectively to provide evidence to support the prognostic significance of burden of marrow disease and potentially guide treatment decisions [31]. Newer methods and technologies to identify metastatic cells in the bone marrow (and blood), such as the detection of neuroblastoma-specific transcripts by reverse transcriptase polymerase chain reaction (RT-PCR) to detect neuroblastoma-specific transcripts are described below.

10.3 Minimum Residual Disease (MRD)-Based Assays to Detect Metastases

Molecular characterization or quantification of tumor cells that have hematogenous spread have been a target of investigation in many tumor types. The targets are generally fusion transcripts, gene mutations, and overexpressed genes. The ideal choice of amplified mRNA should have little or no expression in normal cells and should be specifically amplified in viable tumor cells. The first such target was the discovery of BCR-ABL translocation and its quantification in leukemia [32]. Other fusion transcripts utilized in solid tumors include PAX3−/7-FOXO1 (rhabdomyosarcoma [33]), EWS-FLI (Ewings Sarcoma), and SYT-SSX in synovial sarcoma. Since not all tumors harbor specific gene mutations or rearrangements, the identification of highly expressed mRNA transcript of the tissue of origin is an attractive method for tumor cell quantification. Reverse transcriptase polymerase chain reaction (RT-PCR) for the detection of neuroblastoma mRNA transcripts has been investigated for use in neuroblastoma patients in an effort to improve risk classification, assessment of response, and to be utilized as a prognostic biomarker. For these studies, mRNA has been isolated from blood, bone marrow aspirates, and autologous peripheral blood stem cell apharesis products. The specific mRNA transcript(s) used in published studies has varied [34–44], but has most commonly included both *Tyrosine hydroxylase* (*TH*), the gene that encodes the rate-limiting enzyme required for catecholamines synthesis, and *paired like homeobox 2B* (*PHOX2B*), which is highly expressed in neural crest-derived cells. *TH* and *PHOX2B* were included in the consensus guidelines for assessing bone marrow response [14]. In addition, since neuroblastoma is heterogenous, the addition of multiple genes detected in an RT-PCR-based assay may improve the predictive value of these assays. Additional genes used by investigators include *DCX*, *DDC*, *CHGA*, *CCND1*, B4GALNT1 (*GD2 synthase*), *ISL2*, *CHCRNA3*, and *GAB43* [45–48]. The genes used in RT-PCR-based assays to detect metastatic disease by different cooperative groups and investigators are summarized in Table 10.1.

For newly diagnosed patients, high levels of expression of neuroblastoma-specific mRNA transcripts are predictive of poorer outcome at diagnosis and end of induction [49, 50] and suggest that the detection of MRD by RT-PCR may be useful in pre-treatment risk classification schema. The detection of decreased levels of MRD during therapy is also prognostic [42, 46] in

Table 10.1 Neuroblastoma detection genes used in various MRD assays

Author (Centre, group)/Gene	PHOX2B	TH	DCX	DDC	CHGA	CCND1 GD2 synthase ISL2	CHCRNA3 and GAB43
Burchill (SIOPEN)	x	x	X				
Tytgat (DUTCH/GERMAN)	x	x		x			x
Chung (MSKCC)	x					x	
Yanez (SPAIN)		x	X				
Asgharzadeh, Seeger (CHLA)	x	x	X	x	x		

bone marrow and peripheral stem cell product [45]. In the minimal residual disease setting following completion of therapy, the detection of bone marrow disease by RT-PCR predicted poor outcome [51, 52] and detection of mRNA specifically at the end of immunotherapy was also prognostic (*Advances in Neuroblastoma Research meeting,* Cologne, 2014). The presence or absence of mRNA transcripts was also prognostic for patients with relapsed/refractory disease [53].

While the sensitivity of mRNA detection in blood is inferior to bone marrow [53], sampling of the blood is a more convenient way of assessing disease, especially when frequent monitoring is required or when patients are off therapy. Data regarding the independent prognostic significance of detectable neuroblastoma mRNA transcripts in the blood and/or bone marrow continues to be an area of active research. Prospective studies aimed at determining whether patients with RT-PCR detected neuroblastoma-specific mRNA transcripts overlap with those with relatively high Curie scores will provide additional important data to support the independent prognostic role for MRD in detecting metastatic disease burden at diagnosis, during or following therapy.

10.4 Next Generation Assays to Detect Metastatic Disease

There have been additional attempts to measure tumor cells circulating in the peripheral blood and/or the nucleic acids (mainly circulating DNA and miRNA) released by tumor cells. The most promising recent data involves isolation of nucleic acids, including cell free DNA (cfDNA), in the serum of patients with cancer, including neuroblastoma. In certain cases, cfDNA has also been isolated from other body fluids, including cerebrospinal fluid, saliva, urine, and pleural fluid. cfDNA can be detected in the serum of all individuals, but higher levels are detected in patients with cancer and a large proportion of this cfDNA is from tumor cells and is referred to as circulating tumor DNA (ctDNA). Early studies demonstrated the ability to detect specific known mutant alleles (and their allele frequencies) in the serum of patients with colon and lung cancers, initially using techniques such as digital PCR (dPCR) (reviewed in [54, 55]). For neuroblastoma patients, techniques including dPCR have previously been used to detect copy number aberrations for known neuroblastoma-associated oncogenes, including *ALK* and *MYCN,* in serum suggesting potential utility for this method for the diagnosis and monitoring of disease status and/or response to therapy [56–58]. More recently, studies have shown that the level of ctDNA detected in the plasma of neuroblastoma patients is highest when compared to samples from children with other solid tumors such as Wilm's tumor, osteosarcoma, and Ewings sarcoma [59]. A review summarizing studies to date analyzing ctDNA in pediatric cancer patients was recently published by Abbou et al. [60].

CtDNA, often referred to as a 'liquid biopsy', has many potential applications in neuroblastoma. Relevant to this chapter is its potential role as a method to detect disease burden, including metastatic burden, since ctDNA includes tumor cell DNA from primary and metastatic cells. In addition to its utility in monitoring disease burden and response to therapy, ctDNA can also be used to detect MRD—both at the end of therapy and prior to imaging or histologic-detectable recurrence. Finally, ctDNA represents the spatial and temporal heterogeneity of the tumor and metastases, including the ability to reflect clonal evolution of single nucleotide variants (SNVs) or copy number alterations (CNAs). Genomic copy number alterations have been detected using arrayCGH, and whole genome sequencing (WGS) of ctDNA from neuroblastoma patients [61, 62]. In addition, SNVs have also been identified in neuroblastoma patients' ctDNA [63], including specific clonal variation of SNVs in relapse–diagnosis paired samples. Although mRNA is less stable than DNA in the serum, microRNA (miRNA) can be reliably isolated from cell-free nucleic acids in the serum. miRNA profiles of neuroblastoma tumors have been shown to have prognostic significance [64, 65] and it is likely that future studies will focus on isolating and detecting these miRNAs in the serum of patients with neuroblastoma. Ultimately, quantification of DNA SNVs and CNVs (and miRNAs) from sera of neuroblastoma patients could provide another non-invasive method for MRD, and may be useful as another method to measure primary tumor and metastatic disease burden at diagnosis, during treatment and following its completion.

The analytic and clinical validity of ctDNA in neuroblastoma to detect disease burden and as a surrogate biomarker for genetic aberrations in the primary tumor and/or metastatic lesions is currently being studied retrospectively and in early phase trials. This includes use of ctDNA for assessing ALK mutations in trials examining the efficacy of inhibitors of the tyrosine kinase ALK. A recent joint review written by the American Society of Clinical oncology and College of American Pathologists outlined the issues of incorporating ctDNA into clinical use [66] and these guidelines, together with early findings in neuroblastoma, will lay the groundwork to incorporate these techniques in future neuroblastoma clinical trials.

10.5 Conclusion

As methods become more sensitive to detect metastatic disease, it will be important to determine whether all metastatic diseases are created equal. In other words, as the sensitivity to detect metastatic disease improves, we may identify higher proportions of patients with metastatic disease. Whether these patients, potentially with low levels of burden of disease, historically would have been considered INRG stage M or not, will be important to consider. This would be similar to the changes that occurred when MIBG scans were routinely integrated into clinical practice since they often detected disease not identified on cross-sectional imaging or technetium bone scans. Will more sensitive methods facilitate early detection of relapsed disease, which most often presents in metastatic sites? While previous studies that relied on surveillance imaging to detect relapse did not detect improved outcomes in patients with neuroblastoma (and other pediatric tumors) for whom relapse was detected earlier [67–70], it is possible that with newer therapies and the increasing ability to more deeply interrogate the relapsed tumor genome, early detection could have some impact on overall outcome. Moreover, by integrating newer and complementary methods to identify metastatic burden, the ability to determine the response to novel therapies and combination regimens aimed at treating MRD or relapsed disease may be further enhanced. Finally, there is no question that these newer methods such as ctDNA may lead to discoveries about the genome of neuroblastoma, and in particular, that of metastatic and recurrent neuroblastoma, which should ultimately translate into better therapies and potentially less invasive surveillance methods for all patients with neuroblastoma, but in particular those with high-risk disease.

References

1. Irwin MS, Park JR. Neuroblastoma: pediatric paradigm for precision medicine. Pediatr Clin N Am. 2015;62(1):225–56.
2. Park JR, Bagatell R, Cohn SL, Pearson AD, Villablanca JG, Berthold F, et al. Revisions to the international neuroblastoma response criteria: a consensus statement from the National Cancer Institute clinical trials planning meeting. J Clin Oncol. 2017;35(22):2580–7. https://doi.org/10.1200/JCO.2016.72.0177.

3. Brodeur GM, Pritchard J, Berthold F, Carlsen NL, Castel V, Castelberry RP, et al. Revisions of the international criteria for neuroblastoma diagnosis, staging, and response to treatment. J Clin Oncol. 1993;11(8):1466–77.
4. Cohn SL, Pearson AD, London WB, Monclair T, Ambros PF, Brodeur GM, et al. The International Neuroblastoma Risk Group (INRG) classification system: an INRG task force report. J Clin Oncol. 2009;27(2):289–97.
5. Pinto NR, Applebaum MA, Volchenboum SL, Matthay KK, London WB, Ambros PF, et al. Advances in risk classification and treatment strategies for neuroblastoma. J Clin Oncol. 2015;33(27):3008–17. https://doi.org/10.1200/JCO.2014.59.4648.
6. Park JR, Bagatell R, London WB, Maris JM, Cohn SL, Mattay KM, et al. Children's oncology group's 2013 blueprint for research: neuroblastoma. Pediatr Blood Cancer. 2013;60(6):985–93. https://doi.org/10.1002/pbc.24433.
7. Baker DL, Schmidt ML, Cohn SL, Maris JM, London WB, Buxton A, et al. Outcome after reduced chemotherapy for intermediate-risk neuroblastoma. N Engl J Med. 2010;363(14):1313–23. https://doi.org/10.1056/NEJMoa1001527.
8. Matthay KK, Atkinson JB, Stram DO, Selch M, Reynolds CP, Seeger RC. Patterns of relapse after autologous purged bone marrow transplantation for neuroblastoma: a childrens cancer group pilot study. J Clin Oncol. 1993;11(11):2226–33. https://doi.org/10.1200/jco.1993.11.11.2226.
9. Kramer K, Kushner B, Heller G, Cheung NK. Neuroblastoma metastatic to the central nervous system. The Memorial Sloan-Kettering Cancer Center experience and a literature review. Cancer. 2001;91(8):1510–9.
10. Matthay KK, Brisse H, Couanet D, Couturier J, Benard J, Mosseri V, et al. Central nervous system metastases in neuroblastoma: radiologic, clinical, and biologic features in 23 patients. Cancer. 2003;98(1):155–65. https://doi.org/10.1002/cncr.11448.
11. Morgenstern DA, London WB, Stephens D, Volchenboum SL, Hero B, Di Cataldo A, et al. Metastatic neuroblastoma confined to distant lymph nodes (stage 4N) predicts outcome in patients with stage 4 disease: a study from the international neuroblastoma risk group database. J Clin Oncol. 2014;32(12):1228–35. https://doi.org/10.1200/JCO.2013.53.6342.
12. Morgenstern DA, London WB, Stephens D, Volchenboum SL, Simon T, Nakagawara A, et al. Prognostic significance of pattern and burden of metastatic disease in patients with stage 4 neuroblastoma: a study from the international neuroblastoma risk group database. Eur J Cancer. 2016;65:1–10. https://doi.org/10.1016/j.ejca.2016.06.005.
13. Parikh NS, Howard SC, Chantada G, Israels T, Khattab M, Alcasabas P, et al. SIOP-PODC adapted risk stratification and treatment guidelines: recommendations for neuroblastoma in low- and middle-income settings. Pediatr Blood Cancer. 2015;62(8):1305–16. https://doi.org/10.1002/pbc.25501.
14. Burchill SA, Beiske K, Shimada H, Ambros PF, Seeger R, Tytgat GA, et al. Recommendations for the standardization of bone marrow disease assessment and reporting in children with neuroblastoma on behalf of the international neuroblastoma response criteria bone marrow working group. Cancer. 2017;123(7):1095–105. https://doi.org/10.1002/cncr.30380.
15. Bagatell R, McHugh K, Naranjo A, Van Ryn C, Kirby C, Brock P, et al. Assessment of primary site response in children with high-risk neuroblastoma: an international multicenter study. J Clin Oncol. 2016;34(7):740–6. https://doi.org/10.1200/JCO.2015.63.2042.
16. Matthay KK, Shulkin B, Ladenstein R, Michon J, Giammarile F, Lewington V, et al. Criteria for evaluation of disease extent by (123) I-metaiodobenzylguanidine scans in neuroblastoma: a report for the International Neuroblastoma Risk Group (INRG) task force. Br J Cancer. 2010;102(9):1319–26. https://doi.org/10.1038/sj.bjc.6605621.
17. Matthay KK, Edeline V, Lumbroso J, Tanguy ML, Asselain B, Zucker JM, et al. Correlation of early metastatic response by 123I-metaiodobenzylguanidine scintigraphy with overall response and event-free survival in stage IV neuroblastoma. J Clin Oncol. 2003;21(13):2486–91. https://doi.org/10.1200/JCO.2003.09.122.
18. Suc A, Lumbroso J, Rubie H, Hattchouel JM, Boneu A, Rodary C, et al. Metastatic neuroblastoma in children older than one year: prognostic significance of the initial metaiodobenzylguanidine scan and proposal for a scoring system. Cancer. 1996;77(4):805–11.
19. Yanik GA, Levine JE, Matthay KK, Sisson JC, Shulkin BL, Shapiro B, et al. Pilot study of iodine-131-metaiodobenzylguanidine in combination with myeloablative chemotherapy and autologous stem-cell support for the treatment of neuroblastoma. J Clin Oncol. 2002;20(8):2142–9.
20. Kushner BH, Yeh SD, Kramer K, Larson SM, Cheung NK. Impact of metaiodobenzylguanidine scintigraphy on assessing response of high-risk neuroblastoma to dose-intensive induction chemotherapy. J Clin Oncol. 2003;21(6):1082–6. https://doi.org/10.1200/JCO.2003.07.142.
21. Ady N, Zucker JM, Asselain B, Edeline V, Bonnin F, Michon J, et al. A new 123I-MIBG whole body scan scoring method—application to the prediction of the response of metastases to induction chemotherapy in stage IV neuroblastoma. Eur J Cancer. 1995;31A(2):256–61.
22. Boubaker A, Bischof DA. MIBG scintigraphy for the diagnosis and follow-up of children with neuroblastoma. Q J Nucl Med Mol Imaging. 2008;52(4):388–402.
23. Ladenstein R, Lambert B, Potschger U, Castellani MR, Lewington V, Bar-Sever Z, et al. Validation of the mIBG skeletal SIOPEN scoring method in two

independent high-risk neuroblastoma populations: the SIOPEN/HR-NBL1 and COG-A3973 trials. Eur J Nucl Med Mol Imaging. 2018;45(2):292–305. https://doi.org/10.1007/s00259-017-3829-7.
24. Schmidt M, Simon T, Hero B, Schicha H, Berthold F. The prognostic impact of functional imaging with (123)I-mIBG in patients with stage 4 neuroblastoma >1 year of age on a high-risk treatment protocol: results of the German neuroblastoma trial NB97. Eur J Cancer. 2008;44(11):1552–8. https://doi.org/10.1016/j.ejca.2008.03.013.
25. Yanik GA, Parisi MT, Naranjo A, Nadel H, Gelfand MJ, Park JR, et al. Validation of post-induction curie scores in high risk neuroblastoma. A children's oncology group (COG) and SIOPEN group report on SIOPEN/HR-NBL1. J Nucl Med. 2017;59:502. https://doi.org/10.2967/jnumed.117.195883.
26. Yanik GA, Parisi MT, Shulkin BL, Naranjo A, Kreissman SG, London WB, et al. Semiquantitative mIBG scoring as a prognostic indicator in patients with stage 4 neuroblastoma: a report from the children's oncology group. J Nucl Med. 2013;54:541. https://doi.org/10.2967/jnumed.112.112334.
27. Sharp SE, Shulkin BL, Gelfand MJ, Salisbury S, Furman WL. 123I-MIBG scintigraphy and 18F-FDG PET in neuroblastoma. J Nucl Med. 2009;50(8):1237–43. https://doi.org/10.2967/jnumed.108.060467.
28. Papathanasiou ND, Gaze MN, Sullivan K, Aldridge M, Waddington W, Almuhaideb A, et al. 18F-FDG PET/CT and 123I-metaiodobenzylguanidine imaging in high-risk neuroblastoma: diagnostic comparison and survival analysis. J Nucl Med. 2011;52(4):519–25. https://doi.org/10.2967/jnumed.110.083303.
29. Sato Y, Kurosawa H, Sakamoto S, Kuwashima S, Hashimoto T, Okamoto K, et al. Usefulness of 18F-fluorodeoxyglucose positron emission tomography for follow-up of 13-cis-retinoic acid treatment for residual neuroblastoma after myeloablative chemotherapy. Medicine (Baltimore). 2015;94(31):e1290. https://doi.org/10.1097/MD.0000000000001290.
30. Liu YL, Lu MY, Chang HH, Lu CC, Lin DT, Jou ST, et al. Diagnostic FDG and FDOPA positron emission tomography scans distinguish the genomic type and treatment outcome of neuroblastoma. Oncotarget. 2016;7(14):18774–86. https://doi.org/10.18632/oncotarget.7933.
31. Burchill SA. Micrometastases in neuroblastoma: are they clinically important? J Clin Pathol. 2004;57(1):14–20.
32. Kawasaki ES, Clark SS, Coyne MY, Smith SD, Champlin R, Witte ON, et al. Diagnosis of chronic myeloid and acute lymphocytic leukemias by detection of leukemia-specific mRNA sequences amplified in vitro. Proc Natl Acad Sci U S A. 1988;85(15):5698–702.
33. Kelly KM, Womer RB, Barr FG. Minimal disease detection in patients with alveolar rhabdomyosarcoma using a reverse transcriptase-polymerase chain reaction method. Cancer. 1996;78(6):1320–7. https://doi.org/10.1002/(sici)1097-0142(19960915)78:6<1320::aid-cncr22>3.0.co;2-1.
34. Carlin S, Mairs RJ, McCluskey AG, Tweddle DA, Sprigg A, Estlin C, et al. Development of a real-time polymerase chain reaction assay for prediction of the uptake of meta-[(131)I]iodobenzylguanidine by neuroblastoma tumors. Clin Cancer Res. 2003;9(9):3338–44.
35. Cheung IY, Lo Piccolo MS, Kushner BH, Kramer K, Cheung NK. Quantitation of GD2 synthase mRNA by real-time reverse transcriptase polymerase chain reaction: clinical utility in evaluating adjuvant therapy in neuroblastoma. J Clin Oncol. 2003;21(6):1087–93. https://doi.org/10.1200/jco.2003.02.055.
36. Cheung IY, Sahota A, Cheung NK. Measuring circulating neuroblastoma cells by quantitative reverse transcriptase-polymerase chain reaction analysis. Cancer. 2004;101(10):2303–8. https://doi.org/10.1002/cncr.20660
37. Beiske K, Ambros PF, Burchill SA, Cheung IY, Swerts K. Detecting minimal residual disease in neuroblastoma patients-the present state of the art. Cancer Lett. 2005;228(1–2):229–40. https://doi.org/10.1016/j.canlet.2005.02.053.
38. Cheung IY, Feng Y, Gerald W, Cheung NK. Exploiting gene expression profiling to identify novel minimal residual disease markers of neuroblastoma. Clin Cancer Res. 2008;14(21):7020–7. https://doi.org/10.1158/1078-0432.ccr-08-0541.
39. Stutterheim J, Gerritsen A, Zappeij-Kannegieter L, Kleijn I, Dee R, Hooft L, et al. PHOX2B is a novel and specific marker for minimal residual disease testing in neuroblastoma. J Clin Oncol. 2008;26(33):5443–9. https://doi.org/10.1200/jco.2007.13.6531.
40. Beiske K, Burchill SA, Cheung IY, Hiyama E, Seeger RC, Cohn SL, et al. Consensus criteria for sensitive detection of minimal neuroblastoma cells in bone marrow, blood and stem cell preparations by immunocytology and QRT-PCR: recommendations by the international neuroblastoma risk group task force. Br J Cancer. 2009;100(10):1627–37. https://doi.org/10.1038/sj.bjc.6605029.
41. Stutterheim J, Gerritsen A, Zappeij-Kannegieter L, Yalcin B, Dee R, van Noesel MM, et al. Detecting minimal residual disease in neuroblastoma: the superiority of a panel of real-time quantitative PCR markers. Clin Chem. 2009;55(7):1316–26. https://doi.org/10.1373/clinchem.2008.117945.
42. Stutterheim J, Zappeij-Kannegieter L, Versteeg R, Caron HN, van der Schoot CE, Tytgat GA. The prognostic value of fast molecular response of marrow disease in patients aged over 1 year with stage 4 neuroblastoma. Eur J Cancer. 2011;47(8):1193–202. https://doi.org/10.1016/j.ejca.2011.02.003.
43. Garcia I, Mayol G, Rios J, Domenech G, Cheung NK, Oberthuer A, et al. A three-gene expression signature model for risk stratification of patients with neuroblastoma. Clin Cancer Res. 2012;18(7):2012–23. https://doi.org/10.1158/1078-0432.ccr-11-2483.

44. Stutterheim J, Zappeij-Kannegieter L, Ora I, van Sluis PG, Bras J, den Ouden E, et al. Stability of PCR targets for monitoring minimal residual disease in neuroblastoma. J Mol Diagn. 2012;14(2):168–75. https://doi.org/10.1016/j.jmoldx.2011.12.002.
45. Kreissman SG, Seeger RC, Matthay KK, London WB, Sposto R, Grupp SA, et al. Purged versus non-purged peripheral blood stem-cell transplantation for high-risk neuroblastoma (COG A3973): a randomised phase 3 trial. Lancet Oncol. 2013;14(10):999–1008. https://doi.org/10.1016/s1470-2045(13)70309-7.
46. van Wezel EM, Stutterheim J, Vree F, Zappeij-Kannegieter L, Decarolis B, Hero B, et al. Minimal residual disease detection in autologous stem cell grafts from patients with high risk neuroblastoma. Pediatr Blood Cancer. 2015;62(8):1368–73. https://doi.org/10.1002/pbc.25507.
47. van Wezel EM, Decarolis B, Stutterheim J, Zappeij-Kannegieter L, Berthold F, Schumacher-Kuckelkorn R, et al. Neuroblastoma messenger RNA is frequently detected in bone marrow at diagnosis of localised neuroblastoma patients. Eur J Cancer. 2016;54:149–58. https://doi.org/10.1016/j.ejca.2015.11.007.
48. Brownhill SC, Burchill SA. PCR-based amplification of circulating RNAs as prognostic and predictive biomarkers—focus on neuroblastoma. Pract Lab Med. 2017;7:41–4. https://doi.org/10.1016/j.plabm.2016.04.003.
49. Viprey VF, Gregory WM, Corrias MV, Tchirkov A, Swerts K, Vicha A, et al. Neuroblastoma mRNAs predict outcome in children with stage 4 neuroblastoma: a European HR-NBL1/SIOPEN study. J Clin Oncol. 2014;32(10):1074–83. https://doi.org/10.1200/jco.2013.53.3604.
50. Yanez Y, Hervas D, Grau E, Oltra S, Perez G, Palanca S, et al. TH and DCX mRNAs in peripheral blood and bone marrow predict outcome in metastatic neuroblastoma patients. J Cancer Res Clin Oncol. 2016;142(3):573–80. https://doi.org/10.1007/s00432-015-2054-7.
51. Cheung IY, Feng Y, Cheung NK. Early negative minimal residual disease in bone marrow after immunotherapy is less predictive of late or non-marrow relapse among patients with high-risk stage 4 neuroblastoma. Pediatr Blood Cancer. 2013;60(7):E32–4. https://doi.org/10.1002/pbc.24469.
52. Cheung IY, Lo Piccolo MS, Kushner BH, Cheung NK. Early molecular response of marrow disease to biologic therapy is highly prognostic in neuroblastoma. J Clin Oncol. 2003;21(20):3853–8. https://doi.org/10.1200/jco.2003.11.077.
53. Marachelian A, Villablanca JG, Liu CW, Liu B, Goodarzian F, Lai HA, et al. Expression of five neuroblastoma genes in bone marrow or blood of patients with relapsed/refractory neuroblastoma provides a new biomarker for disease and prognosis. Clin Cancer Res. 2017;23(18):5374–83. https://doi.org/10.1158/1078-0432.ccr-16-2647.
54. Wan JCM, Massie C, Garcia-Corbacho J, Mouliere F, Brenton JD, Caldas C, et al. Liquid biopsies come of age: towards implementation of circulating tumour DNA. Nat Rev Cancer. 2017;17(4):223–38. https://doi.org/10.1038/nrc.2017.7.
55. Bardelli A, Pantel K. Liquid biopsies, what we do not know (yet). Cancer Cell. 2017;31(2):172–9. https://doi.org/10.1016/j.ccell.2017.01.002.
56. Combaret V, Audoynaud C, Iacono I, Favrot MC, Schell M, Bergeron C, et al. Circulating MYCN DNA as a tumor-specific marker in neuroblastoma patients. Cancer Res. 2002;62(13):3646–8.
57. Lodrini M, Sprussel A, Astrahantseff K, Tiburtius D, Konschak R, Lode HN, et al. Using droplet digital PCR to analyze MYCN and ALK copy number in plasma from patients with neuroblastoma. Oncotarget. 2017;8(49):85234–51. https://doi.org/10.18632/oncotarget.19076.
58. Yagyu S, Iehara T, Tanaka S, Gotoh T, Misawa-Furihata A, Sugimoto T, et al. Serum-based quantification of MYCN gene amplification in young patients with neuroblastoma: potential utility as a surrogate biomarker for neuroblastoma. PLoS One. 2016;11(8):e0161039. https://doi.org/10.1371/journal.pone.0161039.
59. Klega KI-TA, Ha G, Clapp AN, Meyer S, Ward A, Clinton C, Nag A, Van Allen E, Mullen E, DuBois SG, Janeway K, Meyerson M, Thorner AR, Crompton BD. Detection of somatic structural variants enables quantification and characterization of circulating tumor DNA in children with solid tumors. JCO Precis Oncol. 2018;1:1.
60. Abbou SD, Shulman DS, DuBois SG, Crompton BD. Assessment of circulating tumor DNA in pediatric solid tumors: the promise of liquid biopsies. Pediatr Blood Cancer. 2019;66:e27595. https://doi.org/10.1002/pbc.27595.
61. Chicard M, Boyault S, Colmet Daage L, Richer W, Gentien D, Pierron G, et al. Genomic copy number profiling using circulating free tumor DNA highlights heterogeneity in neuroblastoma. Clin Cancer Res. 2016;22(22):5564–73. https://doi.org/10.1158/1078-0432.CCR-16-0500.
62. Van Roy N, Van Der Linden M, Menten B, Dheedene A, Vandeputte C, Van Dorpe J, et al. Shallow whole genome sequencing on circulating cell-free DNA allows reliable noninvasive copy-number profiling in neuroblastoma patients. Clin Cancer Res. 2017;23(20):6305–14. https://doi.org/10.1158/1078-0432.CCR-17-0675.
63. Chicard M, Colmet-Daage L, Clement N, Danzon A, Bohec M, Bernard V, et al. Whole-exome sequencing of cell-free DNA reveals temporo-spatial heterogeneity and identifies treatment-resistant clones in neuroblastoma. Clin Cancer Res. 2018;24(4):939–49. https://doi.org/10.1158/1078-0432.CCR-17-1586.
64. Althoff K, Schulte JH, Schramm A. Towards diagnostic application of non-coding RNAs in neuroblastoma. Expert Rev Mol Diagn. 2016;16(12):1307–13. https://doi.org/10.1080/14737159.2016.1256207.
65. Shohet JM, Ghosh R, Coarfa C, Ludwig A, Benham AL, Chen Z, et al. A genome-wide search for promot-

ers that respond to increased MYCN reveals both new oncogenic and tumor suppressor microRNAs associated with aggressive neuroblastoma. Cancer Res. 2011;71(11):3841–51. https://doi.org/10.1158/0008-5472.CAN-10-4391.
66. Merker JD, Oxnard GR, Compton C, Diehn M, Hurley P, Lazar AJ, et al. Circulating tumor DNA analysis in patients with cancer: American Society of Clinical Oncology and College of American pathologists joint review. J Clin Oncol. 2018;36:JCO2017768671. https://doi.org/10.1200/JCO.2017.76.8671.
67. Howell L, Mensah A, Brennan B, Makin G. Detection of recurrence in childhood solid tumors. Cancer. 2005;103(6):1274–9. https://doi.org/10.1002/cncr.20896.
68. Kaste SC. Oncological imaging: tumor surveillance in children. Pediatr Radiol. 2011;41(Suppl 2):505–8. https://doi.org/10.1007/s00247-011-2108-1.
69. Lin JL, Guillerman RP, Russell HV, Lupo PJ, Nicholls L, Okcu MF. Does routine imaging of patients for progression or relapse improve survival in rhabdomyosarcoma? Pediatr Blood Cancer. 2016;63(2):202–5. https://doi.org/10.1002/pbc.25750.
70. Kushner BH, Kramer K, Modak S, Cheung NK. Sensitivity of surveillance studies for detecting asymptomatic and unsuspected relapse of high-risk neuroblastoma. J Clin Oncol. 2009;27(7):1041–6. https://doi.org/10.1200/JCO.2008.17.6107.

Therapeutically Actionable Genetic Aberrations

11

Monica Pomaville and Rani E. George

11.1 Definition of an Actionable Genetic Aberration

A therapeutically actionable genetic aberration is a detectable change in DNA that drives proliferation of tumor cells and is amenable to inhibition. In order to fit these criteria, certain challenges exist. First, oncogenic mutations that confer a proliferative advantage upon tumor cells must be identified, often achieved through next-generation sequencing methods. However, identification of an oncogenic driver does not necessarily translate into an actionable therapeutic target. Such is the case with unsuccessful attempts to target MYCN itself, a predictor of poor prognosis in neuroblastoma. Alternatively, some seemingly rare variations in the genome represent bona fide therapeutic targets and can be applied across tumor types, as exemplified by the successful targeting of BRAF and PARP in other cancers [1]. Therefore, the target must be druggable. Once both of these principles are attained, further challenges exist. Resistance can emerge upon treatment, as shown in the case of some receptor tyrosine kinase inhibitors described later. Another challenge in treating patients with neuroblastoma in particular is relapse. Novel targetable aberrations in this group of patients are under-studied, but can be aided by analyzing tumor cells at relapse through repeat biopsy of either the tumor or through circulating tumor cells or cell-free tumor DNA.

To focus efforts by clinicians, researchers, and the drug development community to produce effective therapies, the determination of genetic aberrations that are therapeutically actionable is of utmost importance [2]. Frameworks to determine the degree to which a therapeutic target is actionable have been developed for adult tumors by multiple groups; however, there is a need for further characterization in pediatric systems. A proposed model, adapted from Carr et al., is described in Fig. 11.1 that incorporates the various inputs necessary to determine a therapeutically actionable genetic aberration, along with a corresponding classification system in Table 11.1 [2]. Divided into class 1 through 5, mutations are described in order of decreasing evidence as therapeutically actionable. Class 1 targets are both detectable and predictive of clinical response with available treatments and have been validated in clinical trials to show a robust response. For the clinician, these are often relatively easy to

M. Pomaville
Department of Pediatric Oncology, Dana-Farber Cancer Institute, Boston, MA, USA

Department of Pediatric Oncology, Children's Hospital of Philadelphia, Philadelphia, USA

R. E. George (✉)
Department of Pediatric Oncology, Dana-Farber Cancer Institute, Boston, MA, USA

Department of Pediatrics, Harvard Medical School, Boston, MA, USA
e-mail: rani_george@dfci.harvard.edu

S. Asgharzadeh, F. Westermann (eds.), *Neuroblastoma*, Pediatric Oncology,
https://doi.org/10.1007/978-3-031-51292-6_11

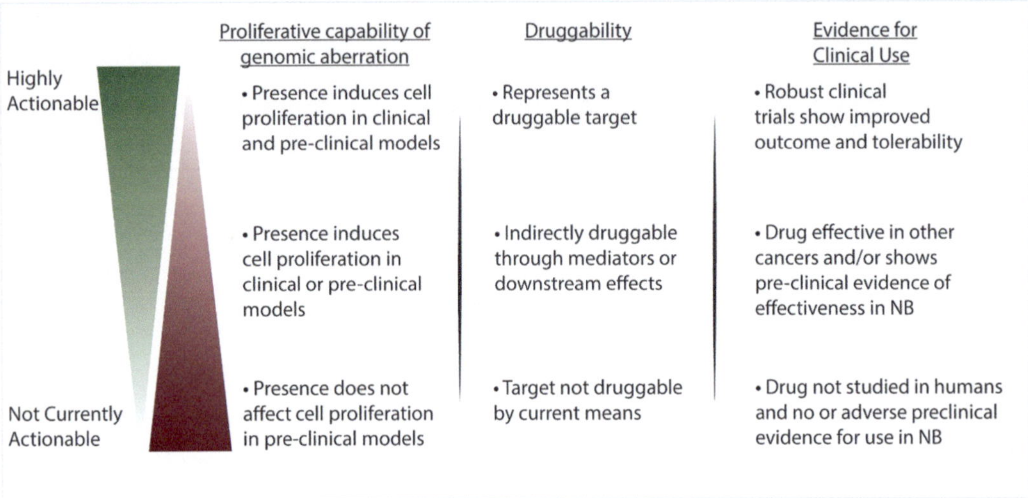

Fig. 11.1 Considerations in the determination of actionable genetic aberrations, modified from Carr et al. [2]

Table 11.1 Classification system for the determination of therapeutically actionable targets in neuroblastoma

Class	Description	Qualifications
Class 1	Highly actionable	• Detectable genomic aberration that induces cell proliferation in human tumors, inhibition of which causes tumor regression • Presence of aberration confers poor prognosis • Inhibitor molecule is available • Robust clinical response seen in validated clinical trials with available treatment • Targeting this aberration either improves outcome in patients or is equally effective as standard therapy with minimization of side effects
Class 2	Actionable	• Detectable genomic aberration that induces cell proliferation • Robust pre-clinical studies show that inhibition induces tumor regression in animal models • Evidence as an effective therapeutic target in other cancers shown by validated clinical trials
Class 3	Likely actionable	• Detectable genomic aberration that induces cell proliferation in neuroblastoma • May or may not have been used to guide treatment decisions in other cancers • Both in vitro and in vivo studies confirm that targeting this aberration leads to inhibition of cell proliferation
Class 4	Potentially actionable	• Detectable genomic aberration in preclinical models that suggests it induces cell proliferation • There may be some evidence that this aberration is druggable • Scientific rationale exists to justify study as a druggable target in neuroblastoma
Class 5	Not currently actionable	• Evidence is lacking to support use of this aberration in guiding patient treatment • Effects of this mutation are benign • No treatment currently exists that targets this aberration • Lack of preclinical data

Table 11.1 (continued)

Target	Therapy	Clinical trial stage and identifier	Cancer type
ALK[a]	Crizotinib	Phase I/II NCT00939770 Phase I NCT01606878	Relapsed or refractory solid tumors or anaplastic large cell lymphoma
	LDK378 (ceritinib)	Phase I NCT01742286 Phase II NCT02559778	Pediatric malignancies with genetic alteration in ALK
	RXDX-101 (entrectinib)	Phase I/II NCT02650401	Recurrent or refractory solid tumors and primary CNS[a] tumors
	PF-06463922 (lorlatinib)	Phase I NCT03107988 Phase III NCT03126916	Patients with ALK-driven relapsed or refractory neuroblastoma, addition to intensive therapy for children with newly diagnosed high-risk neuroblastoma
	Ensartinib	Phase II NCT03213652	Relapsed or refractory advanced solid tumors, non-Hodgkin lymphoma, histiocytic disorders with ALK or ROS genomic alterations
	Brigatinib	Phase I/II NCT04925609	Patients with ALK+ anaplastic large cell lymphoma, inflammatory myofibroblastic tumors or other solid tumors
	Alectinib	Phase II/III NCT05770037	ALK positive cancers
Aurora kinase	MLN8237 (alisertib)	Phase II NCT01154816	Relapsed or refractory solid tumors or leukemia
	MLN8054	Preclinical	
BET Bromodomain	JQ1	Preclinical	
	OTX015 (Oncoethix). MK-8628	Preclinical	
	GSK525762	Phase I NCT01587703	Nut midline carcinoma, MYCN-driven solid tumors, other cancers
	BMS-986158, BMS-986378	Phase I NCT03936465	Relapsed or refractory solid tumors, lymphoma, or CNS tumors
CDK4/6	LEE011 (ribociclib)	Phase I/II NCT05429502	Relapsed or refractory neuroblastoma or other solid tumors
	LY2835219 (abemaciclib)	Phase I NCT02644460	Newly diagnosed DIPG[a], relapsed/refractory/ progressive brain and solid tumors
MDM2	DS-3032b	Phase I	Advanced solid tumors or lymphoma, adult
	RO6839921	Phase I NCT02098967	Advanced neoplasms, including acute myeloid leukemia, adult
ODC[a]	DFMO[a]	Phase I NCT02030964 Phase II NCT02679144	Neuroblastoma
PI3K/MTOR	SF1126	Phase I NCT02337309	Relapsed and refractory neuroblastoma
	BKM120	Phase I/II	Adult advanced non-small cell lung cancer, advanced solid tumors, CNS lymphoma, endometrial cancers, prostate cancer, breast cancer
	NVP-BEZ235	Phase I/II	Adult glioblastoma, HER2 negative breast cancer, pancreatic neuroendocrine tumors

(continued)

Table 11.1 (continued)

Target	Therapy	Clinical trial stage and identifier	Cancer type
	LY3023414	Phase II NCT03213678	Relapsed or refractory advanced solid tumors, non-Hodgkin lymphoma, or histiocytic disorders with TSC or PI3K/mTOR mutations
	Temsirolimus	Phase II NCT00808899	Refractory, relapsed, progressive neuroblastoma
	AZD 6244 hydrogen sulfate (selumetinib)	Phase II NCT03213691	Advanced solid tumors, non-Hodgkin lymphoma, histiocytic disorders with activating MAPK mutations

[a]ALK: Anaplastic lymphoma kinase; DIPG: Diffuse Intrinsic Pontine Glioma; CNS: Central Nervous System, CDK: Cyclin-dependent kinase; ODC: Ornithine decarboxylase; DFMO: Difluoromethylornithine. This list represents a subset of available trials

justify implementing in a patient's plan of treatment and for continued study by pharmaceutical companies and scientists. More difficult to delineate are class 2 and 3 aberrations; these may be promising targets; however, the lack of effective inhibitors or confidence in their specific roles in neuroblastoma make it difficult to implement their inhibition either in the clinic or for further study and drug development. Class 4 aberrations may have some preclinical evidence, and class 5 aberrations are either not druggable or have no preclinical evidence to suggest a therapeutic benefit. Further research in this area is expected to define this classification system more clearly.

11.2 Targeted Treatment Strategies in Neuroblastoma

11.2.1 ALK

Anaplastic lymphoma kinase (ALK) encodes a receptor tyrosine kinase (RTK) normally expressed in the developing central and peripheral nervous systems [3]. A member of the insulin receptor superfamily of RTKs, ALK consists of an extracellular, transmembrane, and intracellular segment that houses its tyrosine kinase catalytic domain. In neuroblastoma, activation of ALK is thought to mediate cell proliferation and survival through its stimulation of the MAPK, PI3K/AKT/mTOR, and JAK/STAT signaling pathways [4]. The discovery of familial and somatically acquired activating mutations in ALK in a significant subset of patients with neuroblastoma resulted in its pursuit as a therapeutic target in the mid-2000s [5–8]. Since then, it has been used in patients with tumor ALK mutations as well as a hallmark model for the identification of targets and the development of therapies for genetic aberrations in pediatric cancer.

ALK mutations occur in approximately 9% of tumors and at similar frequencies in those with favorable and unfavorable prognoses, while ALK amplification occurs in around 1–2% of tumors [9, 10]. Accounting for 2% of all neuroblastoma cases, a common feature found in 50% of familial neuroblastoma is the germline mutation at R1275Q in the tyrosine kinase domain of ALK [4]. ALK^{R1275Q} is also a somatically acquired mutation that, together with ALK^{F1174L}, comprise the most common ALK mutations in sporadic neuroblastoma. The ALK^{F1174L} mutant leads to a greater degree of autophosphorylation and transforming ability in neuroblastoma cells compared to ALK^{R1275Q} and is preferentially found in tumors with MYCN-amplification. The combination of ALK^{F1174L} and MYCN amplification endows patients with a particularly poor outcome [9]. To study this interaction more closely, a transgenic Th-ALK^{F1174L} mouse model was developed that revealed that this mutation is capable of accelerating tumor onset and increasing penetrance in combination with overexpression of MYCN [11]. ALK^{F1174L} with MYCN amplification also increased disease penetrance in a transgenic zebrafish model and showed markedly accelerated tumor onset [12]. Further, expression of ALK^{F1174L} directed to neural crest cells led to the development of tumors that recapitulated human neuroblastoma in a transgenic mouse model and showed that the activating mutation was sufficient to induce neuroblastoma formation [13]. The combination of MYCN and ALK^{F1174L} expression in neural crest cells has also led to neuroblastoma formation in an immunocompetent mouse model [14].

The ability to target ALK arises from the presence of the ATP-binding pocket in its catalytic domain that, when targeted by small-molecule inhibitors, inhibits activation of ALK and its downstream effects [4]. The first of these inhibitors to enter clinical trials was crizotinib, an ATP-competitive dual ALK and c-Met inhibitor used for the treatment of non-small cell lung cancer, a disease that also houses aberrations in ALK [15]. Initial preclinical studies in cell lines with the activating ALK mutation ALK^{R1275Q} and ALK amplification showed sensitivity to the drug with sustained tumor regression in xenografts [16]. By contrast, mice bearing tumors with the F1174L mutation did not show the same level of sensitivity to crizotinib, an effect also seen in a phase 1 trial of patients with neuroblastoma (NCT00939770) [17, 18]. Several other inhibitors have also been developed and have undergone preclinical testing such as TAE684 [19] and its derivative LDK378 (ceritinib, Novartis) [20], which has demonstrated preclinical activity against F1174L and is currently being studied in clinical trials (NCT01742286). PF06463922 (lorlatinib) is a dual ALK/ROS1 inhibitor in a phase 1 clinical trial (NCT03107988) that showed efficacy as a single agent in Th-ALK^{F1174L}/MYCN tumors and patients [21, 22]. Lorlatinib has since supplanted crizotinib in a phase III trial to evaluate ALK inhibition in patients with newly diagnosed high-risk neuroblastoma (NCT03126916). Evolving strategies to impede the function of ALK conjugate these drugs to the cereblon ligand, pomalidomide, to induce chemical degradation of ALK [23]. Additionally, CH-5424802 (alectinib) [24] is being pursued for its ability to inhibit ALK and induce effective clinical responses. RXDX-101 (entrectinib-101, Ignyta), a pan-TRK inhibitor with activity against ALK has produced cytotoxic effects in preclinical models and may be particularly useful in targeting cells with *ALK* amplification [25, 26].

11.2.2 Mediation of Signaling Pathway Molecules

Due to their downstream activation by mutant *ALK* [11, 27] and their identification as independent genomic events in neuroblastoma [28], aberrations in signaling pathways are used to direct targeted treatment strategies. The investigation of inhibitors of the PI3K/AKT/mTOR signaling pathway has provided preclinical evidence for effective use when combined with conventional therapies, as seen with NVP-BEZ235 (dactolisib), a dual PI3K/mTOR inhibitor [29]. An additional study using the pan-PI3K inhibitor, LY294002 led to decreased tumor volume in murine models and induced apoptosis in *MYCN*-amplified neuroblastoma cell lines [30]. Pan-PI3K inhibitors SF1126 and LY3023414 are currently being tested in phase I (NCT02337309) and II (NCT03155620) clinical trials, respectively. Similarly, aberrations in the RAS/MAPK signaling pathway at both diagnosis and relapse support a role for MEK inhibition [31]. A phase II clinical trial of the MEK inhibitor selumetinib (AZD6244, NCT03213691) is underway. The contribution of these signaling pathways, in general, is not completely understood in neuroblastoma and it is clear that there are multiple nodes along them that are targetable, warranting further investigation into their therapeutic potential.

11.3 Targeting MYCN

Amplification of the *MYCN* oncogene is the most common genetic aberration in neuroblastoma and correlates with both high-risk disease and poor prognosis in patients [32, 33]. As a gene encoding a transcription factor involved in many cellular processes such as cell proliferation, maintenance of a stem-like state, and survival, it is not surprising that it promotes aggressive disease and confers dependency of neuroblastoma cells. These features make MYCN an attractive therapeutic target in neuroblastoma. However, attempts at targeting MYCN directly over the years has proved difficult. Its composition of primarily alpha helices with no available surface for small molecule binding provides a structural rationale for this impediment [34]. Thus, treatment has been aimed at targeting molecules that affect the expression, activation, and stability, as well as downstream effects of amplified *MYCN*.

11.3.1 Aurora Kinase

One of the approaches to circumvent direct inhibition of MYCN has been to target Aurora A kinase, the expression of which correlates with poor outcomes in neuroblastoma [35]. Aurora kinase is known to stabilize MYCN in a kinase-independent manner by interacting with MYCN and preventing its degradation [36]. Aurora A kinase also plays a crucial role in the regulation of mitotic checkpoint complexes, and when overexpressed, can lead to genomic instability, suppression of TP53 function and subsequent resistance to apoptosis [37]. Initial pre-clinical testing with the Aurora A inhibitor MLN8237 showed promise in cell line xenograft models and was shown to both destabilize MYCN and induce G2/M cell cycle arrest [37]. However, phase I clinical trials provided little evidence of efficacy as a single agent [38]. Better objective responses were seen when MLN8237 was combined with irinotecan and temozolomide, resulting in an overall 31.8% response rate as defined by the International Neuroblastoma Response Criteria [35].

11.3.2 BET Bromodomain Inhibition

An emerging strategy of targeting MYCN has been to disrupt its transcriptional program by affecting the chromatin structural modifications responsible for its expression. A multitude of molecules participate in the so-called 'reading' and 'writing' of epigenetic marks that govern expression of genes, and inhibition of some regulatory molecules has been effective for certain cancers [39]. Important modulators of epigenetic regulation are the bromodomain and extra-terminal domain (BET) family, a highly conserved set of proteins which consist of BRD2, BRD3, BRD4, and BRDT. Known as "readers," they are able to recognize and subsequently bind to acetylated lysine residues on histone tails of chromatin, the signal for active transcription.

One particular member of the family, BRD4, regulates RNA polymerase II (Pol II)-mediated transcriptional elongation by recruiting positive transcription elongation factor P-TEFb to transcription pause sites [40]. Tumor cells that rely on expression of oncogenes such as amplified *MYCN* in neuroblastoma, are anticipated to be sensitive to BRD4 inhibition. This has been demonstrated by the use of BRD4 inhibitors JQ1 [41] and OTX015 [42] in preclinical models of neuroblastoma. Upon treatment with either agent, transcription of MYCN was decreased in *MYCN*-amplified cell lines, which also showed greater sensitivity to the compounds. Treatment of xenograft models demonstrated prolonged survival and decreased tumor volume in *MYCN*-amplified tumors [41, 42]. An additional inhibitor, I-BET726, is a small molecule that binds with high affinity to BRD2, BRD3, and BRD4 that downregulated expression of MYCN and BCL2, resulting in tumor growth inhibition [43]. One of the major concerns with this type of strategy is how inhibition of chromatin regulators will affect global transcription, with concerns of toxicity in humans. BRD4 inhibition, in particular, has shown surprising specificity for oncogenic drivers such as MYCN, likely due to the transcription addiction exhibited by these tumors, thereby providing some hope for limited toxicity. Accordingly, clinical trials for BRD4 inhibitors are underway for children with advanced solid tumors (NCT03936465).

11.3.3 Transcription-Associated CDK Inhibition

RNA polymerase II-mediated transcription is regulated by cyclin-dependent kinases (CDKs) that are critical to transcription initiation, promotor-proximal pausing and elongation [44]. These CDKs, that are different from their cell cycle regulation counterparts, represent ideal targets for cancers reliant on amplified transcriptional programs such as that of MYCN. In neuroblastoma, prolonged and irreversible inhibition of CDK7/12/13 was achieved with THZ1 with subsequent downregulation of MYCN and its transcriptional program [45]. Super-enhancers (SEs), often acquired through gene amplification and found associated with key oncogenes, represent clusters of enhancers that upregulate transcription to serve as key regulatory hubs that bind to and recruit regulatory units [46]. Due to its perturbation of SEs associated with aberrant MYCN activity, THZ1 was selective for *MYCN*-amplified cells and treatment resulted in decreased tumor volume with minimal toxicity in mouse models of high-risk neuroblastoma [45]. THZ531, a more selective covalent CDK12/13 inhibitor was used to understand the function of these kinases in neuroblastoma. Cytotoxicity was accompanied by aberrant expression of genes involved in the DNA damage response and mRNA processing. CDK12 suppression specifically, led to an elongation defect with premature cleavage and polyadenylation of long (>45 kb) genes that led to their early termination [47, 48].

11.3.4 Other MYCN Targets

In addition to their effects on growth and proliferation alone, targeting certain signaling pathways in neuroblastoma are also thought to affect the function of MYCN. An indirect member of the PI3K/AKT pathway, glycogen synthase kinase-3β (GSK3β) regulates the phosphorylation of the MYCN protein prior to its degradation by the ubiquitin-proteasome system [49]. Inactivated in the presence of PI3K pathway member AKT, GSK3β is no longer functional and MYCN is stabilized. Disruption of this pathway with a PI3K inhibitor led to decreased MYCN protein expression [30]. Downstream targets of MYCN are also pursued as targets. P53, a direct transcriptional target of MYCN, though rarely mutated in neuroblastoma, is often inactivated in presence of *MDM2* amplification, and is thought to decrease p53-mediated apoptosis in this disease [50]. Upon treatment with MDM2 antagonists Nutlin-3 and MI-63, cells with *MYCN* amplification or overexpression were particularly sensitive to both compounds [50]. Ornithine decarboxylase, the rate-limiting enzyme in polyamine synthesis whose gene is a target of MYCN, has also been targeted by the anti-protozoal drug difluoromethylornithene (DFMO) [51]. Shown to inhibit proliferation in neuroblastoma cell lines [52], clinical trials tested DFMO as extended maintenance therapy with initial evidence suggesting its association with high event-free survival (EFS) and overall survival (OS) [53] (NCT02679144, NCT02030964). DFMO has been granted FDA approval for use (NDA215500).

11.4 Overcoming Resistance

While ALK has served as a classic example of an actionable genetic event in neuroblastoma, it has also revealed a challenge that emerges when attempting to provide target-directed therapy—innate or acquired resistance. As preclinical studies have demonstrated, tumors with certain biological features, namely, the ALK^{F1174L}-activating mutation, have been less amenable to ALK inhibition by currently available drugs. Further, resistance to ALK inhibitors is acquired even when they are initially effective, seen previously with crizotinib treatment of EML4-ALK-translocated lung cancer and in an RANBP2-ALK translocated inflammatory myofibroblastic tumor [4]. In neuroblastoma, *ALK* mutations that may have been undetected at diagnosis due to their subclonal nature are identified at relapse [54]. This demonstrates yet another reason warranting further investigation toward therapies that both overcome resistance to ALK inhibitors and show activity in presence of a broad range of activating mutations. The assessment of alternative second- and third-generation ALK inhibitors in addition to the study of combinatorial approaches could achieve this goal. New ALK inhibitors have overcome primary resistance in preclinical neuroblastoma models, most recently the dual ALK/ROS1 smallmoleculeinhibitorlorlatinib(NCT03107988, NCT04753658) [55]. Originally tested in ALK-driven lung cancer, this drug showed activity as a single-agent in ALK^{F1174L}, ALK^{F1245C}, and

ALK^{R1275Q}-mutated neuroblastoma xenograft models, suggesting efficacy in a broad range of ALK variants, possibly due to increased affinity for ALK [56]. Multiple studies of targeted therapies suggest that resistance mechanisms can be predicted in the preclinical setting, thereby enabling the improved design of newer generation inhibitors, or identifying activated kinases that compensate for inhibition of the primary mutation. In MYCN nonamplified neuroblastoma cells with acquired resistance to TAE684 and LDK378, both initially active against ALK^{F1174L}, resistance has been linked to alterations of AXL tyrosine kinase signaling that was overcome with AXL or HSP90 inhibition [57]. Alternatively, in neuroblastoma cells expressing both amplified MYCN and mutated ALK, resistance to ALK inhibition occurred through chromatin remodeling and transcriptional reprogramming that led to the loss of expression of these two oncogenes and a phenotype sustained by aberrantly expressed transcription factors that were regulated by the CTCF paralog, CTCFL (BORIS) [58]. Further studies will determine the prevalence of such phenotypic plasticity as a mechanism of resistance in neuroblastoma.

As development of second-generation ALK inhibitors proceed, focus has also shifted to combinatorial approaches with the intent of inhibiting molecules downstream of ALK. Tumor regression was seen in vivo when crizotinib was combined with an mTOR inhibitor, Torin2 in Th-ALK^{F1174L}/MYCN mice [11]. In *MYCN*-nonamplified cell lines, similar targeting of the PI3K pathway was effective in the presence of the activating ALK^{F1174L} mutation. By using an inhibitor of both PI3K and mTOR combined with crizotinib, synergy together with downregulation of key signaling pathway molecules was seen [27].

Acquired resistance to traditional chemotherapies also emerges during induction therapy that can lead to relapse of the tumor, and patients who do not respond to initial induction therapy face long-term survival rates of less than 20% [37]. Explanations underlying this unfortunate occurrence need further characterization so that new molecular targets can be discovered that can be used to bypass development of resistance. In a preclinical model assessing the development of resistance to the differentiation agent retinoic acid (RA), low levels of the tumor suppressor NF1 and the retinoic acid (RA) receptor co-activator ZNF423 were linked to poor outcome in patients, and inhibition of MEK signaling was able to restore RA differentiation in vitro [59].

Such experience has guided investigation into resistance mechanisms of therapies that alter the transcriptional program in neuroblastoma. Resistance models of THZ1 showed upregulation of the ABC transporter as a major mechanism of resistance in THZ1-treated neuroblastoma cells [60]. Resistance to BET bromodomain inhibition with JQ1 saw upregulation of the PI3K pathway, and prolonged sensitivity to JQ1 in neuroblastoma was aided by concomitant PI3K inhibition [61].

11.5 Treating the High-Risk and Relapsed Patient

Advanced presentation of disease at diagnosis is common in neuroblastoma. Though progress has been made in targeting specific aberrations, key gains to be made in neuroblastoma treatment lie in the ability to treat high-risk, even relapsed disease. With survival of patients with high-risk neuroblastoma at approximately 61%, focus on this group is essential in developing future therapeutic strategies [62]. Though a well-established treatment strategy has not been broadly accepted for patients at relapse, certain treatment strategies are common among many institutions. These typically have included salvage treatment with a series of cytotoxic agents with different mechanisms of action than initially used, anti-GD2 antibody (dinutuximab), chimeric antigen receptor-positive T cell therapy, and ^{131}I-MIBG infusions [37]. However, as our knowledge of targeted treatment strategies increases, so does their integration into treatment at relapse, aided by an understanding of the biological features of the relapsed tumor. One such example in a recent work shows a distinct difference in the tumor genomics in 23 pairs of tumor samples at relapse compared at diagnosis [31]. Whole exome sequencing revealed a median of 29 unique

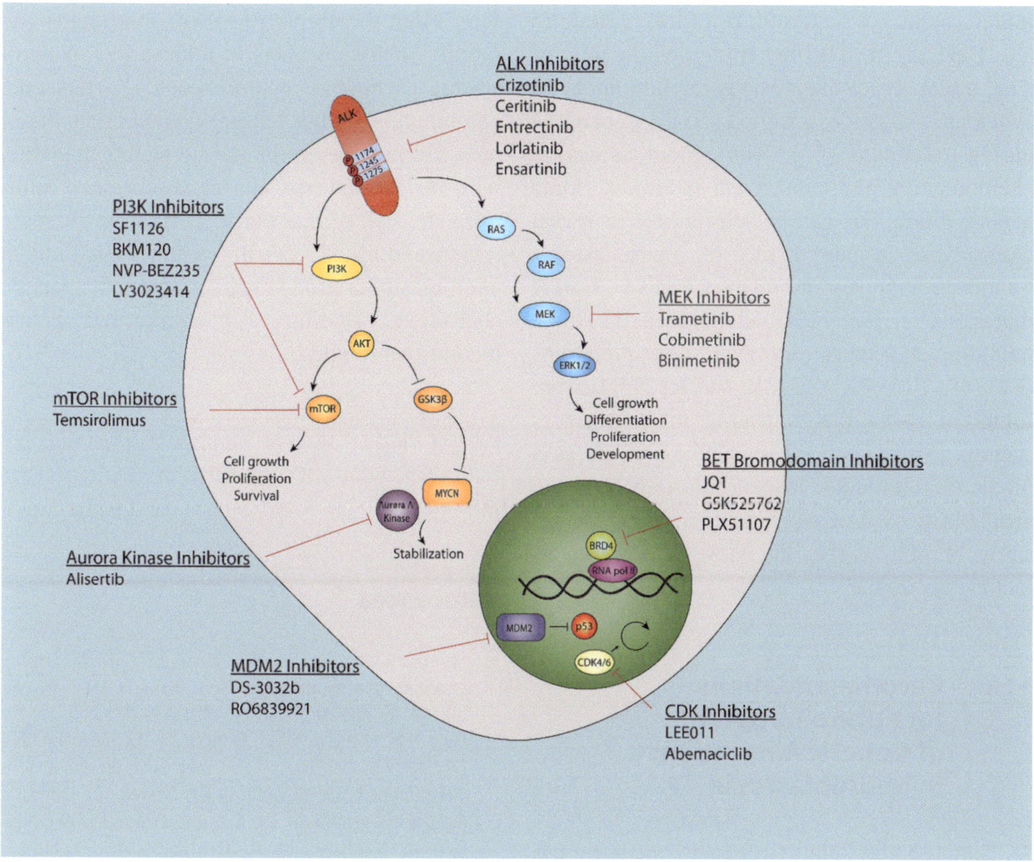

Fig. 11.2 Clinically available therapies that target genetic aberrations in neuroblastoma

somatic mutations at relapse. A significant portion of the tumors at relapse showed mutations in members of the RAS-MAPK pathway MEK inhibition did indeed show sensitivity in RAS/RAF mutated cell lines compared to cell lines with alternative mutational status [31]. Thus, MEK1/2 inhibitors offer a potential treatment strategy for relapsed neuroblastoma with MAPK pathway aberrations. Aberrations in the cyclin D1/CDK4/CDK6/RB axis of cell cycle regulation is also a feature found in relapsed neuroblastoma. While rare at diagnosis, the increased expression and kinase activity of CDK4/CDK6 driven by genetic aberrations are thought to drive cell cycle progression and amplification of cyclin D1. Inhibition of the CDK4/6 axis in neuroblastoma using a small molecule inhibitor resulted in cell cycle arrest and induced cellular senescence in a MYCN amplification-dependent manner [63].

Additional studies and current clinical trials are aimed at using targeted therapies as frontline treatment and at relapse (Fig. 11.2). Crizotinib, the first ALK inhibitor available, has been studied as single-agent therapy and in combination with topotecan and cyclophosphamide in patients with solid tumors. This study, initially in phase I with progression into phase II for evaluation in recurrent neuroblastomas, aimed to test this regimen in patients with somatically acquired mutations in *ALK* (NCT00939770). The objective response for patients with ALK-positive neuroblastoma using crizotinib as a single agent was 15% (95% CI, 3.3–34.3), and crizotinib was preferentially effective in treating tumors with the R1275Q mutation [18]. Crizotinib was under use in a phase-3 trial in patients with high-risk neuroblastoma at diagnosis, however the superior efficacy noted with lorlatinib has led to the replacement of crizotinib with lorlatinib (NCT03126916). Distinct from identification of *ALK* mutations at diagnosis is the possibility of subclonal and newly acquired somatic mutations during treatment [64]. Throughout induction chemotherapy and subsequent treatment, some genetic alterations can be selected for or reveal themselves. In paired sets of neuroblastoma tumors at diagnosis and relapse, cases with *ALK* mutations at diagnosis had retained the same mutation at relapse; however, new mutations (F1174L, F1174S, Y1278S, and R1275Q) were found in cases that appeared to be relapse-specific [54]. Given the role of ALK role as a predictive biomarker in neuroblastoma and the availability of ALK-specific inhibitors, further study of relapse-specific ALK inhibitor treatment is justifiable.

11.6 Recommendations for Future Targeting of Genetic Aberrations in Neuroblastoma

As depicted, the field of pediatric oncology has shown great advances in the ability to treat patients with neuroblastoma. However, those classified as having high-risk and/or relapsed neuroblastoma are still suffering from extremely low long-term survival rates. This selected group of patients is where efforts should be focused to make therapeutic gains in our treatment strategies and ultimate survival. We recommend that in trying to achieve this goal, repeat biopsies should be considered as the standard of care, in the case of relapse, when they are commonly avoided due to concerns for discomfort and uncertain benefit to the patient. However, studies using paired tumor samples at diagnosis and relapse have shown relapse-specific alterations that have actionable potential. Evidence of clonal evolution, accrual of new *ALK* mutations, and new oncogenic mutations in the RAS pathway at relapse justify the use of repeat biopsy, especially if provided with the possibility of targeting the new aberration. With the increased ease and efficiency of performing genetic studies, it seems that the ability to act on aberrations and modify treatment plans at relapse in a patient-specific manner is within reach. To this end, combination studies with new and classic therapies will help determine which agents, together, will provide the best chance of cure and minimize the risk of resistance. Further, to increase understanding of recurring genetic mutations in neuroblastoma and to identify actionable genetic aberrations, sharing of genomic data across institutions should be a goal.

Acknowledgements This work was supported by a Howard Hughes Medical Institute Medical Research Fellowship award (MP) and NIH/NCI 2RO1CA148688 (REG).

References

1. Hyman DM, Taylor BS, Baselga J. Implementing genome-driven oncology. Cell. 2017;168(4):584–99. https://doi.org/10.1016/j.cell.2016.12.015.
2. Carr TH, McEwen R, Dougherty B, Johnson JH, Dry JR, Lai Z, Ghazoui Z, Laing NM, Hodgson DR, Cruzalegui F, Hollingsworth SJ, Barrett JC. Defining actionable mutations for oncology therapeutic development. Nat Rev Cancer. 2016;16(5):319–29. https://doi.org/10.1038/nrc.2016.35.
3. Iwahara T, Fujimoto J, Wen D, Cupples R, Bucay N, Arakawa T, Mori S, Ratzkin B, Yamamoto T. Molecular characterization of ALK, a receptor tyrosine kinase expressed specifically in the nervous system. Oncogene. 1997;14(4):439–49. https://doi.org/10.1038/sj.onc.1200849.
4. Azarova AM, Gautam G, George RE. Emerging importance of ALK in neuroblastoma. Semin Cancer Biol. 2011;21(4):267–75. https://doi.org/10.1016/j.semcancer.2011.09.005.
5. George RE, Sanda T, Hanna M, Fröhling S, Luther W, Zhang J, Ahn Y, Zhou W, London WB, McGrady P, Xue L, Zozulya S, Gregor VE, Webb TR, Gray NS, Gilliland DG, Diller L, Greulich H, Morris SW, Meyerson M, Look AT. Activating mutations in ALK provide a therapeutic target in neuroblastoma. Nature. 2008;455(7215):975–8. https://doi.org/10.1038/nature07397.
6. Mosse YP, Laudenslager M, Longo L, Cole KA, Wood A, Attiyeh EF, Laquaglia MJ, Sennett R, Lynch JE, Perri P, Laureys G, Speleman F, Kim C, Hou C, Hakonarson H, Torkamani A, Schork NJ, Brodeur GM, Tonini GP, Rappaport E, Devoto M, Maris JM. Identification of ALK as a major familial neuroblastoma predisposition gene. Nature. 2008;455(7215):930–5. https://doi.org/10.1038/nature07261.

7. Janoueix-Lerosey I, Lequin D, Brugieres L, Ribeiro A, de Pontual L, Combaret V, Raynal V, Puisieux A, Schleiermacher G, Pierron G, Valteau-Couanet D, Frebourg T, Michon J, Lyonnet S, Amiel J, Delattre O. Somatic and germline activating mutations of the ALK kinase receptor in neuroblastoma. Nature. 2008;455(7215):967–70. https://doi.org/10.1038/nature07398.
8. Chen Y, Takita J, Choi YL, Kato M, Ohira M, Sanada M, Wang L, Soda M, Kikuchi A, Igarashi T, Nakagawara A, Hayashi Y, Mano H, Ogawa S. Oncogenic mutations of ALK kinase in neuroblastoma. Nature. 2008;455(7215):971–4. https://doi.org/10.1038/nature07399.
9. De Brouwer S, De Preter K, Kumps C, Zabrocki P, Porcu M, Westerhout EM, Lakeman A, Vandesompele J, Hoebeeck J, Van Maerken T, De Paepe A, Laureys G, Schulte JH, Schramm A, Van Den Broecke C, Vermeulen J, Van Roy N, Beiske K, Renard M, Noguera R, Delattre O, Janoueix-Lerosey I, Kogner P, Martinsson T, Nakagawara A, Ohira M, Caron H, Eggert A, Cools J, Versteeg R, Speleman F. Meta-analysis of neuroblastomas reveals a skewed ALK mutation spectrum in tumors with MYCN amplification. Clin Cancer Res. 2010;16(17):4353–62. https://doi.org/10.1158/1078-0432.CCR-09-2660.
10. Pugh TJ, Morozova O, Attiyeh EF, Asgharzadeh S, Wei JS, Auclair D, Carter SL, Cibulskis K, Hanna M, Kiezun A, Kim J, Lawrence MS, Lichenstein L, McKenna A, Pedamallu CS, Ramos AH, Shefler E, Sivachenko A, Sougnez C, Stewart C, Ally A, Birol I, Chiu R, Corbett RD, Hirst M, Jackman SD, Kamoh B, Khodabakshi AH, Krzywinski M, Lo A, Moore RA, Mungall KL, Qian J, Tam A, Thiessen N, Zhao Y, Cole KA, Diamond M, Diskin SJ, Mosse YP, Wood AC, Ji L, Sposto R, Badgett T, London WB, Moyer Y, Gastier-Foster JM, Smith MA, Guidry Auvil JM, Gerhard DS, Hogarty MD, Jones SJ, Lander ES, Gabriel SB, Getz G, Seeger RC, Khan J, Marra MA, Meyerson M, Maris JM. The genetic landscape of high-risk neuroblastoma. Nat Genet. 2013;45(3):279–84. https://doi.org/10.1038/ng.2529.
11. Berry T, Luther W, Bhatnagar N, Jamin Y, Poon E, Sanda T, Pei D, Sharma B, Vetharoy WR, Hallsworth A, Ahmad Z, Barker K, Moreau L, Webber H, Wang W, Liu Q, Perez-Atayde A, Rodig S, Cheung NK, Raynaud F, Hallberg B, Robinson SP, Gray NS, Pearson AD, Eccles SA, Chesler L, George RE. The ALK(F1174L) mutation potentiates the oncogenic activity of MYCN in neuroblastoma. Cancer Cell. 2012;22(1):117–30. https://doi.org/10.1016/j.ccr.2012.06.001.
12. Zhu S, Lee JS, Guo F, Shin J, Perez-Atayde AR, Kutok JL, Rodig SJ, Neuberg DS, Helman D, Feng H, Stewart RA, Wang W, George RE, Kanki JP, Look AT. Activated ALK collaborates with MYCN in neuroblastoma pathogenesis. Cancer Cell. 2012;21(3):362–73. https://doi.org/10.1016/j.ccr.2012.02.010.
13. Heukamp LC, Thor T, Schramm A, De Preter K, Kumps C, De Wilde B, Odersky A, Peifer M, Lindner S, Spruessel A, Pattyn F, Mestdagh P, Menten B, Kuhfittig-Kulle S, Kunkele A, Konig K, Meder L, Chatterjee S, Ullrich RT, Schulte S, Vandesompele J, Speleman F, Buttner R, Eggert A, Schulte JH. Targeted expression of mutated ALK induces neuroblastoma in transgenic mice. Sci Transl Med. 2012;4(141):141ra91. https://doi.org/10.1126/scitranslmed.3003967.
14. Cohen MA, Zhang S, Sengupta S, Ma H, Bell GW, Horton B, Sharma B, George RE, Spranger S, Jaenisch R. Formation of human neuroblastoma in mouse-human neural crest chimeras. Cell Stem Cell. 2020;26(4):579–592.e576. https://doi.org/10.1016/j.stem.2020.02.001.
15. Zou HY, Li Q, Lee JH, Arango ME, McDonnell SR, Yamazaki S, Koudriakova TB, Alton G, Cui JJ, Kung PP, Nambu MD, Los G, Bender SL, Mroczkowski B, Christensen JG. An orally available small-molecule inhibitor of c-met, PF-2341066, exhibits cytoreductive antitumor efficacy through antiproliferative and antiangiogenic mechanisms. Cancer Res. 2007;67(9):4408–17. https://doi.org/10.1158/0008-5472.CAN-06-4443.
16. Bresler SC, Wood AC, Haglund EA, Courtright J, Belcastro LT, Plegaria JS, Cole K, Toporovskaya Y, Zhao H, Carpenter EL, Christensen JG, Maris JM, Lemmon MA, Mosse YP. Differential inhibitor sensitivity of anaplastic lymphoma kinase variants found in neuroblastoma. Sci Transl Med. 2011;3(108):108ra114. https://doi.org/10.1126/scitranslmed.3002950.
17. Mosse YP, Lim MS, Voss SD, Wilner K, Ruffner K, Laliberte J, Rolland D, Balis FM, Maris JM, Weigel BJ, Ingle AM, Ahern C, Adamson PC, Blaney SM. Safety and activity of crizotinib for paediatric patients with refractory solid tumours or anaplastic large-cell lymphoma: a children's oncology group phase 1 consortium study. Lancet Oncol. 2013;14(6):472–80. https://doi.org/10.1016/S1470-2045(13)70095-0.
18. Foster JH, Voss SD, Hall DC, Minard CG, Balis FM, Wilner K, Berg SL, Fox E, Adamson PC, Blaney SM, Weigel BJ, Mosse YP. Activity of crizotinib in patients with ALK-aberrant relapsed/refractory neuroblastoma: a children's oncology group study (ADVL0912). Clin Cancer Res. 2021;27(13):3543–8. https://doi.org/10.1158/1078-0432.CCR-20-4224.
19. Galkin AV, Melnick JS, Kim S, Hood TL, Li N, Li L, Xia G, Steensma R, Chopiuk G, Jiang J, Wan Y, Ding P, Liu Y, Sun F, Schultz PG, Gray NS, Warmuth M. Identification of NVP-TAE684, a potent, selective, and efficacious inhibitor of NPM-ALK. Proc Natl Acad Sci U S A. 2007;104(1):270–5. https://doi.org/10.1073/pnas.0609412103.
20. Chen J, Jiang C, Wang S. LDK378: a promising anaplastic lymphoma kinase (ALK) inhibitor. J Med Chem. 2013;56(14):5673–4. https://doi.org/10.1021/jm401005u.
21. Guan J, Tucker ER, Wan H, Chand D, Danielson LS, Ruuth K, El Wakil A, Witek B, Jamin Y, Umapathy G, Robinson SP, Johnson TW, Smeal T, Martinsson

T, Chesler L, Palmer RH, Hallberg B. The ALK inhibitor PF-06463922 is effective as a single agent in neuroblastoma driven by expression of ALK and MYCN. Dis Model Mech. 2016;9(9):941–52. https://doi.org/10.1242/dmm.024448.
22. Goldsmith KC, Park JR, Kayser K, Malvar J, Chi Y-Y, Groshen SG, Villablanca JG, Krytska K, Lai LM, Acharya PT, Goodarzian F, Pawel B, Shimada H, Ghazarian S, States L, Marshall L, Chesler L, Granger M, Desai AV, Mody R, Morgenstern DA, Shusterman S, Macy ME, Pinto N, Schleiermacher G, Vo K, Thurm HC, Chen J, Liyanage M, Peltz G, Matthay KK, Berko ER, Maris JM, Marachelian A, Mossé YP. Lorlatinib with or without chemotherapy in ALK-driven refractory/relapsed neuroblastoma: phase 1 trial results. Nat Med. 2023;29(5):1092–102. PMID: 37012551.
23. Powell CE, Gao Y, Tan L, Donovan KA, Nowak RP, Loehr A, Bahcall M, Fischer ES, Janne PA, George RE, Gray NS. Chemically induced degradation of anaplastic lymphoma kinase (ALK). J Med Chem. 2018;61(9):4249–55. https://doi.org/10.1021/acs.jmedchem.7b01655.
24. Song Z, Wang M, Zhang A. Alectinib: a novel second generation anaplastic lymphoma kinase (ALK) inhibitor for overcoming clinically-acquired resistance. Acta Pharm Sin B. 2015;5(1):34–7. https://doi.org/10.1016/j.apsb.2014.12.007.
25. Aveic S, Pantile M, Seydel A, Esposito MR, Zanon C, Li G, Tonini GP. Combating autophagy is a strategy to increase cytotoxic effects of novel ALK inhibitor entrectinib in neuroblastoma cells. Oncotarget. 2016;7(5):5646–63. https://doi.org/10.18632/oncotarget.6778.
26. Sano R, Krytska K, Larmour CE, Raman P, Martinez D, Ligon GF, Lillquist JS, Cucchi U, Orsini P, Rizzi S, Pawel BR, Alvarado D, Mossé YP. An antibody-drug conjugate directed to the ALK receptor demonstrates efficacy in preclinical models of neuroblastoma. Sci Transl Med. 2019;11(483):eaau9732. PMID: 30867324.
27. Moore NF, Azarova AM, Bhatnagar N, Ross KN, Drake LE, Frumm S, Liu QS, Christie AL, Sanda T, Chesler L, Kung AL, Gray NS, Stegmaier K, George RE. Molecular rationale for the use of PI3K/AKT/mTOR pathway inhibitors in combination with crizotinib in ALK-mutated neuroblastoma. Oncotarget. 2014;5(18):8737–49. https://doi.org/10.18632/oncotarget.2372.
28. Shukla N, Ameur N, Yilmaz I, Nafa K, Lau CY, Marchetti A, Borsu L, Barr FG, Ladanyi M. Oncogene mutation profiling of pediatric solid tumors reveals significant subsets of embryonal rhabdomyosarcoma and neuroblastoma with mutated genes in growth signaling pathways. Clin Cancer Res. 2012;18(3):748–57. https://doi.org/10.1158/1078-0432.CCR-11-2056.
29. Westhoff MA, Faham N, Marx D, Nonnenmacher L, Jennewein C, Enzenmuller S, Gonzalez P, Fulda S, Debatin KM. Sequential dosing in chemosensitization: targeting the PI3K/Akt/mTOR pathway in neuroblastoma. PLoS One. 2013;8(12):e83128. https://doi.org/10.1371/journal.pone.0083128.
30. Chesler L, Schlieve C, Goldenberg DD, Kenney A, Kim G, McMillan A, Matthay KK, Rowitch D, Weiss WA. Inhibition of phosphatidylinositol 3-kinase destabilizes MYCN protein and blocks malignant progression in neuroblastoma. Cancer Res. 2006;66(16):8139–46. https://doi.org/10.1158/0008-5472.CAN-05-2769.
31. Eleveld TF, Oldridge DA, Bernard V, Koster J, Daage LC, Diskin SJ, Schild L, Bentahar NB, Bellini A, Chicard M, Lapouble E, Combaret V, Legoix-Né P, Michon J, Pugh TJ, Hart LS, Rader J, Attiyeh EF, Wei JS, Zhang S, Naranjo A, Gastier-Foster JM, Hogarty MD, Asgharzadeh S, Smith MA, Guidry Auvil JM, Watkins TB, Zwijnenburg DA, Ebus ME, van Sluis P, Hakkert A, van Wezel E, van der Schoot CE, Westerhout EM, Schulte JH, Tytgat GA, Dolman ME, Janoueix-Lerosey I, Gerhard DS, Caron HN, Delattre O, Khan J, Versteeg R, Schleiermacher G, Molenaar JJ, Maris JM. Relapsed neuroblastomas show frequent RAS-MAPK pathway mutations. Nat Genet. 2015;47(8):864–71. https://doi.org/10.1038/ng.3333.
32. Brodeur GM, Seeger RC, Schwab M, Varmus HE, Bishop JM. Amplification of N-myc in untreated human neuroblastomas correlates with advanced disease stage. Science. 1984;224(4653):1121–4.
33. Seeger RC, Brodeur GM, Sather H, Dalton A, Siegel SE, Wong KY, Hammond D. Association of multiple copies of the N-myc oncogene with rapid progression of neuroblastomas. N Engl J Med. 1985;313(18):1111–6. https://doi.org/10.1056/NEJM198510313131802.
34. Huang M, Weiss WA. Neuroblastoma and MYCN. Cold Spring Harb Perspect Med. 2013;3(10):a014415. https://doi.org/10.1101/cshperspect.a014415.
35. DuBois SG, Marachelian A, Fox E, Kudgus RA, Reid JM, Groshen S, Malvar J, Bagatell R, Wagner L, Maris JM, Hawkins R, Courtier J, Lai H, Goodarzian F, Shimada H, Czarnecki S, Tsao-Wei D, Matthay KK, Mosse YP. Phase I study of the Aurora a kinase inhibitor alisertib in combination with irinotecan and temozolomide for patients with relapsed or refractory neuroblastoma: a NANT (new approaches to neuroblastoma therapy) trial. J Clin Oncol. 2016;34(12):1368–75. https://doi.org/10.1200/JCO.2015.65.4889.
36. Otto T, Horn S, Brockmann M, Eilers U, Schuttrumpf L, Popov N, Kenney AM, Schulte JH, Beijersbergen R, Christiansen H, Berwanger B, Eilers M. Stabilization of N-Myc is a critical function of Aurora a in human neuroblastoma. Cancer Cell. 2009;15(1):67–78. https://doi.org/10.1016/j.ccr.2008.12.005.
37. Whittle SB, Smith V, Doherty E, Zhao S, McCarty S, Zage PE. Overview and recent advances in the treatment of neuroblastoma. Expert Rev Anticancer Ther. 2017;17(4):369–86. https://doi.org/10.1080/14737140.2017.1285230.

38. Mosse YP, Lipsitz E, Fox E, Teachey DT, Maris JM, Weigel B, Adamson PC, Ingle MA, Ahern CH, Blaney SM. Pediatric phase I trial and pharmacokinetic study of MLN8237, an investigational oral selective small-molecule inhibitor of Aurora kinase A: a children's oncology group phase I consortium study. Clin Cancer Res. 2012;18(21):6058–64. https://doi.org/10.1158/1078-0432.CCR-11-3251.
39. Filippakopoulos P, Qi J, Picaud S, Shen Y, Smith WB, Fedorov O, Morse EM, Keates T, Hickman TT, Felletar I, Philpott M, Munro S, McKeown MR, Wang Y, Christie AL, West N, Cameron MJ, Schwartz B, Heightman TD, La Thangue N, French CA, Wiest O, Kung AL, Knapp S, Bradner JE. Selective inhibition of BET bromodomains. Nature. 2010;468(7327):1067–73. https://doi.org/10.1038/nature09504.
40. Jang MK, Mochizuki K, Zhou M, Jeong HS, Brady JN, Ozato K. The bromodomain protein Brd4 is a positive regulatory component of P-TEFb and stimulates RNA polymerase II-dependent transcription. Mol Cell. 2005;19(4):523–34. https://doi.org/10.1016/j.molcel.2005.06.027.
41. Puissant A, Frumm SM, Alexe G, Bassil CF, Qi J, Chanthery YH, Nekritz EA, Zeid R, Gustafson WC, Greninger P, Garnett MJ, McDermott U, Benes CH, Kung AL, Weiss WA, Bradner JE, Stegmaier K. Targeting MYCN in neuroblastoma by BET bromodomain inhibition. Cancer Discov. 2013;3(3):308–23. https://doi.org/10.1158/2159-8290.CD-12-0418.
42. Henssen A, Althoff K, Odersky A, Beckers A, Koche R, Speleman F, Schafers S, Bell E, Nortmeyer M, Westermann F, De Preter K, Florin A, Heukamp L, Spruessel A, Astrahanseff K, Lindner S, Sadowski N, Schramm A, Astorgues-Xerri L, Riveiro ME, Eggert A, Cvitkovic E, Schulte JH. Targeting MYCN-driven transcription by BET-bromodomain inhibition. Clin Cancer Res. 2016;22(10):2470–81. https://doi.org/10.1158/1078-0432.CCR-15-1449.
43. Wyce A, Ganji G, Smitheman KN, Chung CW, Korenchuk S, Bai Y, Barbash O, Le B, Craggs PD, McCabe MT, Kennedy-Wilson KM, Sanchez LV, Gosmini RL, Parr N, McHugh CF, Dhanak D, Prinjha RK, Auger KR, Tummino PJ. BET inhibition silences expression of MYCN and BCL2 and induces cytotoxicity in neuroblastoma tumor models. PLoS One. 2013;8(8):e72967. https://doi.org/10.1371/journal.pone.0072967.
44. Larochelle S, Amat R, Glover-Cutter K, Sanso M, Zhang C, Allen JJ, Shokat KM, Bentley DL, Fisher RP. Cyclin-dependent kinase control of the initiation-to-elongation switch of RNA polymerase II. Nat Struct Mol Biol. 2012;19(11):1108–15. https://doi.org/10.1038/nsmb.2399.
45. Chipumuro E, Marco E, Christensen CL, Kwiatkowski N, Zhang T, Hatheway CM, Abraham BJ, Sharma B, Yeung C, Altabef A, Perez-Atayde A, Wong KK, Yuan GC, Gray NS, Young RA, George RE. CDK7 inhibition suppresses super-enhancer-linked oncogenic transcription in MYCN-driven cancer. Cell. 2014;159(5):1126–39. https://doi.org/10.1016/j.cell.2014.10.024.
46. Lovén J, Hoke HA, Lin CY, Lau A, Orlando DA, Vakoc CR, Bradner JE, Lee TI, Young RA. Selective inhibition of tumor oncogenes by disruption of super-enhancers. Cell. 2013;153(2):320–34. https://doi.org/10.1016/j.cell.2013.03.036.
47. Krajewska M, Dries R, Grassetti AV, Dust S, Gao Y, Huang H, Sharma B, Day DS, Kwiatkowski N, Pomaville M, Dodd O, Chipumuro E, Zhang T, Greenleaf AL, Yuan GC, Gray NS, Young RA, Geyer M, Gerber SA, George RE. CDK12 loss in cancer cells affects DNA damage response genes through premature cleavage and polyadenylation. Nat Commun. 2019;10(1):1757. https://doi.org/10.1038/s41467-019-09703-y.
48. Zhang T, Kwiatkowski N, Olson CM, Dixon-Clarke SE, Abraham BJ, Greifenberg AK, Ficarro SB, Elkins JM, Liang Y, Hannett NM, Manz T, Hao M, Bartkowiak B, Greenleaf AL, Marto JA, Geyer M, Bullock AN, Young RA, Gray NS. Covalent targeting of remote cysteine residues to develop CDK12 and CDK13 inhibitors. Nat Chem Biol. 2016;12(10):876–84. https://doi.org/10.1038/nchembio.2166.
49. Sjostrom SK, Finn G, Hahn WC, Rowitch DH, Kenney AM. The Cdk1 complex plays a prime role in regulating N-myc phosphorylation and turnover in neural precursors. Dev Cell. 2005;9(3):327–38. https://doi.org/10.1016/j.devcel.2005.07.014.
50. Gamble LD, Kees UR, Tweddle DA, Lunec J. MYCN sensitizes neuroblastoma to the MDM2-p53 antagonists Nutlin-3 and MI-63. Oncogene. 2012;31(6):752–63. https://doi.org/10.1038/onc.2011.270.
51. Hogarty MD, Norris MD, Davis K, Liu X, Evageliou NF, Hayes CS, Pawel B, Guo R, Zhao H, Sekyere E, Keating J, Thomas W, Cheng NC, Murray J, Smith J, Sutton R, Venn N, London WB, Buxton A, Gilmour SK, Marshall GM, Haber M. ODC1 is a critical determinant of MYCN oncogenesis and a therapeutic target in neuroblastoma. Cancer Res. 2008;68(23):9735–45. https://doi.org/10.1158/0008-5472.CAN-07-6866.
52. Saulnier Sholler GL, Gerner EW, Bergendahl G, MacArthur RB, VanderWerff A, Ashikaga T, Bond JP, Ferguson W, Roberts W, Wada RK, Eslin D, Kraveka JM, Kaplan J, Mitchell D, Parikh NS, Neville K, Sender L, Higgins T, Kawakita M, Hiramatsu K, Moriya SS, Bachmann AS. A phase I trial of DFMO targeting polyamine addiction in patients with relapsed/refractory neuroblastoma. PLoS One. 2015;10(5):e0127246. https://doi.org/10.1371/journal.pone.0127246.
53. Sholler GLS, Ferguson W, Bergendahl G, Bond JP, Neville K, Eslin D, Brown V, Roberts W, Wada RK, Oesterheld J, Mitchell D, Foley J, Parikh NS, Eshun F, Zage P, Rawwas J, Sencer S, Pankiewicz D, Quinn M, Rich M, Junewick J, Kraveka JM. Maintenance DFMO increases survival in high risk neuroblastoma. Sci Rep. 2018;8(1):14445. https://doi.org/10.1038/s41598-018-32659-w.

54. Schleiermacher G, Javanmardi N, Bernard V, Leroy Q, Cappo J, Rio Frio T, Pierron G, Lapouble E, Combaret V, Speleman F, de Wilde B, Djos A, Ora I, Hedborg F, Träger C, Holmqvist BM, Abrahamsson J, Peuchmaur M, Michon J, Janoueix-Lerosey I, Kogner P, Delattre O, Martinsson T. Emergence of new ALK mutations at relapse of neuroblastoma. J Clin Oncol. 2014;32(25):2727–34. https://doi.org/10.1200/JCO.2013.54.0674.
55. Zou HY, Friboulet L, Kodack DP, Engstrom LD, Li Q, West M, Tang RW, Wang H, Tsaparikos K, Wang J, Timofeevski S, Katayama R, Dinh DM, Lam H, Lam JL, Yamazaki S, Hu W, Patel B, Bezwada D, Frias RL, Lifshits E, Mahmood S, Gainor JF, Affolter T, Lappin PB, Gukasyan H, Lee N, Deng S, Jain RK, Johnson TW, Shaw AT, Fantin VR, Smeal T. PF-06463922, an ALK/ROS1 inhibitor, overcomes resistance to first and second generation ALK inhibitors in preclinical models. Cancer Cell. 2015;28(1):70–81. https://doi.org/10.1016/j.ccell.2015.05.010.
56. Infarinato NR, Park JH, Krytska K, Ryles HT, Sano R, Szigety KM, Li Y, Zou HY, Lee NV, Smeal T, Lemmon MA, Mosse YP. The ALK/ROS1 inhibitor PF-06463922 overcomes primary resistance to crizotinib in ALK-driven neuroblastoma. Cancer Discov. 2016;6(1):96–107. https://doi.org/10.1158/2159-8290.CD-15-1056.
57. Debruyne DN, Bhatnagar N, Sharma B, Luther W, Moore NF, Cheung NK, Gray NS, George RE. ALK inhibitor resistance in ALK(F1174L)-driven neuroblastoma is associated with AXL activation and induction of EMT. Oncogene. 2016;35(28):3681–91. https://doi.org/10.1038/onc.2015.434.
58. Debruyne DN, Dries R, Sengupta S, Seruggia D, Gao Y, Sharma B, Huang H, Moreau L, McLane M, Day DS, Marco E, Chen T, Gray NS, Wong KK, Orkin SH, Yuan GC, Young RA, George RE. BORIS promotes chromatin regulatory interactions in treatment-resistant cancer cells. Nature. 2019;572(7771):676–80. https://doi.org/10.1038/s41586-019-1472-0.
59. Holzel M, Huang S, Koster J, Ora I, Lakeman A, Caron H, Nijkamp W, Xie J, Callens T, Asgharzadeh S, Seeger RC, Messiaen L, Versteeg R, Bernards R. NF1 is a tumor suppressor in neuroblastoma that determines retinoic acid response and disease outcome. Cell. 2010;142(2):218–29. https://doi.org/10.1016/j.cell.2010.06.004.
60. Gao Y, Zhang T, Terai H, Ficarro SB, Kwiatkowski N, Hao MF, Sharma B, Christensen CL, Chipumuro E, Wong KK, Marto JA, Hammerman PS, Gray NS, George RE. Overcoming resistance to the THZ series of covalent transcriptional CDK inhibitors. Cell Chem Biol. 2017;25:135. https://doi.org/10.1016/j.chembiol.2017.11.007.
61. Iniguez AB, Alexe G, Wang EJ, Roti G, Patel S, Chen L, Kitara S, Conway A, Robichaud AL, Stolte B, Bandopadhayay P, Goodale A, Pantel S, Lee Y, Cheff DM, Hall MD, Guha R, Davis MI, Menard M, Nasholm N, Weiss WA, Qi J, Beroukhim R, Piccioni F, Johannessen C, Stegmaier K. Resistance to epigenetic-targeted therapy engenders tumor cell vulnerabilities associated with enhancer remodeling. Cancer Cell. 2018;34(6):922–938.e927. https://doi.org/10.1016/j.ccell.2018.11.005.
62. Irwin MS, Naranjo A, Zhang FF, Cohn SL, London WB, Gastier-Foster JM, Ramirez NC, Pfau R, Reshmi S, Wagner E, Nuchtern J, Asgharzadeh S, Shimada H, Maris JM, Bagatell R, Park JR, Hogarty MD. Revised neuroblastoma risk classification system: a report from the Children's Oncology Group. J Clin Oncol. 2021;39(29):3229–41. PMID: 34319759.
63. Rader J, Russell MR, Hart LS, Nakazawa MS, Belcastro LT, Martinez D, Li Y, Carpenter EL, Attiyeh EF, Diskin SJ, Kim S, Parasuraman S, Caponigro G, Schnepp RW, Wood AC, Pawel B, Cole KA, Maris JM. Dual CDK4/CDK6 inhibition induces cell-cycle arrest and senescence in neuroblastoma. Clin Cancer Res. 2013;19(22):6173–82. https://doi.org/10.1158/1078-0432.CCR-13-1675.
64. Landau DA, Carter SL, Stojanov P, McKenna A, Stevenson K, Lawrence MS, Sougnez C, Stewart C, Sivachenko A, Wang L, Wan Y, Zhang W, Shukla SA, Vartanov A, Fernandes SM, Saksena G, Cibulskis K, Tesar B, Gabriel S, Hacohen N, Meyerson M, Lander ES, Neuberg D, Brown JR, Getz G, Wu CJ. Evolution and impact of subclonal mutations in chronic lymphocytic leukemia. Cell. 2013;152(4):714–26. https://doi.org/10.1016/j.cell.2013.01.019.

12 Re-Engaging the Immune System: Immunotherapy for Neuroblastoma

Miho Nakajima and Nai-Kong V. Cheung

12.1 Introduction: Rationale of Immunotherapy for Neuroblastoma

Neuroblastoma (NB) has a unique biology characterized by two divergent phenotypes, spontaneously regressing (e.g., stage 4 s, s for special) versus multiple resistant lethal outcome (e.g., stage 4). Historically, stage 4 biology is early dissemination to bones and bone marrow that usually recur after initial response to multimodal combination chemoradiotherapy. On the other hand, stage 4 s biology can be widespread to most organs of the body, typically marrow and skin, despite which, predictably maturing into ganglioneuroma or disappearing usually within a year from initial diagnosis during infancy. Stage 4 s biology is now found among NB detected prenatally, as well those diagnosed as stage1 and stage 2 in the infant stage (<18 months of age). Although its mechanism remains unclear, many have proposed an immune-based mechanism. GD2, a disialoganglioside, is a tumor-associated antigen (TAA) expressed on neuroectodermal derived tumors such as NB, retinoblastoma, melanoma, as well as sarcomas, including osteosarcoma, rhabdomyosarcoma, and Ewings sarcoma [1]. Because of its high expression in NB, and restricted expression in normal tissues, GD2 is a near ideal target because of its membrane proximity, homogeneity, and infrequent antigen loss [2, 3]. Even though normal human brain and nerve tissues express GD2, immunoglobulins G (IgGs) cannot cross the blood brain barrier to cause damage, except with peripheral nerve fibers, where pain side effect of anti-GD2 antibody treatment is pronounced. Despite ever-increasing, intensive chemotherapy, surgery, radiation, and myeloablative therapy with stem cell rescue, the long-term outcome is guarded because of late effects even if patients survive the disease. Immunotherapy, with no cross toxicity with genotoxic agents while exploiting death mechanism in tumors different from those of conventional cytotoxic therapies, as well as having the potential of long-term immunity against cancer, is indeed highly desirable if it can fulfill its therapeutic promise.

M. Nakajima
Department of Pediatric Oncology, National Cancer Center Hospital, Tokyo, Japan
e-mail: mihnakaj@ncc.go.jp

N.-K. V. Cheung (✉)
Department of Pediatrics, Memorial Sloan Kettering Cancer Center, New York, NY, USA
e-mail: cheungn@mskcc.org

12.2 Mechanism of Immunotherapy for NB

There are potent effectors that can kill NB. They include complements, natural killer (NK) cells, granulocytes, macrophages, and even T cells. NK

S. Asgharzadeh, F. Westermann (eds.), *Neuroblastoma*, Pediatric Oncology,
https://doi.org/10.1007/978-3-031-51292-6_12

cells kill through antibody-dependent cell-mediated cytotoxicity (ADCC) when an IgG antibody that binds to tumor cells engages the Fc-receptor. Anti-GD2 monoclonal antibodies (mAbs) are classic mediators of NK-ADCC. Similarly, granulocytes are potent killers through myeloid-ADCC when such mAb is present. Phagocytes such as activated macrophages can also be highly effective in ADPC (antibody-dependent phagocyte-mediated cytotoxicity). Complement-mediated cytotoxicity (CMC) is an extremely effective killing mechanism often misunderstood or underrated [4–8]. While all of these effector mechanisms require a functional Fc in the IgG molecule, the absence of Fc receptor (FcR) on T cells have left T cells out of the antibody therapy toolbox. More recently, with the advent of bispecific antibodies which engage T cells, the power of T cells can now be realized. Whatever effector mechanism of killing, it is also increasingly clear that there are built-in immune checkpoints that have been supplanted by tumor cells to inhibit innate and adaptive immunity. These include, among others, human leukocyte antigen (HLA) alleles on tumor cells that engage killer cell immunoglobulin-like receptors (KIRs) to inhibit NK activation [8–12] or to inhibit myeloid-ADCC. Decay-accelerating factor (DAF) or CD59 on the surface of tumor cells can also derail CMC [13–15]. The ability of NB to transdifferentiate using epigenetic mechanisms between the substrate adherent (mesenchymal) phenotype (with HLA expression and DAF expression) and the neuroblastic phenotype (with low or none HLA or DAF expression) allows these tumor cells to wear different protective armors, depending on the "fighters" (innate immunity versus T cell based immunity) sent to confront them [15, 16]. Even upregulation of HLA on NB may be enough to inhibit NK cells, it is not enough to engage classic T cells, given the paucity of mutations in these tumors, severely cutting down tumor-specific T cell clonal frequency [2]. When T cells are redirected with bispecific antibodies or chimeric antigen receptors (CAR) to kill tumors, they come under the influence of immune checkpoints, Tregs, and the suppressive tumor microenvironment [17]. It is important to remember that the immune framework for attacking NB is likely to be complex. However, our understanding has greatly increased in recent years just by focusing on the preclinical and the clinical experience of anti-GD2 antibodies (Fig. 12.1).

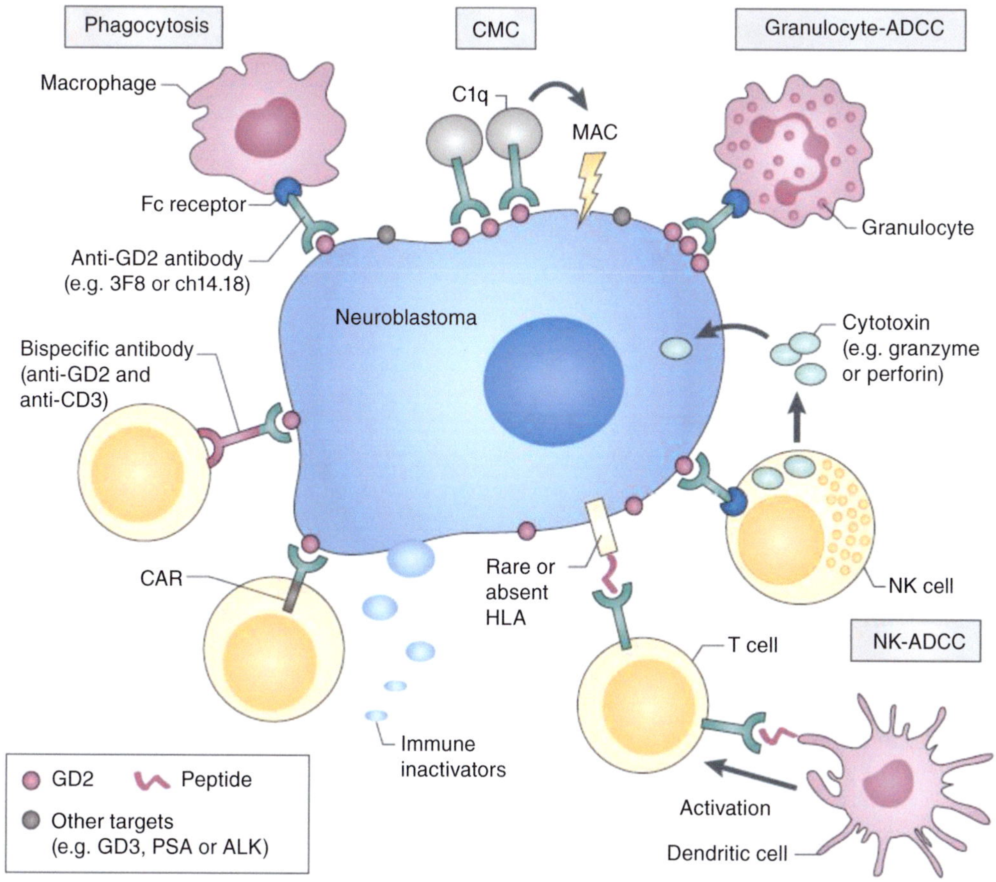

Fig. 12.1 Mechanism of immunotherapy for neuroblastoma. Multiple potent effectors are involved in the mechanism of killing neuroblastoma. Anti-GD2 antibodies such as 3F8 or dinutuximab help to initiate NK cell-mediated antibody-dependent cell-mediated cytotoxicity (NK-ADCC), granulocyte-ADCC, CMC (complement-mediated cytotoxicity) and phagocytosis via its Fc moiety. To obtain the effect of cytotoxic T cells against neuroblastoma, bispecific antibodies are used to retarget polyclonal T cells to kill neuroblastoma similar to CAR T cells, which are genetically engineered T cells to kill neuroblastoma. (Reprinted with permission from Cheung NK and Dyer MA. Neuroblastoma: developmental biology, cancer genomics and immunotherapy. Nature Reviews Cancer 13:397–411, 2013 (PMID: 23702928))

12.3 Development of Anti-GD2 Monoclonal Antibody Therapy (Fig. 12.2, Tables 12.1, 12.2)

In 1987, a phase 1 study of first in-human anti-GD2 therapy using murine IgG3 monoclonal antibody 3F8 was published, confirming the safety and clinical activity against metastatic NB and melanoma with major side effects, including pain, urticaria, and hypertension [18]. Subsequently, the same group introduced the concept of using cytokine GM-CSF to enhance myeloid-ADCC [4]. Since these first-in-human experience, many studies have followed using mouse IgG2a as well as its human-mouse chimeric form (14G2a and ch14.18 [dinutuximab]). Building on the hypothesis that pain was CMC-related, hu14.18-K322A was developed where a single mutation was introduced to eliminate CMC, while the IgG1 was defucosylated to increase NK-ADCC substantially over dinutuximab. In a phase I study, hu14.18-K322A still had significant pain side effects, while the anti-tumor

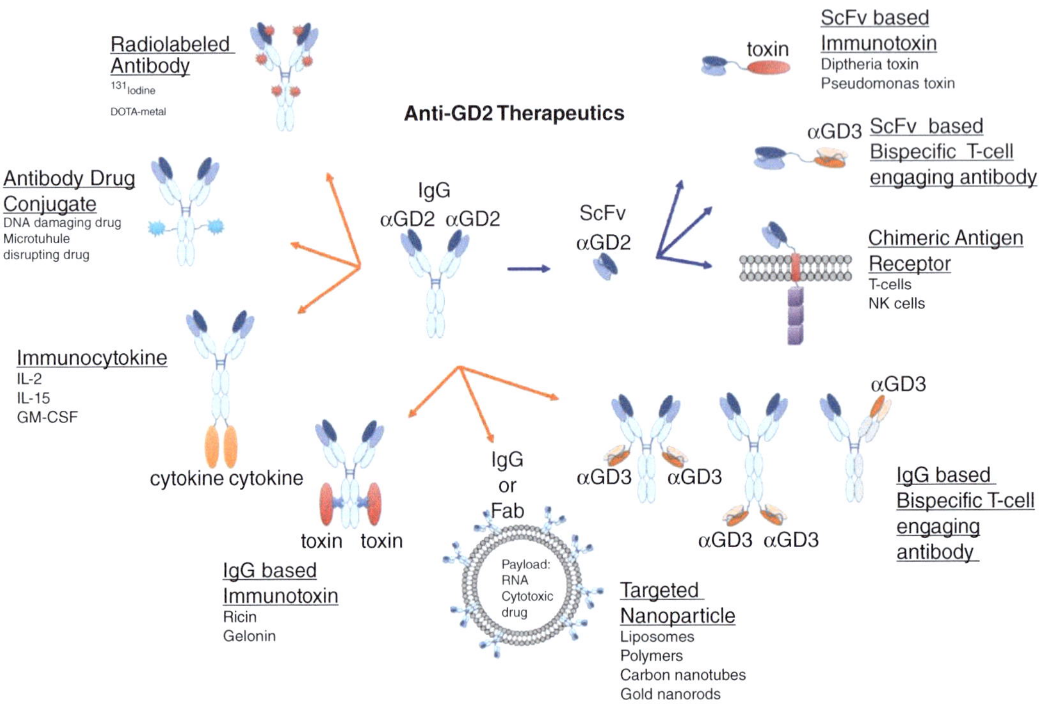

Fig. 12.2 Compilation of anti-GD2 therapeutics. Orange arrows illustrate different types of Anti-GD2 IgG templates, including radiolabeled antibodies, antibody-drug conjugate, immunocytokine, immunotoxin, targeted nanoparticles, and bispecific T cell-engaging antibody. Blue arrows illustrate different types of anti-GD2 scFv fragments such as immunotoxins, bispecific T cell-engaging antibody and chimeric antigen receptors. (Reprinted with permission from Ahmed et al., Ahmed M, and Cheung NK. Engineering anti-GD2 monoclonal antibodies for cancer immunotherapy. FEBS Letters 588:288–297, 2014 [PMID: 24295643])

efficacy was comparable to dinutuximab [19–21]. In contrast, mouse 3F8 possessed exceptional CMC properties (because of its >ten-fold slower k_{off} and higher affinity), but its pain side effects were not worse than dinutuximab. Indeed for a tumor like NB that lacks DAF, this anti-tumor mechanism appears to be crucial. Despite the substantial lower NK-ADCC activity (because of a mouse Fc), the clinical activity of 3F8 was at least comparable to dinutuximab in long-term patient survival.

In 2010, Children's Oncology Group (COG) reported the results of a randomized study using dinutuximab with GM-CSF, interleukin-2, and isotretinoin for high-risk NB patients who responded at least partially to high-dose chemotherapy and stem cell rescue. Compared to standard therapy only with isotretinoin, the patients treated with dinutuximab had significantly prolonged event-free survival (EFS) and overall survival (OS) at 2 years. In a follow-up analysis, EFS was no longer significant, but OS still was [22]. As expected, more than half of the patients in the mAb group had Grade 3 to 4 pain as a main side effect [23]. COG also conducted a phase 2 study of immunocytokine therapy showing that hu14.18-IL2 which consists of humanized 14.18 anti-GD2 antibody linked to IL2 achieved 21.7% CR rate (5 out of 36 patients) for those with bone marrow disease, but not patients with bulky disease [24, 25]. In 2012, Memorial Sloan Kettering Cancer Center (MSK) reported the outcome of 169 patients with high-risk stage 4 NB (diagnosed at ≥18 months of age or *MYCN* amplified) treated between 1988 to 2008 with 3F8 plus GM-CSF, 13-cis retinoic acid, but without IL2 [8]. A recent update of a larger cohort of patients confirmed the survival statistics, suggesting the efficacy of mouse 3F8 against chemotherapy-resistant minimal residual disease

Table 12.1 Completed clinical trials of mAbs, chemoimmunotherapy, radioimmunotherapy and vaccine therapy

Type of immunotherapy	Immunotherapy combination	Phase	Clinical trial
MoAb: Murine 3F8	Murine 3F8	2	NCT00002458
	Murine 3F8 + iv GM-CSF	2	NCT00002560
	Murine 3F8 + chemotherapy+ radiation+ autologous SCT (N7)	2	NCT00002634
	Murine 3F8+ etoposide+ isotretinoin	2	NCT00004110
	Murine 3F8+ barley Beta-glucan	1	NCT00037011
	Murine 3F8 + GM-CSF+ dose intensive chemotherapy (N8)	2	NCT00040872
	Murine 3F8+ sc GM-CSF	2	NCT00072358
	Murine 3F8 + GM-CSF+ barley beta-glucan+ isotretinoin	2	NCT00089258
	Murine 3F8 (dose escalation) + sc GM-CSF	1	NCT00450307
	Murine 3F8+ yeast Beta-glucan	1	NCT00492167
	Murine 3F8+ allogenic NK cells	1	NCT00877110
	Murine 3F8+ GM-CSF+ isotretinoin (first CR with SCT)	2	NCT01183416
	Murine 3F8+ GM-CSF+ isotretinoin (first CR without SCT)	2	NCT01183429
	Murine 3F8+ GM-CSF+ isotretinoin (>second CR)	2	NCT01183884
	Murine 3F8+ GM-CSF+ isotretinoin (refractory disease)	2	NCT01183897
	Murine 3F8+ GM-CSF+ isotretinoin		NCT02100930
MoAb: Naxitamab (hu3F8)	Naxitamab	1	NCT01419834
	Naxitamab+ IL2	1	NCT01662804
MoAb: Dinutuximab (ch14.18)	Dinutuximab+ GM-CSF+ IL2+ isotretinoin	1	NCT00005576
	Dinutuximab+ GM-CSF + IL2+ isotretinoin	3	NCT00026312
	Dinutuximab+ GM-CSF, IL2+ isotretinoin	3	NCT01041638

(continued)

Table 12.1 (continued)

Type of immunotherapy	Immunotherapy combination	Phase	Clinical trial
hu14.18K322A	Humanized 14.18K322A	1	NCT00743496
	Hu14.18K322A+ GM-CSF + IL2+ CD133+ selected autologous stem cell infusion	1	NCT02130869
Immunocytokine	Hu14.18-IL2 fusion protein	1	NCT00003750
	Hu14.18-IL2 fusion protein	2	NCT00082758
Radioimmunotherapy	I-131-Murine 3F8 (intraventricular or intrathecal)	1	NCT00003022
	I-131-Murine 3F8 (systemic) + bevacizumab+ autologous SCT	1	NCT00450827
ICI	Ipilimumab	1	NCT01445379
CAR T cell	GD2-CAR.OX40.28.ICD9	1	NCT02107963
NK cell	NK cell infusion+ RhIL-15	1	NCT01875601
T cell	Donor-derived gene-modified multi-virus-specific cytotoxic T cells against GD2	1	NCT01460901
Vaccine	IL2 gene modified autologous or partially HLA matched allogeneic NB cell vaccine	1	NCT00002748
	Anti-idiotype rat MoAb, A1G4 vaccine with BCG adjuvant	1	NCT00003023
	Autologous NB tumor cell vaccine	1	NCT00048386
	IL2 gene-modified allogenic NB cell vaccine	1	NCT00186862
	Tumor lysate-pulsated DC vaccines + HSCT	2	NCT00405327
	Tumor lysate-pulsed DC vaccine, HSCT	2	NCT00405327
	GD2/GD3-KLH + OPT-821 + oral beta glucan	1/2	NCT00911560
	Autologous DC vaccine	1	NCT01241162

Table 12.2 Ongoing clinical trials of mAbs, chemoimmunotherapy, radioimmunotherapy and vaccine therapy

Types	Immunotherapy combination	Phase	Clinical trial	Status
MoAb: Naxitamab (humanized 3F8, hu3F8)	Naxitamab+ GM-CSF	1/2	NCT01757626	Recruiting
	I-124-Naxitamab for PET imaging	Pilot	NCT02307630	Recruiting
	Naxitamab+ allogenic NK cells+rIL2	1	NCT02650648	Recruiting
	Naxitamab+ GMCSF+ isotretinoin (first CR)	2	NCT03033303	Recruiting
	Naxitamab+ GM-CSF	2	NCT03363373	Recruiting
MoAb: Dinutuximab (ch14.18)	Dinutuximab+ NK cells+ Lenalidomide	1	NCT02573896	Not yet recruiting
	I-131-MIBG or Crizotinib with Dinutuximab+ auto SCT	3	NCT03126916	Recruiting
	Dinutuximab+I-131-MIBG +/− vorinostat	1	NCT03332667	Recruiting
	Hu5F9-G4 (Magrolimab) + Dinutuximab	1	NCT04751383	Not yet recruiting
	Dinutuximab +GM-CSF + isotretinoin	2	NCT 03786783	Active not recruiting
MoAb: Hu14.18K322A	Hu14.18K322A+ allogeneic NK cells	1	NCT01576692	Active not recruit
	Hu14.18K322A + GM-CSF+ IL2+ allogeneic NK cells	2	NCT01857934	Recruiting
Antibody-drug conjugate	Lorvotuzumab Mertansine (anti CD56)	2	NCT02452554	Active not recruit
Immunocytokine	Hu14.18-IL2+ Haploidentical NK cells	1	NCT03209869	Recruiting
Radioimmunotherapy	I-131–8H9 (intrathecal)	1	NCT00089245	Recruiting
	I-131-murine 3F8 (intrathecal)	2	NCT00445965	Active not recruit
	I-131-Omburtamab (intraventricular)	2/3	NCT03275402	Not yet recruiting
Chemoimmunotherapy	Irinotecan +Temozolomide with Dinutuximab vs. Temsirolimus	2	NCT01767194	Active not recruit
	Irinotecan +Temozolomide + Dinutuximab	2	NCT 04385277	Recruiting
	NK cell infusion with irinotecan +Temozolomide + Dinutuximab	1/2	NCT04211675	Not yet recruiting
	Naxitamab + irinotecan + Temozolomide + GM-CSF	1/2	NCT03189706	Recruiting
ICI	Nivolumab ± Iplimumab	1/2	NCT02304458	Recruiting
	GVAX vaccine + Nivolumab ±Iplimumab	1	NCT04239040	Recruiting

(continued)

Table 12.2 (continued)

Types	Immunotherapy combination	Phase	Clinical trial	Status
Bispecific antibody	ATCs armed with GD2 bispecific hu3F8xOKT3 + GM-CSF+ IL2	1/2	NCT02173093	Recruiting
	Hu3F8–BsAb (recombinant)	1/2	NCT03860207	Recruiting
CAR T cells	GD2 CAR and iCaspase suicide switch	1	NCT01822652	Active not recruiting
	CD171 specific CAR T cells expressing EGFRt	1	NCT02311621	Recruiting
	GD2 specific CAR+ IL-15 expressing autologous NKT cells	1	NCT03294954	Recruiting
	GD2 CAR T cells and constitutively active IL7 receptors	1	NCT03635632	Not yet recruiting
	GD2 CAR T cells	1	NCT04539366	Not yet recruiting
Vaccines	Lymphotactin+ IL2 gene-modified NB tumor cell vaccine	1/2	NCT00703222	Active not recruit
	A Study of a Vaccine in Combination With Beta-glucan in People With Neuroblastoma	1/2	NCT06057948	Recruiting
	Allogenic tumor cell vaccines + Oral metronomic cytoxan	1/2	NCT01192555	Active not recruit

in bone marrow, especially when GM-CSF was given subcutaneously [8, 26–28].

Hu3F8 (Naxitamab) was developed to exploit the human Fc to improve NK-ADCC while preserving much of the superior CMC properties of mouse 3F8 [29]. Moreover, humanization reduced the immunogenicity of these antibodies [30]. In phase I and II clinical trials, the anti-tumor activity was substantially improved over mouse 3F8 [31–33]. But most importantly, the toxicity profile appeared to stay manageable despite a 2.5-fold increase (compared to dinutuximab or mouse 3F8) in the dose per cycle, all outpatient treatment in contrast to inpatient treatment for dinutuximab. Naxitamab received FDA breakthrough designation in August 2018 because of its relatively low toxicity profile and exceptional anti-tumor response. Even though mAbs have improved the outcome of high-risk NB, their survival benefits have so far been restricted to patients with minimal residual disease [8, 23]. Relapsed patients, especially those with chemo-resistant and widespread soft tissue involvements, or those with central nervous system (CNS) metastasis, continue to be a challenge.

12.4 Combination Use of mAb: Chemoimmunotherapy and Radioimmunotherapy

12.4.1 Chemoimmunotherapy

Multimodal combination seems an obvious next step if one were to exploit immunotherapy beyond small disease burden [34]. Irinotecan and temozolomide have tolerable toxicities and activity against NB [35, 36], and their combination with anti-GD2 therapy has yielded promising results. In a randomized study using irinotecan, temozolomide plus either temsirolimus or dinutuximab, 9 out of 17 patients assigned to dinutuximab group showed major responses (4 PR and 5 CR), while only one out of 18 patients assigned to temosirolimus group achieved PR [37]. Furthermore, data of expanded cohort of this study was published and showed objective response of 41.5% (22 [11CR and 11PR] out of 53 patients). This additional data also showed that 22 patients continued to have stable disease which resulted in 83.1% of disease control rate for relapsed or refractory NB [38]. Another data was presented at SIOP in 2019 which showed chemoimmunotherapy using Naxitamab, humanized mAb, with 39% overall response rate, including 13 CR and 9PR out of 56 patients. This study included multiply relapsed patients as well as the patients who were previously treated with irinotecan and temozolomide which differed from previous COG study [39]. This strategy using chemoimmunotherapy is expected to become a standard regimen for relapsed or refractory NB.

12.4.2 Radioimmunotherapy

CNS is a sanctuary site of NB because of the blood brain barrier. Akin to acute lymphoblastic leukemia (ALL), CNS relapse is a hurdle to cure at least for a subset of NB patients. The overall incidence of CNS NB reported was 6.3%, which has increased from 1980 to 1999. It is likely to keep increasing during this immunotherapy era when further improvement in survival is expected [40]. In childhood ALL, the addition of intrathecal chemotherapy finally broke the barrier to achieving cure [41]. Intrathecal administration of radiolabeled mAbs have been studied in preclinical and clinical settings for various cancers, including brain tumors [42]. Given that NB is a radiosensitive tumor, its radioimmunotherapy was first tested in the 1990s [43, 44]. Intra-Ommaya ^{131}I-3F8 was evaluated among patients with various GD2(+) brain tumors or GD2(+) metastatic solid tumors in a phase 1 trial, confirming its safety and high therapeutic index, and defining the maximum-tolerated dose [45]. In a phase II study, 21 patients with recurrent metastatic CNS NB were treated with this compartmental radioimmunotherapy (cRIT), consisting of surgery, chemotherapy, craniospinal radiation, intrathecal ^{131}I-3F8 or ^{131}I-8H9 (anti-B7H3) mAbs for CNS disease control, while receiving intravenous 3F8 plus GMCSF for systemic disease control. Seventeen out of 21 patients remained alive at median follow up of 33 months from the date of CNS relapse and all 17 remained free of CNS NB [46]. In a follow-up analysis of 105 patients treated with this strategy since 2003, the median survival was 58 months compared to historical control of less than 6 months [47]. This led to the FDA breakthrough designation for radioiodine-labeled 8H9 (omburtamab) in June 2017.

12.4.3 Vaccine Therapy

The role for vaccines in infectious disease is well known for over 100 years. Cancer vaccines have been tested in various shapes and forms, including whole tumor cells, peptides, glycolipids, anti-idiotypes, viral and bacterial vectors, DNA, RNA, and dendritic cells. However, none so far has proven effective for pediatric malignancies. NB is known to express TAAs such as gangliosides (GD2, GD3, and GM2) and glycoproteins (B7H3, CD56, L1-CAM, and glypican 2) with potentials as tumor vaccine targets [48]. IL2 adenovector-transduced autologous tumor cell vaccines were tested in dose escalation study for advanced NB; local and systemic immunity against autologous tumor cells were found, and 5 out of 10 patients showed clinical responses (including 1 CR and 1 PR) [49]. Whole tumor cell vaccines seem ideal since they carry all potential tumor antigens and could induce an immune response to the entire spectrum of targets. Yet, the complexity of adaptive immunity (antigen dominance, antigen competition, co-stimulatory signals, HLA expression, immune suppression) often derails a meaningful anti-tumor immune response. Whole autologous tumor vaccine adds another level of complexity relating to quality control, cost, and time of manufacture. Tumor lysate-pulsed dendritic cell vaccines showed tumor response in 1 out of 10 patients and stable disease in 5 out of 10 patients [50]. The documented anti-tumor benefit of anti-GD2 antibodies for metastatic NB provides the rationale for GD2-directed NB vaccines. GD2 ganglioside-KLH vaccine was tested as a subcutaneous injection in the presence of the saponin QS21 (OPT821) and oral beta-glucan in a phase I clinical trial [51]. Among 15 patients with high-risk stage 4 with multiple relapsed NB brought back to remission at protocol entry, 12/15 remained alive now past 8 years since the first report [52]. 6 out of 10 patients achieved negative MRD in the BM. The Phase II clinical trial confirmed the survival outcome and the importance of anti-GD2 antibody titer that was induced [53, 54].

12.5 Next Generation of Antibody-Based or Cellular Therapy

12.5.1 Chimeric Antigen Receptor (CAR) Immunotherapy

Due to low or absent expression of human HLA-class I antigens in human tumors, including NB, classic T cell immunotherapy is ineffective [55]. Following the enormous success of genetically engineered CAR T cell therapy against hematologic malignancies, many have attempted to realize its efficacy among solid tumors in adult and children [56, 57]. CAR T cells were generated against NB to carry out major histocompatibility complex (MHC)-independent anti-tumor cytotoxicity. CAR against NB usually consists of three domains: extracellular antigen binding domain, which is single chain variable fragment (scFv) of anti-GD2 (or anti-L1CAM), a transmembrane domain, and an endodomain [58]. Among 6 heavily pre-treated patients receiving first generation CAR targeting glycoprotein antigen L1CAM, 1 patient, who had minimal residual disease at study enrollment, had a partial response on day 56 after cell infusion. In all patients, CAR T cells did not persist, likely because of a host immune response against CE7 [59]. When Epstein-Barr virus (EBV) specific cytotoxic T cells were used as building blocks, the endogenous EBV was able to prolong the persistence of CAR T cells [60, 61]. These CAR cytotoxic T cells (CTLs) retained cytotoxic activities both against EBV target and GD2 target even at 24 weeks post infusions. Of 11 patients treated, 4 out of 8 patients had measurable tumor response or necrosis. In these studies, CAR Ts were safe without any pain or neuropathy side effects. A tumor which responded to CART therapy showed T cell infiltrates, but no PCR signal for CAR-CTLs or CAR-activated T cells (ATCs). Over the ensuing decade, responses to GD2-CAR Ts have been less favorable [62], and new concerns for significant neurotoxicity have been raised in preclinical models when second generation CAR Ts were used [63].

12.5.2 Bispecific Antibodies

For four decades since the advent of hybridoma, therapeutic antibodies have shown clinical benefit as monospecific IgGs [64]. These IgGs include rituximab, trastuzumab, cetuximab, and anti-GD2 antibodies (dinutuximab and naxitamab), among others. Their anti-tumor immune properties require Fc functions, especially their binding to FcR on white cells, a receptor that T cells lack. The concept of bispecific antibody (BsAb), where a single antibody molecule carries dual antigen specificity, is at least 50 years old. When the second specificity is for T cells, the T-cell engaging bispecific antibody concept emerges. Among T cell-based cytotherapy, antibody-driven approaches have advantages over genetic modification of T cells (CAR Ts): being an off-the-shelf drug with no need for genetic manipulation, using standard manufacturing protocols and drug distribution networks. Lower cost is another consideration for antibody-based versus gene-based approaches [65]. Among the various strategies to improve on the standard anti-GD2 IgG mAb, e.g., immunocytokines, immunotoxins, antibody drug conjugates, radiolabeled IgGs, T cell-engaging bispecific antibodies is the most recent strategy to move into the clinic (see Table 12.2) [1, 66]. Of the many BsAb platforms [67], chemical conjugation and hybrid hybridoma (quandroma) are some of the earliest examples (Fig. 12.1) [68, 69]. With increasing sophistication in antibody engineering, second generation bispecific antibodies were developed [67, 70, 71]. Bispecific T-cell engaging antibodies (BITEs) were built on the tandem scFv platform where two scFvs of separate specificities are connected by flexible linker peptide [72, 73]. Despite its short half-life (partly because of its small size), BiTEs showed potent antitumor effects in preclinical studies [74]. Blinatumomab is a BiTE targeting CD19 antigen on ALL cells and engages T cells through its anti-CD3 scFv. In the phase II trial in adult relapsed or refractory B precursor ALL, 81 out of 189 patients (43%) achieved either CR or CR with partial recovery of peripheral blood count and manageable toxicity [75]. In pediatrics, phase I/II study among relapsed/refractory ALL achieved CR among 27 out of 70 patients (39%) within first two cycles, including 14 patients who achieved complete response in their minimal residual disease [76]. Although BiTEs have been tested against a large number of tumor targets (e.g., CEA, EPCAM, and PMSA), its anti-tumor benefit is not as robust as blinatumomab. This experience prompted the development of alternative BsAb platforms. Anti-GD2 BsAbs using a BiTE [77], dimeric BiTE [78], and 2 + 2 (2 binding arms for tumor target and 2 binding arms for CD3) antibody platform [66] have been described. The latter platform showed potent antitumor effects in humanized SCID mice and transgenic mice models when the BsAb was administered intravenously or delivered on T cells [79]. Although these anti-tumor responses were strong enough to overcome the PD1-PDL1 checkpoint in preclinical studies, the immuno-suppressive tumor microenvironment in the patient, including T cells (Treg), could diminish this T-cell-based clinical anti-tumor effect [72, 73, 80].

The concept of antibody-armed T cells was initially established using chemically conjugated bispecific antibodies (BiAb) [81]. ATCs armed with Her2-directed BiAbs lysed Her2(+) cells, not just high HER2 expressors but also low or borderline HER2(+) cells [82–84]. A phase I clinical trial among stage 4 breast cancer patients receiving CD3xHER2 BiAb-armed ATCs in combination with low dose IL2 and GM-CSF showed no dose limiting toxicities [85]. Thirteen out of 22 patients showed some clinical responses

(1 VGPR, 12 SD). Anti-GD2 BiAb demonstrated substantial anti-tumor killing in preclinical NB cell line models, associated with a higher level of circulating Th1 cytokines and chemokines compared to unarmed ATCs [81]. This led to phase I/II clinical study using ATCs armed with anti-GD2 BiAb for recurrent or refractory advanced stage NB patients (NCT02173093).

12.6 Future Directions

Much progress has been made in immunotherapy in NB using the classic IgG approach to engage innate immunity. New targets for neuroblastoma have emerged, such as glypican-2, L1CAM, and PTK7. Novel attempts to engage T cells using CAR and BsAb have shown compelling success in childhood ALL. However, their potentials in solid tumors are still work in progress. The immunosuppressive tumor microenvironment continued to create hurdles for T cell-based approaches, and immune checkpoint inhibitors (ICI) have been particularly disappointing in pediatrics in the attempt to engage T cells in solid tumors [17]. The failures of ICI were unexpected since NB frequently expressed PD-L1 and its expression was correlated with inferior treatment outcome [86–88]. But again the restricted mutation landscape and paucity of HLA in NB could explain the inadequate T cell clonal frequency. Many have proposed combining CAR T and BsAb with ICI. PD-1 blockade-enhanced CAR T cell survival and cytotoxicity against PD-L1 positive tumors. This synergism was tested in the CARPETS phase 1 clinical trials using GD2-specific CAR T cells for metastatic melanoma patients [89, 90]. Similarly, dual blockade of PD-1 and PD-L1 showed they could maximize the tumor killing of CEA/CD3-bispecific T cell-engaging antibody in vitro [91]. Some have also suggested the combination of immunotherapy with local radiation (ASCOPAL effect) or intra-tumoral injection of antibody-based therapies to enhance systemic immunity, or the combination with vaccines to facilitate epitope spread or the vaccination effect [92]. The toolbox for building novel immunotherapy has expanded exponentially in the past decade and further breakthrough is anticipated before this decade ends.

Acknowledgement Supported in part by Enid A. Haupt Endowed Chair Fund.

Conflict of Interest Declaration N.K. Cheung (NKC) reports receiving commercial research grants from Y-mAbs Therapeutics, Inc. in 2015 and Abpro-Labs, Inc. in 2017. Both NKC and Memorial Sloan Kettering Cancer Center have financial interest in Y-mAbs Therapeutics. NKC reported owning stock options in Eureka Therapeutics, Inc. NKC is the inventor of issued patents licensed by Memorial Sloan Kettering Cancer Center to Y-mAbs Therapeutics, and Biotec pharmacon. NKC is a paid consultant for Eureka Therapeutics. MN has no conflicts to declare.

References

1. Ahmed M, Cheung NK. Engineering anti-GD2 monoclonal antibodies for cancer immunotherapy. FEBS Lett. 2014;588(2):288–97. https://doi.org/10.1016/j.febslet.2013.11.030.
2. Cheung NK, Dyer MA. Neuroblastoma: developmental biology, cancer genomics and immunotherapy. Nat Rev Cancer. 2013;13(6):397–411. https://doi.org/10.1038/nrc3526.
3. Kramer K, Gerald WL, Kushner BH, Larson SM, Hameed M, Cheung NK. Disialoganglioside G(D2) loss following monoclonal antibody therapy is rare in neuroblastoma. Clin Cancer Res. 1998;4(9):2135–9.
4. Kushner BH, Cheung NK. GM-CSF enhances 3F8 monoclonal antibody-dependent cellular cytotoxicity against human melanoma and neuroblastoma. Blood. 1989;73(7):1936–41.
5. Kushner BH, Cheung NK. Absolute requirement of CD11/CD18 adhesion molecules, FcRII and the phosphatidylinositol-linked FcRIII for monoclonal antibody-mediated neutrophil antihuman tumor cytotoxicity. Blood. 1992;79(6):1484–90.
6. Metelitsa LS, Gillies SD, Super M, Shimada H, Reynolds CP, Seeger RC. Antidisialoganglioside/granulocyte macrophage-colony-stimulating factor fusion protein facilitates neutrophil antibody-dependent cellular cytotoxicity and depends on FcgammaRII (CD32) and mac-1 (CD11b/CD18) for enhanced effector cell adhesion and azurophil granule exocytosis. Blood. 2002;99(11):4166–73.
7. Cheung NK, Sowers R, Vickers AJ, Cheung IY, Kushner BH, Gorlick R. FCGR2A polymorphism is correlated with clinical outcome after immunotherapy of neuroblastoma with anti-GD2 antibody and granulocyte macrophage colony-stimulating factor. J Clin Oncol. 2006;24(18):2885–90.

8. Cheung NK, Cheung IY, Kushner BH, Ostrovnaya I, Chamberlain E, Kramer K, et al. Murine anti-GD2 monoclonal antibody 3F8 combined with granulocyte-macrophage colony-stimulating factor and 13-cis-retinoic acid in high-risk patients with stage 4 neuroblastoma in first remission. J Clin Oncol. 2012;30(26):3264–70. https://doi.org/10.1200/JCO.2011.41.3807.
9. Delgado DC, Hank JA, Kolesar J, Lorentzen D, Gan J, Seo S, et al. Genotypes of NK cell KIR receptors, their ligands, and Fcgamma receptors in the response of neuroblastoma patients to Hu14.18-IL2 immunotherapy. Cancer Res. 2010;70(23):9554–61.
10. Venstrom JM, Zheng J, Noor N, Danis KE, Yeh AW, Cheung IY, et al. KIR and HLA genotypes are associated with disease progression and survival following autologous hematopoietic stem cell transplantation for high-risk neuroblastoma. Clin Cancer Res. 2009;15(23):7330–4. https://doi.org/10.1158/1078-0432.CCR-09-1720.
11. Leung W, Handgretinger R, Iyengar R, Turner V, Holladay MS, Hale GA. Inhibitory KIR-HLA receptor-ligand mismatch in autologous haematopoietic stem cell transplantation for solid tumour and lymphoma. Br J Cancer. 2007;97(4):539–42. https://doi.org/10.1038/sj.bjc.6603913.
12. Tarek N, Le Luduec JB, Gallagher MM, Zheng J, Venstrom JM, Chamberlain E, et al. Unlicensed NK cells target neuroblastoma following anti-GD2 antibody treatment. J Clin Invest. 2012;122(9):3260–70. https://doi.org/10.1172/JCI62749.
13. Cheung NK, Walter EI, Smith-Mensah WH, Ratnoff WD, Tykocinski ML, Medof ME. Decay-accelerating factor protects human tumor cells from complement-mediated cytotoxicity in vitro. J Clin Invest. 1988;81(4):1122–8.
14. Chen S, Caragine T, Cheung NK, Tomlinson S. CD59 expressed on a tumor cell surface modulates decay-accelerating factor expression and enhances tumor growth in a rat model of human neuroblastoma. Cancer Res. 2000;60(11):3013–8.
15. Chen S, Caragine T, Cheung NK, Tomlinson S. Surface antigen expression and complement susceptibility of differentiated neuroblastoma clones. Am J Pathol. 2000;156(3):1085–91. https://doi.org/10.1016/S0002-9440(10)64976-0.
16. Biedler JL, Spengler BA, Chang TD, Ross RA. Transdifferentiation of human neuroblastoma cells results in coordinate loss of neuronal and malignant properties. In: Evans AE, D'Angio GJ, Knudson AG, Seeger RC, editors. Advances in neuroblastoma research. Prog clin biol res. New York, NY: Alan Liss; 1988. p. 265–76.
17. Park JA, Cheung NV. Limitations and opportunities for immune checkpoint inhibitors in pediatric malignancies. Cancer Treat Rev. 2017;58:22–33. https://doi.org/10.1016/j.ctrv.2017.05.006.
18. Cheung NK, Lazarus H, Miraldi FD, Abramowsky CR, Kallick S, Saarinen UM, et al. Ganglioside GD2 specific monoclonal antibody 3F8: a phase I study in patients with neuroblastoma and malignant melanoma. J Clin Oncol. 1987;5(9):1430–40.
19. Navid F, Sondel PM, Barfield R, Shulkin BL, Kaufman RA, Allay JA, et al. Phase I trial of a novel anti-GD2 monoclonal antibody, Hu14.18K322A, designed to decrease toxicity in children with refractory or recurrent neuroblastoma. J Clin Oncol. 2014;32(14):1445–52. https://doi.org/10.1200/JCO.2013.50.4423.
20. Anghelescu DL, Goldberg JL, Faughnan LG, Wu J, Mao S, Furman WL, et al. Comparison of pain outcomes between two anti-GD2 antibodies in patients with neuroblastoma. Pediatr Blood Cancer. 2015;62(2):224–8. https://doi.org/10.1002/pbc.25280.
21. Cheung NV. Antibody induced pain in children: an opportunity to study pain mechanism, IgG design and analgesics. Pediatr Blood Cancer. 2015;62(2):186–7. https://doi.org/10.1002/pbc.25320.
22. Yu AL, Gilman AL, Ozkaynak MF, Sondel PM, London WB, Cretella S, et al. Update of outcome for high-risk neuroblastoma treated on a randomized trial of chimeric anti-GD2 antibody (ch14.18) + GM-CSF/IL2 immunotherapy in 1st response: a children's oncology group study. Adv Neuroblast Res. 2014;2014:PL013.
23. Yu AL, Gilman AL, Ozkaynak MF, London WB, Kreissman SG, Chen HX, et al. Anti-GD2 antibody with GM-CSF, interleukin-2, and isotretinoin for neuroblastoma. N Engl J Med. 2010;363(14):1324–34. https://doi.org/10.1056/NEJMoa0911123.
24. Shusterman S, London WB, Gillies SD, Hank JA, Voss SD, Seeger RC, et al. Antitumor activity of hu14.18-IL2 in patients with relapsed/refractory neuroblastoma: a children's oncology group (COG) phase II study. J Clin Oncol. 2010;28(33):4969–75. https://doi.org/10.1200/JCO.2009.27.8861.
25. Yang RK, Kalogriopoulos NA, Rakhmilevich AL, Ranheim EA, Seo S, Kim K, et al. Intratumoral hu14.18-IL-2 (IC) induces local and systemic antitumor effects that involve both activated T and NK cells as well as enhanced IC retention. J Immunol. 2012;189(5):2656–64. https://doi.org/10.4049/jimmunol.1200934.
26. Cheung NK, Cheung IY, Kramer K, Modak S, Kuk D, Pandit-Taskar N, et al. Key role for myeloid cells: phase II results of anti-GD2 antibody 3F8 plus granulocyte-macrophage colony-stimulating factor for chemoresistant osteomedullary neuroblastoma. Int J Cancer. 2014;135(9):2199–205. https://doi.org/10.1002/ijc.28851.
27. Kushner BH, Ostrovnaya I, Cheung IY, Kuk D, Kramer K, Modak S, et al. Prolonged progression-free survival after consolidating second or later remissions of neuroblastoma with anti-GD2 immunotherapy and isotretinoin: a prospective phase II study. Onco Targets Ther. 2015;4(7):e1016704. https://doi.org/10.1080/2162402X.2015.1016704.
28. Cheung IY, Hsu K, Cheung NK. Activation of peripheral-blood granulocytes is strongly correlated with patient outcome after immunotherapy with

anti-GD2 monoclonal antibody and granulocyte-macrophage colony-stimulating factor. J Clin Oncol. 2012;30:426–32.
29. Dobrenkov K, Cheung NK. GD2-targeted immunotherapy and radioimmunotherapy. Semin Oncol. 2014;41(5):589–612. https://doi.org/10.1053/j.seminoncol.2014.07.003.
30. Cheung NK, Guo H, Hu J, Tassev DV, Cheung IY. Humanizing murine IgG3 anti-GD2 antibody m3F8 substantially improves antibody-dependent cell-mediated cytotoxicity while retaining targeting in vivo. Onco Targets Ther. 2012;1(4):477–86.
31. Kushner BH, Cheung IY, Basu EM, Modak S, Cheung NK. Phase I study of anti-GD2 humanized 3F8 monoclonal antibody plus GM-CSF: high dosing and major responses in patients with resistant high-risk neuroblastoma advances in neuroblastoma research congress 2016. Cairns, QL; 2016.
32. Cheung IY, Kushner BH, Modak S, Basu EM, Roberts SS, Cheung N-KV. Phase I trial of anti-GD2 monoclonal antibody hu3F8 plus GM-CSF: impact of body weight, immunogenicity and anti-GD2 response on pharmacokinetics and survival. Onco Targets Ther. 2017;6(11):e1358331. https://doi.org/10.1080/2162402X.2017.1358331.
33. Kushner BH, Modak M, Cheung IY, Basu EM, Kudva A, Roberts SS, et al. High-dose humanized-3F8 (hu3F8) plus stepped-up dosing of GM-CSF: outpatient treatment, low immunogenicity, and major responses in a phase II trial advances in neuroblastoma research congress 2018. San Francisco, CA; 2018. p. Abstract #287.
34. Nowak AK, Robinson BW, Lake RA. Synergy between chemotherapy and immunotherapy in the treatment of established murine solid tumors. Cancer Res. 2003;63(15):4490–6.
35. Bagatell R, London WB, Wagner LM, Voss SD, Stewart CF, Maris JM, et al. Phase II study of irinotecan and temozolomide in children with relapsed or refractory neuroblastoma: a children's oncology group study. J Clin Oncol. 2011;29(2):208–13. https://doi.org/10.1200/JCO.2010.31.7107.
36. Kushner BH, Kramer K, Modak S, Cheung NK. Irinotecan plus temozolomide for relapsed or refractory neuroblastoma. J Clin Oncol. 2006;24(33):5271–6. https://doi.org/10.1200/JCO.2006.06.7272.
37. Mody R, Naranjo A, Van Ryn C, Yu AL, London WB, Shulkin BL, et al. Irinotecan-temozolomide with temsirolimus or dinutuximab in children with refractory or relapsed neuroblastoma (COG ANBL1221): an open-label, randomised, phase 2 trial. Lancet Oncol. 2017;18(7):946–57. https://doi.org/10.1016/S1470-2045(17)30355-8.
38. Mody R, Yu AL, Naranjo A, Zhang FF, London WB, Shulkin BL, et al. Irinotecan, temozolomide, and dinutuximab with GM-CSF in children with refractory or relapsed neuroblastoma: a report from the children's oncology group. J Clin Oncol. 2020;38(19):2160–9. https://doi.org/10.1200/JCO.20.00203.
39. Modak SKB, Flores M, et al. Naxitamab-based chemoimmunotherapy for resistant high-risk neuroblastoma: preliminary results of "HITS" pilot/phase II study. Lyon: International Society of Paediatric Oncology (51st); 2019.
40. Kramer K, Kushner B, Heller G, Cheung NK. Neuroblastoma metastatic to the central nervous system. The memorial Sloan-Kettering cancer center experience and a literature review. Cancer. 2001;91(8):1510–9.
41. Pui CH, Evans WE. Acute lymphoblastic leukemia. N Engl J Med. 1998;339(9):605–15.
42. Larson SM, Carrasquillo JA, Cheung N-KV, Press OW. Radioimmunotherapy of human tumours. Nat Rev Cancer. 2015;15:347. https://doi.org/10.1038/nrc3925; https://www.nature.com/articles/nrc3925#supplementary-information.
43. Cheung NK, Kushner BH, LaQuaglia M, Kramer K, Gollamudi S, Heller G, et al. N7: a novel multimodality therapy of high risk neuroblastoma (NB) in children diagnosed over 1 year of age. Med Pediatr Oncol. 2001;36:227–30.
44. Kramer K, Cheung NK, Humm J, DiResta G, Arbit E, Larson S, et al. Pharmacokinetics and acute toxicology of intraventricular 131 I-monoclonal antibody targeting disialoganglioside in non-human primates. J Neuro-Oncol. 1997;35(2):101–11.
45. Kramer K, Humm JL, Souweidane MM, Zanzonico PB, Dunkel IJ, Gerald WL, et al. Phase I study of targeted radioimmunotherapy for leptomeningeal cancers using intra-ommaya 131-I-3F8. J Clin Oncol. 2007;25(34):5465–70.
46. Kramer K, Kushner BH, Modak S, Pandit-Taskar N, Smith-Jones P, Zanzonico P, et al. Compartmental intrathecal radioimmunotherapy: results for treatment for metastatic CNS neuroblastoma. J Neuro-Oncol. 2010;97(3):409–18. https://doi.org/10.1007/s11060-009-0038-7.
47. Kramer K, Kushner BH, Modak S, Pandit-Taskar N, Tomlinson U, Donzelli M, et al. A curative approach for neuroblastoma metastatic to the CNS: safety and efficacy of intraventricular 131I-labeled monoclonal antibody 8H9 targeting the surface glycoprotein B7-H3 advances in neuroblastoma research 2018 (12th). San Francisco, CA; 2018. p. Abstract #273, 20.
48. Nakajima H, Modak S. Cancer vaccines in pediatrics. Immunotherapy for pediatric malignancies. Cham: Springer; 2018. p. 217–42.
49. Bowman L, Grossmann M, Rill D, Brown M, Zhong WY, Alexander B, et al. IL-2 adenovector-transduced autologous tumor cells induce antitumor immune responses in patients with neuroblastoma. Blood. 1998;92(6):1941–9.
50. Geiger JD, Hutchinson RJ, Hohenkirk LF, McKenna EA, Yanik GA, Levine JE, et al. Vaccination of pediatric solid tumor patients with tumor lysate-pulsed dendritic cells can expand specific T cells and mediate tumor regression. Cancer Res. 2001;61(23):8513–9.

51. Durrant LG, Noble P, Spendlove I. Immunology in the clinic review series; focus on cancer: glycolipids as targets for tumour immunotherapy. Clin Exp Immunol. 2012;167(2):206–15. https://doi.org/10.1111/j.1365-2249.2011.04516.x.
52. Kushner BH, Cheung IY, Modak S, Kramer K, Ragupathi G, Cheung NK. Phase I trial of a bivalent gangliosides vaccine in combination with beta-glucan for high-risk neuroblastoma in second or later remission. Clin Cancer Res. 2014;20:1375. https://doi.org/10.1158/1078-0432.CCR-13-1012.
53. Cheung IY, Kushner B, Modak S, Ragupathi G, Roberts S, Basu EM, et al. Phase II trial of GD2-KLH/GD3-KLH vaccine for stage 4 neuroblastoma in ≥2nd remission: induced anti-GD2 titer strongly correlates with survival advances in neuroblastoma research. San Francisco, CA; 2018.
54. Cheung IY, Cheung NV, Modak S, Mauguen A, Feng Y, Basu E, et al. Survival impact of anti-GD2 antibody response in a phase II ganglioside vaccine trial among patients with high-risk neuroblastoma with prior disease progression. J Clin Oncol. 2021;39(3):215–26. https://doi.org/10.1200/JCO.20.01892.
55. Raffaghello L, Prigione I, Bocca P, Morandi F, Camoriano M, Gambini C, et al. Multiple defects of the antigen-processing machinery components in human neuroblastoma: immunotherapeutic implications. Oncogene. 2005;24(29):4634–44.
56. Morgan RA, Dudley ME, Wunderlich JR, Hughes MS, Yang JC, Sherry RM, et al. Cancer regression in patients after transfer of genetically engineered lymphocytes. Science (New York, NY). 2006;314(5796):126–9.
57. Blattman JN, Greenberg PD. Cancer immunotherapy: a treatment for the masses. Science (New York, NY). 2004;305(5681):200–5. https://doi.org/10.1126/science.1100369.
58. Pule MA, Savoldo B, Myers GD, Rossig C, Russell HV, Dotti G, et al. Virus-specific T cells engineered to coexpress tumor-specific receptors: persistence and antitumor activity in individuals with neuroblastoma. Nat Med. 2008;14(11):1264–70.
59. Park JR, Digiusto DL, Slovak M, Wright C, Naranjo A, Wagner J, et al. Adoptive transfer of chimeric antigen receptor re-directed cytolytic T lymphocyte clones in patients with neuroblastoma. Mol Ther. 2007;15(4):825–33.
60. Young LS, Rickinson AB. Epstein-Barr virus: 40 years on. Nat Rev Cancer. 2004;4(10):757–68. https://doi.org/10.1038/nrc1452.
61. O'Reilly RJ. Epstein-Barr virus sustains tumor killers. Nat Med. 2008;14(11):1148–50.
62. Richards RM, Sotillo E, Majzner RG. CAR T cell therapy for neuroblastoma. Front Immunol. 2018;9:2380. https://doi.org/10.3389/fimmu.2018.02380.
63. Richman SA, Nunez-Cruz S, Moghimi B, Li LZ, Gershenson ZT, Mourelatos Z, et al. High-affinity GD2-specific CAR T cells induce fatal encephalitis in a preclinical neuroblastoma model. Cancer Immunol Res. 2018;6(1):36–46. https://doi.org/10.1158/2326-6066.CIR-17-0211.
64. Dobrenkov K, Cheung NK. Therapeutic antibodies and immunologic conjugates. In: Armitage JO, Niederhuber JE, Doroshow JH, Kastan MB, Tepper JE, editors. Abeloff's clinical oncology. 6th ed. Philadelphia, PA: Elsevier Churchill Livingstone; 2017. p. Chapter 30.
65. Suzuki M, Curran KJ, Cheung NK. Chimeric antigen receptors and bispecific antibodies to retarget T cells in pediatric oncology. Pediatr Blood Cancer. 2015;62:1326. https://doi.org/10.1002/pbc.25513.
66. Xu H, Cheng M, Guo H, Chen Y, Huse M, Cheung NK. Retargeting T cells to GD2 pentasaccharide on human tumors using bispecific humanized antibody. Cancer Immunol Res. 2015;3(3):266–77. https://doi.org/10.1158/2326-6066.CIR-14-0230-T.
67. Wu Z, Cheung NV. T cell engaging bispecific antibody (T-BsAb): from technology to therapeutics. Pharmacol Ther. 2017;182:161. https://doi.org/10.1016/j.pharmthera.2017.08.005.
68. Milstein C, Cuello AC. Hybrid hybridomas and their use in immunohistochemistry. Nature. 1983;305(5934):537–40.
69. Staerz UD, Kanagawa O, Bevan MJ. Hybrid antibodies can target sites for attack by T-cells. Nature. 1985;314(6012):628–31. https://doi.org/10.1038/314628a0.
70. Satta A, Mezzanzanica D, Turatti F, Canevari S, Figini M. Redirection of T-cell effector functions for cancer therapy: bispecific antibodies and chimeric antigen receptors. Future Oncol. 2013;9(4):527–39. https://doi.org/10.2217/fon.12.203.
71. Kontermann RE, Brinkmann U. Bispecific antibodies. Drug Discov Today. 2015;20(7):838–47. https://doi.org/10.1016/j.drudis.2015.02.008.
72. Baeuerle PA, Reinhardt C. Bispecific T-cell engaging antibodies for cancer therapy. Cancer Res. 2009;69(12):4941–4. https://doi.org/10.1158/0008-5472.CAN-09-0547.
73. Wolf E, Hofmeister R, Kufer P, Schlereth B, Baeuerle PA. BiTEs: bispecific antibody constructs with unique anti-tumor activity. Drug Discov Today. 2005;10(18):1237–44. https://doi.org/10.1016/S1359-6446(05)03554-3.
74. Mack M, Riethmuller G, Kufer P. A small bispecific antibody construct expressed as a functional single-chain molecule with high tumor cell cytotoxicity. Proc Natl Acad Sci U S A. 1995;92(15):7021–5.
75. Topp MS, Gokbuget N, Stein AS, Zugmaier G, O'Brien S, Bargou RC, et al. Safety and activity of blinatumomab for adult patients with relapsed or refractory B-precursor acute lymphoblastic leukaemia: a multicentre, single-arm, phase 2 study. Lancet Oncol. 2015;16(1):57–66. https://doi.org/10.1016/S1470-2045(14)71170-2.
76. von Stackelberg A, Locatelli F, Zugmaier G, Handgretinger R, Trippett TM, Rizzari C, et al. Phase I/phase II study of blinatumomab in pediatric patients

with relapsed/refractory acute lymphoblastic leukemia. J Clin Oncol. 2016;34(36):4381–9.
77. Cheng M, Ahmed M, Xu H, Cheung NK. Structural design of disialoganglioside GD2 and CD3-bispecific antibodies to redirect T cells for tumor therapy. Int J Cancer. 2014;136:476. https://doi.org/10.1002/ijc.29007.
78. Ahmed M, Cheng M, Cheung IY, Cheung NK. Human derived dimerization tag enhances tumor killing potency of a T-cell engaging bispecific antibody. Onco Targets Ther. 2015;4(4):e989776. https://doi.org/10.4161/2162402X.2014.989776.
79. Nakajima M, Guo HF, Hoseini SS, Suzuki M, Xu H, Cheung NV. Potent antitumor effect of T cells armed with anti-GD2 bispecific antibody. Pediatr Blood Cancer. 2021;68(7):e28971. https://doi.org/10.1002/pbc.28971.
80. Choi BD, Gedeon PC, Sanchez-Perez L, Bigner DD, Sampson JH. Regulatory T cells are redirected to kill glioblastoma by an EGFRvIII-targeted bispecific antibody. Onco Targets Ther. 2013;2(12):e26757. https://doi.org/10.4161/onci.26757.
81. Yankelevich M, Kondadasula SV, Thakur A, Buck S, Cheung NK, Lum LG. Anti-CD3 x anti-GD2 bispecific antibody redirects T-cell cytolytic activity to neuroblastoma targets. Pediatr Blood Cancer. 2012;59(7):1198–205. https://doi.org/10.1002/pbc.24237.
82. Sen M, Wankowski DM, Garlie NK, Siebenlist RE, Van Epps D, LeFever AV, et al. Use of anti-CD3 x anti-HER2/neu bispecific antibody for redirecting cytotoxicity of activated T cells toward HER2/neu+ tumors. J Hematother Stem Cell Res. 2001;10(2):247–60. https://doi.org/10.1089/15258160151134944.
83. Lum HE, Miller M, Davol PA, Grabert RC, Davis JB, Lum LG. Preclinical studies comparing different bispecific antibodies for redirecting T cell cytotoxicity to extracellular antigens on prostate carcinomas. Anticancer Res. 2005;25(1A):43–52.
84. Grabert RC, Cousens LP, Smith JA, Olson S, Gall J, Young WB, et al. Human T cells armed with Her2/neu bispecific antibodies divide, are cytotoxic, and secrete cytokines with repeated stimulation. Clin Cancer Res. 2006;12(2):569–76.
85. Lum LG, Thakur A. Targeting T cells with bispecific antibodies for cancer therapy. BioDrugs. 2011;25(6):365–79. https://doi.org/10.2165/11595950-000000000-00000.
86. Dondero A, Pastorino F, Della Chiesa M, Corrias MV, Morandi F, Pistoia V, et al. PD-L1 expression in metastatic neuroblastoma as an additional mechanism for limiting immune surveillance. Onco Targets Ther. 2016;5(1):e1064578. https://doi.org/10.1080/2162402X.2015.1064578.
87. Melaiu O, Mina M, Chierici M, Boldrini R, Jurman G, Romania P, et al. PD-L1 is a therapeutic target of the bromodomain inhibitor JQ1 and, combined with HLA class I, a promising prognostic biomarker in neuroblastoma. Clin Cancer Res. 2017;23(15):4462–72. https://doi.org/10.1158/1078-0432.CCR-16-2601.
88. Majzner RG, Simon JS, Grosso JF, Martinez D, Pawel BR, Santi M, et al. Assessment of programmed death-ligand 1 expression and tumor-associated immune cells in pediatric cancer tissues. Cancer. 2017;123(19):3807–15. https://doi.org/10.1002/cncr.30724.
89. Gargett T, Yu W, Dotti G, Yvon ES, Christo SN, Hayball JD, et al. GD2-specific CAR T cells undergo potent activation and deletion following antigen encounter but can be protected from activation-induced cell death by PD-1 blockade. Mol Ther. 2016;24(6):1135–49. https://doi.org/10.1038/mt.2016.63.
90. Heczey A, Louis CU. Advances in chimeric antigen receptor immunotherapy for neuroblastoma. Discov Med. 2013;16(90):287–94.
91. Osada T, Patel SP, Hammond SA, Osada K, Morse MA, Lyerly HK. CEA/CD3-bispecific T cell-engaging (BiTE) antibody-mediated T lymphocyte cytotoxicity maximized by inhibition of both PD1 and PD-L1. Cancer immunology, immunotherapy: CII; 2015. https://doi.org/10.1007/s00262-015-1671-y.
92. Voeller J, Erbe AK, Slowinski J, Rasmussen K, Carlson PM, Hoefges A, et al. Combined innate and adaptive immunotherapy overcomes resistance of immunologically cold syngeneic murine neuroblastoma to checkpoint inhibition. J Immunother Cancer. 2019;7(1):344. https://doi.org/10.1186/s40425-019-0823-6.

13 Future of Clinical Trials and Application of Precision Medicine

Theresa Thole and Angelika Eggert

13.1 Introduction

Neuroblastoma is one of the most complex and challenging malignancies the pediatric oncologist faces, and serves as a paradigm for three major applications in precision medicine: (1) exploring the prognostic benefit of combining molecular data with clinically defined risk factors; (2) testing the potential to tailor therapy for patient subgroups according to their individual risk for recurrence; and (3) evaluating molecular targeted therapies. Despite tremendous progress in understanding the molecular mechanisms behind neuroblastoma, prognosis for patients with advanced disease remains poor, with long-term event-free survival (EFS) below 50%. Polychemotherapy, radiation therapy, and immunotherapy remain the standard approach to treat high-risk disease, as only a few druggable genetic aberrations are identified at diagnosis. In recent years, only one new drug (the anti-GD2 antibody dinutuxumab) has been introduced into first-line therapy [1]. However, recent studies indicate that actionable aberrations are far more common in relapsed neuroblastoma, possibly as a result of clonal expansion.

T. Thole
Charité University Medicine, Berlin, Germany

A. Eggert (✉)
Charité University Medicine, Berlin, Germany

DKTK Site Berlin, DKFZ, Heidelberg, Germany
e-mail: angelika.eggert@charite.de

Response to induction chemotherapy correlates with outcome and remains insufficient in 1/3 of children with high-risk neuroblastoma [2–4]. High-risk neuroblastoma patients who relapse or progress quickly during frontline therapy have a dismal prognosis. Early treatment with novel therapies could be realized with the early identification of these ultra-high-risk patients. Earlier events in the high-risk population correlate with *MYCN* amplification, high lactate dehydrogenase (LDH), and liver metastases at diagnosis among other clinical variables [4, 5]. However, improved molecular and imaging tools are needed to unequivocally identify ultra-high-risk patients as early as possible. Earlier unequivocal identification of these patients would drive the switch from the current 'one-fits-all' treatment to a 'precision medicine' therapeutic approach.

In patients who experience neuroblastoma relapse, 5-year overall survival (OS) is 20% [6] with outcomes dependent on the time of relapse and initial patient tumor stage [4, 6, 7]. A recently published meta-analysis of three phase II clinical trials run by the SIOPEN group in Europe reported median progression-free survival of 12.5% and 5.7% for patients with refractory and relapsed disease, respectively [8]. Although a robust pipeline of potential new therapeutic approaches for high-risk and relapsed neuroblastoma inspires optimism, it also brings substantial challenges needing appropriate and systematic address in a precision medicine approach (Fig. 13.1):

S. Asgharzadeh, F. Westermann (eds.), *Neuroblastoma*, Pediatric Oncology,
https://doi.org/10.1007/978-3-031-51292-6_13

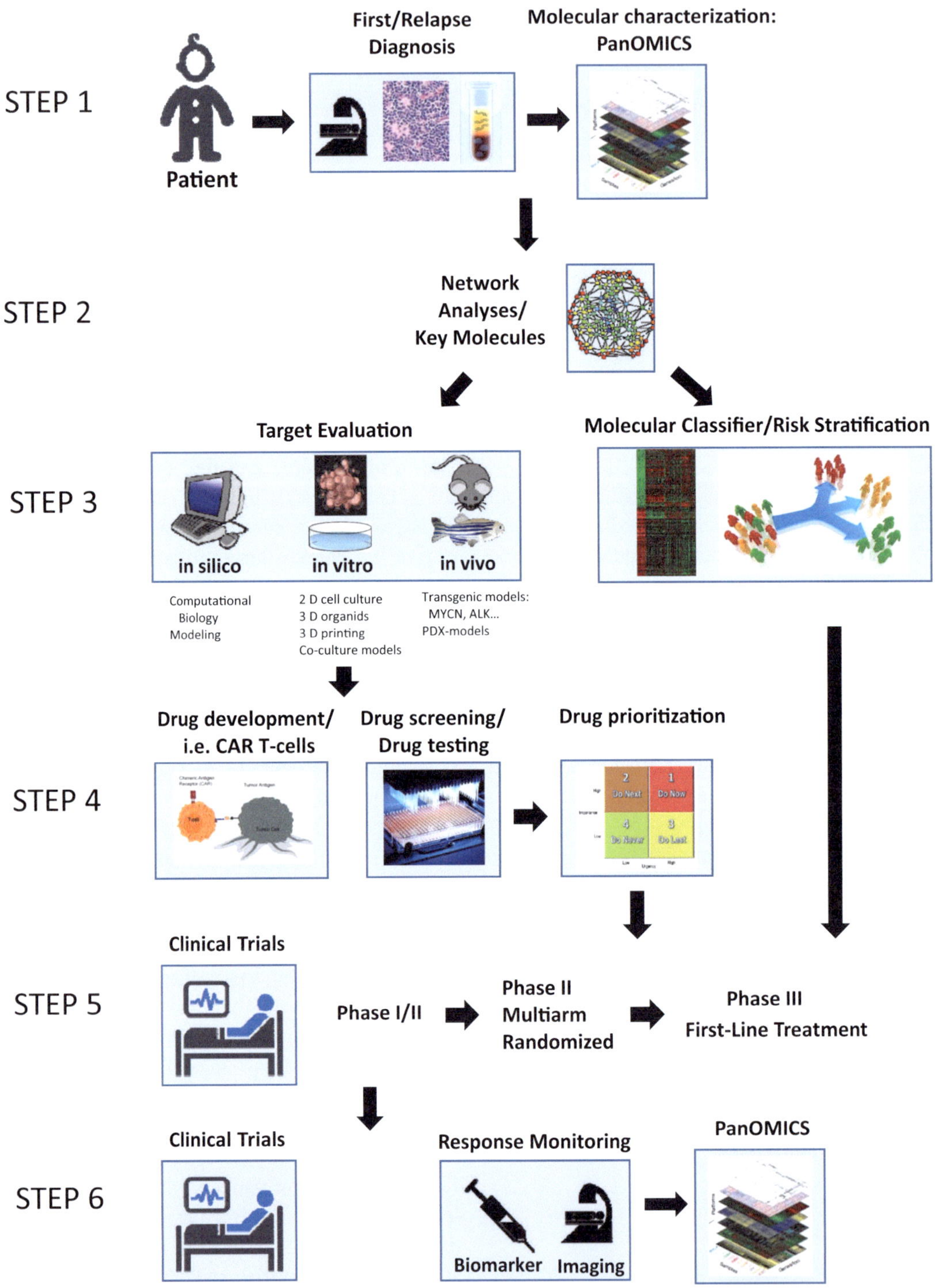

Fig. 13.1 Model for a systematic and stepwise precision medicine approach in neuroblastoma

- Adequate risk-based patient selection for molecularly targeted therapies both at diagnosis and relapse.
- Robust and reproducible identification of molecular targets in pan-omics approaches considering both spatial and temporal tumor heterogeneity.
- Functional evaluation of molecular targets and the respective drugs in predictive preclinical models that recapitulate the complexity of human tumor behavior including the influence of the tumor microenvironment.
- Appropriate prioritization of drugs for phase I/II trials in a fairly rare cancer.
- Application of new statistical methods and trial designs in phase I/II trials that minimize the requested patient number to speed evaluation.
- Selection of best-performing drugs for phase III trials and introduction of promising drugs into first-line treatment.
- Intensifying international cooperation for phase III trials to speed patient accrual.

This chapter summarizes key aspects of future patient selection, drug development, clinical trial design, and personalized medicine approaches. We point out their impact on opening new avenues for risk stratification and targeted therapies in neuroblastoma.

13.2 Risk Stratification and Patient Selection Based on Molecular Signatures

A patient's age at diagnosis, stage of disease, and whether neuroblastoma cells harbor a *MYCN* amplification are the three strongest determinants of clinical outcome [9]. These determinants, combined with chromosome 11q loss, tumor histology, ploidy, and grade of differentiation, formed the foundations of risk-group stratification for neuroblastoma patients, and resulted in the current International Neuroblastoma Risk Group (INRG) staging system [9]. However, neuroblastoma is much more heterogeneous when examined at the molecular level. Numerous studies suggest that the new technologies available for genomic, epigenomic, and proteomic analyses can further refine neuroblastoma patient-risk stratification. Chromosomal structural analyses and gene expression profiles have been shown to add critical prognostic information to individual genetic aberrations, but some results still need prospective validation in larger multinational patient cohorts.

For patients with low- and intermediate-risk neuroblastoma, molecular classifiers will help to identify rare patients who still require therapy as treatment intensity continues to be reduced in this population. For patients with high-risk disease, early identification of patients at highest risk of treatment failure, and ultimately of disease recurrence (= ultra-high-risk patients), is needed to introduce experimental therapies and improve survival rates. Trials could be designed to treat these poorly responding patients with a different window-of-opportunity therapy before consolidation with stem cell transplantation [10]. This approach would lead to more meaningful drug testing earlier in the disease process before tumors become even more resistant to therapy, thus enhancing the likelihood of response.

No individual mRNA expression marker is currently widely accepted as clinically significant enough for incorporation into a risk-stratification scheme [11], but extensive effort has been devoted to developing multigene classifiers. The evolution of microarray and RNA sequencing technology has driven development of specific mRNA expression signatures supporting outcome prediction. Several robust mRNA classifiers ranging from 39- to 144-gene expression signatures have been identified and validated in large independent test sets [12–18]. The first mRNA-based classifier has very recently been incorporated as a clinical stratification tool in the new German trial for low- and intermediate-risk neuroblastoma (Fig. 13.2). Whole-genome-based molecular risk classifications have also been proposed [19–23]. Whole-genome and whole-exome sequencing (WGS/WES) approaches aim primarily for new classifications and target discov-

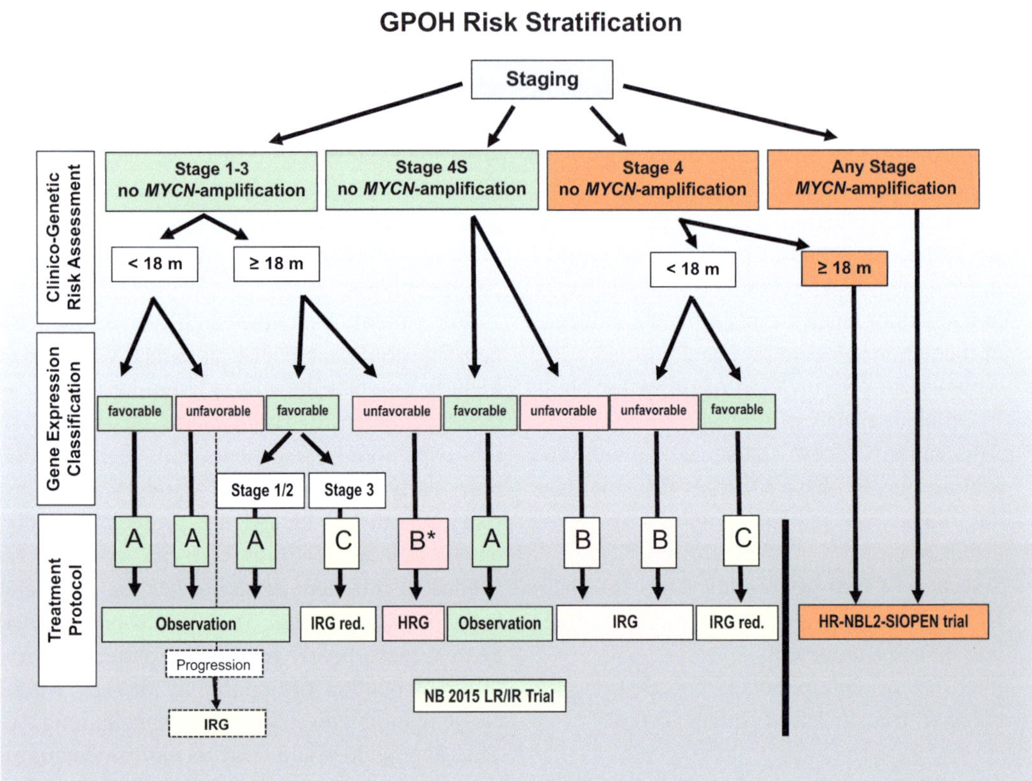

Fig. 13.2 Current risk stratification scheme of the German neuroblastoma trials

eries and not risk assessment. No commercially available assays have yet been validated for use in neuroblastoma risk stratification. However, custom-made panel sequencing is certain to be of use in standardized assessments of risk factors and druggable targets. International neuroblastoma researchers at a SIOPEN genomics meeting in 2015 defined a consensus gene panel (from among all available genomic data) for mutational assessment in high-risk neuroblastoma [24]. The use of a common next-generation sequencing (NGS) profile is the first step toward clinically applied and cost-efficient molecular profiling supporting precision medicine approaches.

MicroRNA-based classifiers can also achieve accurate outcome prediction [25, 26]. A combination signature employing mRNA, microRNA, WGS, and comparative genomic hybridization (CGH) array data is being prospectively evaluated within clinical trials to better define prognostic signatures and provide further insight about the molecular basis of clinical heterogeneity [27, 28]. Optimal risk stratification is likely to require a comprehensive analysis that includes both mRNA and microRNA expression; epigenetic modifications and genomic, proteomic, and metabolomic analyses, which will each require technologies capable of generating rapid and reproducible results [6]. Integrating data from different *-omics* platforms will provide a more thorough and comprehensive understanding of how biological processes are regulated at different layers.

Molecular detection of minimal residual disease (MRD) is considered an important prognostic factor in metastatic neuroblastoma. Many studies have been performed to identify suitable targets for MRD detection. Tyrosine hydroxylase (*TH*), doublecortin (*DCX*), and *PHOX2B* genes are good candidates for detecting circulating neuroblastoma cells and could be considered in new pretreatment risk-stratification strategies for metastatic neuroblastoma [29, 30]. More sophisticated WGS-based technologies for neuroblastoma MRD monitoring are currently being assessed.

To remain clinically relevant, the INRG classification system will need continued modification as new molecular information is identified in the clinical setting and confirmed to be prognostic in prospective studies [6]. With the identification of smaller cohorts of biologically distinct neuroblastoma patients, the need for international consensus will become even more crucial. Future studies must include more refined risk classifications and more individualized treatments based on molecular and genetic aberrations specific to the patient.

13.3 Systematic Identification of New Therapy Targets

Efficient drug development requires (1) identification of molecular alterations in biopsied neuroblastoma cells from each individual patient; (2) functional evaluation of new target molecules and their roles in tumorigenesis, progression, metastasis, or drug resistance; and (3) exploitation of therapeutic targets based on drug screening approaches or new chemical drug development. This strategy is limited in neuroblastoma by a striking paucity of recurrent mutations when compared to adult cancers [31–33]. While initial WGS studies revealed relatively low mutation rates in neuroblastoma at diagnosis [34], more recent studies highlight clonal mutation selection during disease progression and higher mutational burden in the relapsing tumors [35–37]. Therefore, performing a new biopsy at relapse is of utmost importance to support optimal individualized treatment strategies [38]. Ideally, any subclonal actionable mutation would be identified in the tumor at diagnosis and guide pre-emptive targeting before clonal expansion [10]. Achieving this ideal will depend on sequencing tumor samples at sufficient depth or application of single-cell analysis techniques [39]. Practical implementation of genomics-based therapy at early time points will require a turnaround time that is clinically relevant for a disease which is often rapidly progressing. Furthermore, it will require the ability to reliably identify subclonal aberrations and to trace the relationships among multiple clones to prioritize targets.

Neuroblastoma evolution from diagnosis to relapse [36, 37], the increased spectrum of actionable mutations in relapsed tumors [40], the spatiotemporal heterogeneity of mutations observed in individual patients [35], and the recently described phenomenon of plasticity with respect to transcriptional circuitries in neuroblastoma cells [41], all suggest that treatment decisions will be better informed if they are based on molecular profiling conducted at the time of treatment, rather than simply at diagnosis, and by genomic assessment of tumor cells from multiple sites [10]. Several recent studies highlight the importance of spatial intratumor heterogeneity in neuroblastoma. Abbasi et al. demonstrated subclonal heterogeneity between the primary tumor and metastases at diagnosis [39]. The presence of 1q, 19q, or *ATRX* deletion in metastases, but not the primary tumor, was associated with increased risk for relapse. Detailed analysis of a single patient at multiple time points through the course of initial treatment and subsequent relapse demonstrated a loss of subclones identified in the primary tumor but expansion of metastatic subclones that were present at diagnosis [39].

Liquid biopsy approaches for genomic profiling using circulating tumor DNA are rapidly developing, and have the potential to provide insights into tumor heterogeneity and clonal evolution that cannot be achieved from traditional biopsies [2, 42]. Tumor evolution, resistance mechanisms, and therapeutic response biomarkers can be more accurately monitored with these non-invasive procedures [43, 44]. Recent studies support the feasibility of liquid biopsy approaches to monitor *MYCN* or *ALK* genomic status [45] or genomic copy number profiles [46] in neuroblastoma patients.

Relevant alterations in the tumor microenvironment (TME), especially signaling from other types of cells, might not be identified by examining neuroblastoma samples alone. TME effects can be investigated through computational techniques that model paracrine signaling, elucidate TME contributions to disease and treatment resistance, and propose treatments targeting the tumor-stroma interface [47–49]. The contributions of immune and vascular cells in the TME should particularly be considered, and can be studied by flow cytometric sorting and subsequent single-cell analyses.

While panomics approaches systematically identify patient-individual drug targets via hypothesis-free models not relying on prior biological knowledge, molecular targeted drug development can also focus on previously identified key oncogenic drivers. *MYCN* amplification and activating *ALK* mutations are key oncogenic drivers in neuroblastoma pathogenesis [50]. An integrated genome, exome, and transcriptome sequencing study of 240 primary high-risk neuroblastomas conducted as part of the TARGET initiative identified somatic mutations at significant frequency in only three additional genes also showing detectable expression: *PTPN11* (2.9%), *ATRX* (2.5%), and *NRAS* (0.8%) [51]. Currently, the only directly druggable protein encoded by a gene mutated in neuroblastoma is ALK, which has been extensively validated. However, activating mutations in proteins in the MAPK pathway (PTPN11 and NRAS) might potentially be indirectly targeted by inhibiting MEK [37]. Other aberrations occurring at low frequency that may be directly or indirectly targetable include *BRAF* and *NF1*; *ARID1A/B; RPTOR* amplification; the TP53 ubiquitin ligase, *MDM2,* and the *CDK4* and *CDK6* cyclin-dependent kinases as well as their negative regulator, *CDKN2A* (formerly p16INK4A) [40, 51–56]. Chromosomal rearrangements that activate the *TERT* telomerase reverse transcriptase have recently been identified in ~23% of high-stage neuroblastomas lacking *MYCN* amplifications, but with very poor patient prognoses [57, 58]. Overall, however, validated actionable aberrations are present in only a small proportion of high-risk patients at diagnosis.

Functional genetic regulators of neuroblastoma development and progression also include microRNAs [59–61], long non-coding RNAs (lncRNAs) [62], alternative splicing programs [63], fragile sites [64] and genome-wide methylation [65–71]. MicroRNAs have been implicated in neuroblastoma metastasis, *MYCN* regulation and cell differentiation, and may, thus, serve as novel therapeutic targets [72].

13.4 Systematic Preclinical Evaluation and Target and Drug Prioritization

Prioritization is necessary to identify targets and drugs which may be of potential benefit to neuroblastoma patients due to the large number of potential targets and drugs becoming available for evaluation and the genetic heterogeneity of neuroblastoma with few recurrently altered genes. Several European initiatives are systematically obtaining molecular data with the aim to discover novel drug targets by routinely profiling tumors at relapse: MOlecular Screening for CAncer Treatment Optimisation (MOSCATO-01) [73], MoleculAr Profiling for Pediatric and Young Adult Cancer Treatment Stratification (MAPPYACTS), Individualized Therapy for Relapsed Malignancies in Childhood (INFORM) [38], Individualised Therapy (iTHER), and Stratified Medicine Paediatrics (SM-PAEDS), comparable to the TARGET project in the USA, which analyzes both primary and relapsed neuroblastomas [54, 74]. The first pivotal evaluation step should be to prioritize targets according to the level of existing biological evidence. Then drugs available for the target should be defined. Finally, those drugs available for pediatric use should be established, and the agents prioritized for testing in early-phase clinical trials.

One important bottleneck in systematic preclinical evaluation is translating results from preclinical cell culture or animal models to the patient. This translation can only succeed if robust predictive preclinical models are used that adequately recapitulate the complexity of human tumor biology [75, 76]. Although preclinical assessment of targeted agents in a small number of transgenic and xenograft models of neuroblastoma is commonplace, the more thorough preclinical assessment of efficacy using larger numbers of models is uncommon. The National Cancer Institute (NCI) Pediatric Preclinical

Testing Consortium (PPTC) led the way >10 years ago by initiating systematic testing of up to 12 promising agents or combinations in panels of cell lines and xenograft models for pediatric cancers, including neuroblastoma [77]. However, the use of conventional 2D cell cultures and xenografts from established cell lines has limited the predictive value of these initial analyses. Recent initiatives have brought together large collections of more reliable 3D organoid and patient-derived xenograft (PDX) models that better represent the diversity in neuroblastoma (i.e., the European IMI2 consortium ITCC P4) [78]. Braekeveldt et al. have established orthotopic PDX models from high-risk neuroblastomas that retain the specific chromosomal aberrations and metastatic patterns from the original tumors, which could be relevant for studying neuroblastoma invasion and metastasis in vivo [79, 80]. These more complex models create new opportunities for a more thorough preclinical evaluation of drug efficacy through phase II-like trials conducted in mice, which may also accelerate biomarker development.

Transgenic animal models can be the basis for high volume and velocity data [47]. The distinctly important advantage of animal models for neuroblastoma is the veracity in simulating the developmental context of neuroblastoma onset and progression. Unlike cell lines, which lack vascularity, immune involvement and paracrine signaling from other cell types, animal models can better recapitulate human disease [81, 82]. Neuroblastoma has several animal models, the most notable being *MYCN*- and *ALK*-expressing mice and zebrafish [83, 84]. Additionally, neuroblastomas from patients can be xenografted into zebrafish and mice, providing a way to capture the heterogeneity of human disease [77, 85–87]. Zebrafish have an advantage over mouse models due to their small size, high fecundity, and ease of maintenance. Their transparent embryos allow easy observation of cancer progression and metastasis [88, 89]. Conversely, mice more closely mimic human biology, and can be better analogs for investigating epigenetics and drug therapies. Preclinical models for neuroblastoma must also consider the use of clinically achievable doses guided by rigorous pharmacokinetic data. The multiagent and multimodal treatment in patients must be modeled. The relevance of post-treatment mutations for cure must also be validated and the understanding of drug resistance mechanisms advanced. Applying these measures will bring preclinical drug testing in animal models nearer to and better prepare for clinical testing.

Although the number of early-phase clinical trials in pediatric cancer has increased as a result of the European Pediatric Medicine Regulation, the development of drugs for neuroblastoma is still driven by the adult drug market and not by prioritization based on the molecular characteristics of the disease. The fragmented drug development process has resulted in the clinical evaluation of drugs without a strong biological rationale and with multiple phase II trials performed for the same drug target [90]. New targets in neuroblastoma should rather be prioritized based on their biology. Specifically, target expression, target dependency and validation, and preclinical data for efficacy, potential combinations, and biomarker availability should drive prioritization. To this end, the European ITCC consortium, in combination with the SIOPEN group, has established the Neuroblastoma New Drug Development Strategy (NDDS) to accelerate the development of new drugs [90]. The targets given top priority by NDDS, based on available data and potentially available inhibitors, were ALK, MEK, CDK4/6, MDM2, MYCN, BIRC5, and checkpoint kinase 1 (CHEK1). The critical importance of combinations has been highlighted, as these may overcome resistance and enhance efficacy where dysregulation of more than one biological pathway is driving disease. However, the mechanism of action and cumulative toxicities of additional agents must be carefully considered when designing treatment regimens.

A substantial logistical challenge lies in the systematic evaluation of the numerous possible permutations of combinations in a clinical setting [91]. In view of the limited number of children available for early-phase studies, a rational preclinical approach is needed to select combinations based on neuroblastoma biology and data obtained in tumors treated with one agent from the combination [90]. A proposed combination should only be evaluated clinically following preclinical evaluation of the combinations in a range of well-characterized models.

13.5 Current Approaches for Relapsed Neuroblastoma

Internationally, a large number of early-phase trials for single agents, including difluoromethylornithine (DFMO) or inhibitors of ALK, aurora kinases, mTOR or CDK4/6 have been completed in children with relapsed high-risk neuroblastoma [92–105]. A number of additional targets, including *MYCN* and mutations in the RAS-MAPK pathway have been identified and are the subject of ongoing studies to identify appropriate targeted therapeutic agents. A detailed overview of promising preclinical investigations and ongoing clinical trials for major drug targets in high-risk and relapsed neuroblastomas can be found elsewhere [6, 10, 106].

Most recently, there have been promising response rates in trials focused on combining novel agents, including alisertib, dinutuximab, and temsirolimus, with an effective chemotherapy backbone (i.e., irinotecan/temozolomide) [94, 107], suggesting these combinations should be moved more quickly to the frontline setting. Although the effective integration of novel therapies with toxic chemotherapeutic agents presents a challenge, it has been achieved in the relapse setting [94, 107]. Allocation to trial arms could be determined by patient randomization for drugs lacking predictive biomarkers. The promising combination of sirolimus/dasatinib + irinotecan/temozolomide is currently being tested biomarker-independently in a phase II clinical trial (RIST) in Germany following several objective responses in a retrospective compassionate use program [108].

Approximately 90% of neuroblastomas are MIBG-avid, and infusions of 131I-MIBG allow targeted delivery of radiation therapy directly to the sites of active disease. Initial studies showed overall response rates of 21–47% in patients with neuroblastoma [6, 109–111]. Subsequent studies have used autologous stem cell rescue after MIBG treatment, allowing for administration of higher radiation doses. In a large phase II study, 164 patients with relapsed neuroblastoma were treated with 131I-MIBG. Of the treated patients, 34% had stable disease for a median of 6 months [112], spurring efforts to include 131I-MIBG therapy as part of upfront consolidation treatment for high-risk neuroblastoma. Additional clinical trials are ongoing through the NANT consortium to identify the best anticancer agents to combine with MIBG therapy.

The efficacy of immunotherapy has been demonstrated in neuroblastoma patients with minimal residual disease. The role of immunotherapy in patients with relapsed disease is the focus of ongoing studies. A recent trial combining chemotherapy with dinutuximab demonstrated promising results. Dinutuximab plus irinotecan/temozolomide showed a significantly higher objective response rate (53%) than irinotecan/temozolomide alone (15%) [107], leading to a current COG trial combining dinutuximab with irinotecan/temozolomide (NCT01767194). Mismatches between the human natural killer cell Ig-like receptors, KIR, and their ligand genotypes as well as polymorphisms in the Fcγ receptor have been associated with better responses to anti-GD2 immunotherapy in further analyses [6, 113, 114]. The significant side effects of anti-GD2 immunotherapy have sparked evaluation of many other immunological approaches, including immunomodulatory CTLA4 checkpoint inhibitors [115], anti-tumor vaccines [116, 117], and cell-based immunotherapy using either natural killer cells [118] or anti-GD2-targeted autologous T cells [119], which demonstrate anti-tumor activity [120, 121]. Next-generation chimeric antigen receptor (CAR)-T cells are also currently in development, in which the constructs include costimulatory domains to activate the T cell [122–128].

13.6 Future Clinical Trial Design and Personalized Medicine Trials

Opportunities to improve outcomes are presented by the increased prevalence of potentially actionable targets at relapse, the development of new agents, and an increased understanding of molecular mechanisms driving neuroblastoma pathogenesis. However, major challenges for trialists and clinicians are also created [10]. A key consideration is identifying the most beneficial time point to conduct trials of the novel agents. To date, clinical trials for neuroblastoma have largely followed the traditional drug development pathway [10]. Novel agents are first shown to be safe in adults and then enter phase I safety trials in children, usually as a single agent. Phase I combination studies follow, leading to progression to phase II trials and ultimately (for a small number of agents) to testing in large randomized phase III clinical trials. Using this strategy, most novel agents are tested extensively in phase I and II trials on children with relapsed disease [10]. However, once safety and activity have been demonstrated, further testing should rapidly move to ultra-high-risk, newly diagnosed patients who still have a chance of cure. Early stopping rules should be used to monitor safety and inferior efficacy to mitigate any risk.

The objective of an early-phase clinical trial is not only to determine the pediatric-recommended phase II dose (RP2D), safety profile, pharmacokinetics, and pharmacodynamics of a drug but also to assess preliminary signals of activity [90]. The pediatric RP2D remains very close to the equivalent adult RP2D, and toxicity profiles are class-related and similar to adult drugs [129]. Thus, for drugs with a wide therapeutic index, it is recommended that the pediatric early-phase clinical trial start at the adult RP2D corrected for body surface area. A dose escalation study is required for drugs with narrow therapeutic indices. Existing dose escalation designs, such as 3 + 3, were developed to evaluate toxic chemotherapeutics. The use of these conventional dose escalation designs for the less toxic molecularly targeted agents tests more dose levels than necessary and extends study durations [90, 130].

New dose escalation designs, such as the Bayesian logistic regression model (BLRM) or continuous reassessment method (CRM), maximize efficiency by shortening trial duration and less exposing patients to doses below the maximum tolerated dose (MTD) [90, 131]. Relatively small expansion cohorts can inform statistical go/no-go decisions, such as the Ensign 3-stage design [132], where 10 patients are recruited at the RP2D. Further evaluation of the drug is postponed or abandoned if no response occurs in the first 10 patients. If a response occurs in the first 10 patients, then 16 further patients are enrolled. If preliminary evidence of activity is documented, then the drug is evaluated further in neuroblastoma-specific, adaptive-design, parallel, randomized, or multi-arm/multistage phase II trials. Evaluation in randomized trials is essential, as a comparison with historical controls will overestimate drug efficacy [133].

To compensate for small patient numbers and long recruitment times, statistical designs can be amended to allow for less stringent comparisons among different trial arms [134, 135]. The traditional view is that trials should be powered at 80% with a type 1 error rate of 5% (equal to a P value of 0.05). It is feasible, however, to raise the error rate to 10%, and still have meaningful results from substantially smaller patient numbers and a faster trial. This approach increases the risk of selecting a treatment that is not as effective as thought, but has been shown to be highly unlikely to choose an inferior treatment [134]. COG has successfully demonstrated that a randomized clinical trial design can be used to simultaneously select a 'winner' and drop an ineffective treatment regimen in the setting of relapsed neuroblastoma [10, 107]. Single agents or combinations, which show activity in the randomized phase II trials, are then introduced into frontline therapy and evaluated further—a three-stage process from first-in-child studies to frontline therapy. For phase III trials, intensified international cooperation is needed to eliminate redundant trials and speed accrual.

The capacity to incorporate phase II elements within large phase III trials will likely increase access to novel therapies. However, it also relates to the difficulty in gaining access to novel agents for rare cancer types from pharmaceutical companies. There is little commercial gain in developing new treatments for high-risk neuroblastoma patients. Regulations introduced in Europe and the USA to provide incentives for pharmaceutical companies to test drugs in children have provided some progress in this area, but are not without their problems [75]. Recently proposed initiatives, including the suppression of regulations allowing product-specific waivers where the associated disease does not occur in children [136], would be welcome advances, particularly in the context of precision medicine.

More recent clinical trials have focused on the potential of personalized therapy for children with relapsed neuroblastoma, using genomic information to direct molecularly targeted therapies against the tumors in cases most likely to derive clinical benefit. Pilot studies have demonstrated the feasibility of generating therapeutic treatment plans based on genomic profiling in less than 12 days [137]. A national, multi-institutional phase I trial showed clinical benefit in 64% of patients (defined as disease stabilization for at least one therapy cycle or partial response), with an overall response rate of 7% and progression-free survival time of 59 days [138]. A subsequent single-institution study demonstrated that incorporating tumor DNA sequencing data into clinical patient management was feasible, and revealed potentially actionable findings in nearly half the patients that, in some, directly led to changes in treatment [139]. Although these results demonstrate the feasibility and safety of performing real-time genomic profiling to guide treatment decision-making for neuroblastoma patients, the lack of control groups has limited assessment of whether improved outcomes resulted from the targeted therapy approach or that, which would have occurred with standard care. Ongoing national studies are underway to better determine the efficacy of molecularly guided therapy in these patient populations (NCT02162732, NCT02520713).

In summary, a reconsideration of clinical trial design and early identification of patients at ultra-high-risk of treatment failure as well as the identification of targetable, subclonal aberrations at diagnosis will shift testing of novel agents from relapsed patients, where they are less likely to be effective, to newly diagnosed patients, where they are more likely to improve patient outcomes.

References

1. Yu AL, Gilman AL, Ozkaynak MF, London WB, Kreissman SG, Chen HX, Smith M, Anderson B, Villablanca JG, Matthay KK, Shimada H, Grupp SA, Seeger R, Reynolds CP, Buxton A, Reisfeld RA, Gillies SD, Cohn SL, Maris JM, Sondel PM, Children's Oncology G. Anti-GD2 antibody with GM-CSF, interleukin-2, and isotretinoin for neuroblastoma. N Engl J Med. 2010;363(14):1324–34. https://doi.org/10.1056/NEJMoa0911123.
2. Berlanga P, Canete A, Castel V. Advances in emerging drugs for the treatment of neuroblastoma. Expert Opin Emerg Drugs. 2017;22(1):63–75. https://doi.org/10.1080/14728214.2017.1294159.
3. Castel V, Canete A, Navarro S, Garcia-Miguel P, Melero C, Acha T, Navajas A, Badal MD. Outcome of high-risk neuroblastoma using a dose intensity approach: improvement in initial but not in long-term results. Med Pediatr Oncol. 2001;37(6):537–42. https://doi.org/10.1002/mpo.1248.
4. London WB, Castel V, Monclair T, Ambros PF, Pearson AD, Cohn SL, Berthold F, Nakagawara A, Ladenstein RL, Iehara T, Matthay KK. Clinical and biologic features predictive of survival after relapse of neuroblastoma: a report from the international neuroblastoma risk group project. J Clin Oncol. 2011;29(24):3286–92. https://doi.org/10.1200/JCO.2010.34.3392.
5. Moreno L, Pearson AD, Guo D, Morgenstern D, Pasqualini C, Ash S, Valteau-Couanet D, Cohn S, London WB. Predicting "early" relapse/progression/death in children with INRGSS stage M neuroblastoma using clinical and biologic factors: an INRG database analysis. Cairns, QL: Paper presented at the Advances in Neuroblastoma Research Congress ANR; 2016.
6. Whittle SB, Smith V, Doherty E, Zhao S, McCarty S, Zage PE. Overview and recent advances in the treatment of neuroblastoma. Expert Rev Anticancer Ther. 2017;17(4):369–86. https://doi.org/10.1080/14737140.2017.1285230.

7. Garaventa A, Parodi S, De Bernardi B, Dau D, Manzitti C, Conte M, Casale F, Viscardi E, Bianchi M, D'Angelo P, Zanazzo GA, Luksch R, Favre C, Tamburini A, Haupt R. Outcome of children with neuroblastoma after progression or relapse. A retrospective study of the Italian neuroblastoma registry. Eur J Cancer. 2009;45(16):2835–42. https://doi.org/10.1016/j.ejca.2009.06.010.
8. Moreno L, Rubie H, Varo A, Le Deley MC, Amoroso L, Chevance A, Garaventa A, Gambart M, Bautista F, Valteau-Couanet D, Geoerger B, Vassal G, Paoletti X, Pearson AD. Outcome of children with relapsed or refractory neuroblastoma: a meta-analysis of ITCC/SIOPEN European phase II clinical trials. Pediatr Blood Cancer. 2017;64(1):25–31. https://doi.org/10.1002/pbc.26192.
9. Cohn SL, Pearson AD, London WB, Monclair T, Ambros PF, Brodeur GM, Faldum A, Hero B, Iehara T, Machin D, Mosseri V, Simon T, Garaventa A, Castel V, Matthay KK, Force IT. The International Neuroblastoma Risk Group (INRG) classification system: an INRG task force report. J Clin Oncol. 2009;27(2):289–97. https://doi.org/10.1200/JCO.2008.16.6785.
10. Fletcher JI, Ziegler DS, Trahair TN, Marshall GM, Haber M, Norris MD. Too many targets, not enough patients: rethinking neuroblastoma clinical trials. Nat Rev Cancer. 2018;18(6):389–400. https://doi.org/10.1038/s41568-018-0003-x.
11. Ohira M, Nakagawara A. Global genomic and RNA profiles for novel risk stratification of neuroblastoma. Cancer Sci. 2010;101(11):2295–301. https://doi.org/10.1111/j.1349-7006.2010.01681.x.
12. Wei JS, Greer BT, Westermann F, Steinberg SM, Son CG, Chen QR, Whiteford CC, Bilke S, Krasnoselsky AL, Cenacchi N, Catchpoole D, Berthold F, Schwab M, Khan J. Prediction of clinical outcome using gene expression profiling and artificial neural networks for patients with neuroblastoma. Cancer Res. 2004;64(19):6883–91. https://doi.org/10.1158/0008-5472.CAN-04-0695.
13. Schramm A, Schulte JH, Klein-Hitpass L, Havers W, Sieverts H, Berwanger B, Christiansen H, Warnat P, Brors B, Eils J, Eils R, Eggert A. Prediction of clinical outcome and biological characterization of neuroblastoma by expression profiling. Oncogene. 2005;24(53):7902–12. https://doi.org/10.1038/sj.onc.1208936.
14. Ohira M, Oba S, Nakamura Y, Isogai E, Kaneko S, Nakagawa A, Hirata T, Kubo H, Goto T, Yamada S, Yoshida Y, Fuchioka M, Ishii S, Nakagawara A. Expression profiling using a tumor-specific cDNA microarray predicts the prognosis of intermediate risk neuroblastomas. Cancer Cell. 2005;7(4):337–50. https://doi.org/10.1016/j.ccr.2005.03.019.
15. Oberthuer A, Berthold F, Warnat P, Hero B, Kahlert Y, Spitz R, Ernestus K, Konig R, Haas S, Eils R, Schwab M, Brors B, Westermann F, Fischer M. Customized oligonucleotide microarray gene expression-based classification of neuroblastoma patients outperforms current clinical risk stratification. J Clin Oncol. 2006;24(31):5070–8. https://doi.org/10.1200/JCO.2006.06.1879.
16. Schramm A, Vandesompele J, Schulte JH, Dreesmann S, Kaderali L, Brors B, Eils R, Speleman F, Eggert A. Translating expression profiling into a clinically feasible test to predict neuroblastoma outcome. Clin Cancer Res. 2007;13(5):1459–65. https://doi.org/10.1158/1078-0432.CCR-06-2032.
17. Oberthuer A, Kaderali L, Kahlert Y, Hero B, Westermann F, Berthold F, Brors B, Eils R, Fischer M. Subclassification and individual survival time prediction from gene expression data of neuroblastoma patients by using CASPAR. Clin Cancer Res. 2008;14(20):6590–601. https://doi.org/10.1158/1078-0432.CCR-07-4377.
18. De Preter K, Vermeulen J, Brors B, Delattre O, Eggert A, Fischer M, Janoueix-Lerosey I, Lavarino C, Maris JM, Mora J, Nakagawara A, Oberthuer A, Ohira M, Schleiermacher G, Schramm A, Schulte JH, Wang Q, Westermann F, Speleman F, Vandesompele J. Accurate outcome prediction in neuroblastoma across independent data sets using a multigene signature. Clin Cancer Res. 2010;16(5):1532–41. https://doi.org/10.1158/1078-0432.CCR-09-2607.
19. Tomioka N, Oba S, Ohira M, Misra A, Fridlyand J, Ishii S, Nakamura Y, Isogai E, Hirata T, Yoshida Y, Todo S, Kaneko Y, Albertson DG, Pinkel D, Feuerstein BG, Nakagawara A. Novel risk stratification of patients with neuroblastoma by genomic signature, which is independent of molecular signature. Oncogene. 2008;27(4):441–9. https://doi.org/10.1038/sj.onc.1210661.
20. Bilke S, Chen QR, Westerman F, Schwab M, Catchpoole D, Khan J. Inferring a tumor progression model for neuroblastoma from genomic data. J Clin Oncol. 2005;23(29):7322–31. https://doi.org/10.1200/JCO.2005.03.2821.
21. Michels E, Vandesompele J, De Preter K, Hoebeeck J, Vermeulen J, Schramm A, Molenaar JJ, Menten B, Marques B, Stallings RL, Combaret V, Devalck C, De Paepe A, Versteeg R, Eggert A, Laureys G, Van Roy N, Speleman F. ArrayCGH-based classification of neuroblastoma into genomic subgroups. Genes Chromosomes Cancer. 2007;46(12):1098–108. https://doi.org/10.1002/gcc.20496.
22. Schleiermacher G, Michon J, Huon I, d'Enghien CD, Klijanienko J, Brisse H, Ribeiro A, Mosseri V, Rubie H, Munzer C, Thomas C, Valteau-Couanet D, Auvrignon A, Plantaz D, Delattre O, Couturier J, Societe Francaise des Cancers de lE. Chromosomal CGH identifies patients with a higher risk of relapse in neuroblastoma without MYCN amplification. Br J Cancer. 2007;97(2):238–46. https://doi.org/10.1038/sj.bjc.6603820.
23. Schleiermacher G, Janoueix-Lerosey I, Ribeiro A, Klijanienko J, Couturier J, Pierron G, Mosseri V, Valent A, Auger N, Plantaz D, Rubie H, Valteau-Couanet D, Bourdeaut F, Combaret V, Bergeron C, Michon J, Delattre O. Accumulation of segmental

alterations determines progression in neuroblastoma. J Clin Oncol. 2010;28(19):3122–30. https://doi.org/10.1200/JCO.2009.26.7955.
24. Esposito M, Aveic S, Seydel A, Tonini G. The role of omics in neuroblastoma: patient's risk classification and personalised therapy. Adv Modern Oncol. 2016;2:271–8.
25. Bray I, Bryan K, Prenter S, Buckley PG, Foley NH, Murphy DM, Alcock L, Mestdagh P, Vandesompele J, Speleman F, London WB, McGrady PW, Higgins DG, O'Meara A, O'Sullivan M, Stallings RL. Widespread dysregulation of MiRNAs by MYCN amplification and chromosomal imbalances in neuroblastoma: association of miRNA expression with survival. PLoS One. 2009;4(11):e7850. https://doi.org/10.1371/journal.pone.0007850.
26. De Preter K, Mestdagh P, Vermeulen J, Zeka F, Naranjo A, Bray I, Castel V, Chen C, Drozynska E, Eggert A, Hogarty MD, Izycka-Swieszewska E, London WB, Noguera R, Piqueras M, Bryan K, Schowe B, van Sluis P, Molenaar JJ, Schramm A, Schulte JH, Stallings RL, Versteeg R, Laureys G, Van Roy N, Speleman F, Vandesompele J. miRNA expression profiling enables risk stratification in archived and fresh neuroblastoma tumor samples. Clin Cancer Res. 2011;17(24):7684–92. https://doi.org/10.1158/1078-0432.CCR-11-0610.
27. Wang Q, Diskin S, Rappaport E, Attiyeh E, Mosse Y, Shue D, Seiser E, Jagannathan J, Shusterman S, Bansal M, Khazi D, Winter C, Okawa E, Grant G, Cnaan A, Zhao H, Cheung NK, Gerald W, London W, Matthay KK, Brodeur GM, Maris JM. Integrative genomics identifies distinct molecular classes of neuroblastoma and shows that multiple genes are targeted by regional alterations in DNA copy number. Cancer Res. 2006;66(12):6050–62. https://doi.org/10.1158/0008-5472.CAN-05-4618.
28. Fischer M, Bauer T, Oberthur A, Hero B, Theissen J, Ehrich M, Spitz R, Eils R, Westermann F, Brors B, Konig R, Berthold F. Integrated genomic profiling identifies two distinct molecular subtypes with divergent outcome in neuroblastoma with loss of chromosome 11q. Oncogene. 2010;29(6):865–75. https://doi.org/10.1038/onc.2009.390.
29. Yanez Y, Hervas D, Grau E, Oltra S, Perez G, Palanca S, Bermudez M, Marquez C, Canete A, Castel V. TH and DCX mRNAs in peripheral blood and bone marrow predict outcome in metastatic neuroblastoma patients. J Cancer Res Clin Oncol. 2016;142(3):573–80. https://doi.org/10.1007/s00432-015-2054-7.
30. Viprey VF, Gregory WM, Corrias MV, Tchirkov A, Swerts K, Vicha A, Dallorso S, Brock P, Luksch R, Valteau-Couanet D, Papadakis V, Laureys G, Pearson AD, Ladenstein R, Burchill SA. Neuroblastoma mRNAs predict outcome in children with stage 4 neuroblastoma: a European HR-NBL1/SIOPEN study. J Clin Oncol. 2014;32(10):1074–83. https://doi.org/10.1200/JCO.2013.53.3604.
31. Adamson PC, Houghton PJ, Perilongo G, Pritchard-Jones K. Drug discovery in paediatric oncology: roadblocks to progress. Nat Rev Clin Oncol. 2014;11(12):732–9. https://doi.org/10.1038/nrclinonc.2014.149.
32. Lawrence MS, Stojanov P, Polak P, Kryukov GV, Cibulskis K, Sivachenko A, Carter SL, Stewart C, Mermel CH, Roberts SA, Kiezun A, Hammerman PS, McKenna A, Drier Y, Zou L, Ramos AH, Pugh TJ, Stransky N, Helman E, Kim J, Sougnez C, Ambrogio L, Nickerson E, Shefler E, Cortes ML, Auclair D, Saksena G, Voet D, Noble M, DiCara D, Lin P, Lichtenstein L, Heiman DI, Fennell T, Imielinski M, Hernandez B, Hodis E, Baca S, Dulak AM, Lohr J, Landau DA, Wu CJ, Melendez-Zajgla J, Hidalgo-Miranda A, Koren A, McCarroll SA, Mora J, Crompton B, Onofrio R, Parkin M, Winckler W, Ardlie K, Gabriel SB, Roberts CWM, Biegel JA, Stegmaier K, Bass AJ, Garraway LA, Meyerson M, Golub TR, Gordenin DA, Sunyaev S, Lander ES, Getz G. Mutational heterogeneity in cancer and the search for new cancer-associated genes. Nature. 2013;499(7457):214–8. https://doi.org/10.1038/nature12213.
33. Speleman F, De Preter K, Vandesompele J. Neuroblastoma genetics and phenotype: a tale of heterogeneity. Semin Cancer Biol. 2011;21(4):238–44. https://doi.org/10.1016/j.semcancer.2011.07.003.
34. Vogelstein B, Papadopoulos N, Velculescu VE, Zhou S, Diaz LA Jr, Kinzler KW. Cancer genome landscapes. Science. 2013;339(6127):1546–58. https://doi.org/10.1126/science.1235122.
35. Schleiermacher G, Javanmardi N, Bernard V, Leroy Q, Cappo J, Rio Frio T, Pierron G, Lapouble E, Combaret V, Speleman F, de Wilde B, Djos A, Ora I, Hedborg F, Trager C, Holmqvist BM, Abrahamsson J, Peuchmaur M, Michon J, Janoueix-Lerosey I, Kogner P, Delattre O, Martinsson T. Emergence of new ALK mutations at relapse of neuroblastoma. J Clin Oncol. 2014;32(25):2727–34. https://doi.org/10.1200/JCO.2013.54.0674.
36. Schramm A, Koster J, Assenov Y, Althoff K, Peifer M, Mahlow E, Odersky A, Beisser D, Ernst C, Henssen AG, Stephan H, Schroder C, Heukamp L, Engesser A, Kahlert Y, Theissen J, Hero B, Roels F, Altmuller J, Nurnberg P, Astrahantseff K, Gloeckner C, De Preter K, Plass C, Lee S, Lode HN, Henrich KO, Gartlgruber M, Speleman F, Schmezer P, Westermann F, Rahmann S, Fischer M, Eggert A, Schulte JH. Mutational dynamics between primary and relapse neuroblastomas. Nat Genet. 2015;47(8):872–7. https://doi.org/10.1038/ng.3349.
37. Eleveld TF, Oldridge DA, Bernard V, Koster J, Colmet Daage L, Diskin SJ, Schild L, Bentahar NB, Bellini A, Chicard M, Lapouble E, Combaret V, Legoix-Ne P, Michon J, Pugh TJ, Hart LS, Rader J, Attiyeh EF, Wei JS, Zhang S, Naranjo A, Gastier-Foster JM, Hogarty MD, Asgharzadeh S, Smith MA, Guidry Auvil JM, Watkins TB, Zwijnenburg DA,

Ebus ME, van Sluis P, Hakkert A, van Wezel E, van der Schoot CE, Westerhout EM, Schulte JH, Tytgat GA, Dolman ME, Janoueix-Lerosey I, Gerhard DS, Caron HN, Delattre O, Khan J, Versteeg R, Schleiermacher G, Molenaar JJ, Maris JM. Relapsed neuroblastomas show frequent RAS-MAPK pathway mutations. Nat Genet. 2015;47(8):864–71. https://doi.org/10.1038/ng.3333.

38. Worst BC, van Tilburg CM, Balasubramanian GP, Fiesel P, Witt R, Freitag A, Boudalil M, Previti C, Wolf S, Schmidt S, Chotewutmontri S, Bewerunge-Hudler M, Schick M, Schlesner M, Hutter B, Taylor L, Borst T, Sutter C, Bartram CR, Milde T, Pfaff E, Kulozik AE, von Stackelberg A, Meisel R, Borkhardt A, Reinhardt D, Klusmann JH, Fleischhack G, Tippelt S, Dirksen U, Jurgens H, Kramm CM, von Bueren AO, Westermann F, Fischer M, Burkhardt B, Wossmann W, Nathrath M, Bielack SS, Fruhwald MC, Fulda S, Klingebiel T, Koscielniak E, Schwab M, Tremmel R, Driever PH, Schulte JH, Brors B, von Deimling A, Lichter P, Eggert A, Capper D, Pfister SM, Jones DT, Witt O. Next-generation personalised medicine for high-risk paediatric cancer patients—the INFORM pilot study. Eur J Cancer. 2016;65:91–101. https://doi.org/10.1016/j.ejca.2016.06.009.
39. Abbasi MR, Rifatbegovic F, Brunner C, Mann G, Ziegler A, Potschger U, Crazzolara R, Ussowicz M, Benesch M, Ebetsberger-Dachs G, Chan GCF, Jones N, Ladenstein R, Ambros IM, Ambros PF. Impact of disseminated neuroblastoma cells on the identification of the relapse-seeding clone. Clin Cancer Res. 2017;23(15):4224–32. https://doi.org/10.1158/1078-0432.CCR-16-2082.
40. Chmielecki J, Bailey M, He J, Elvin J, Vergilio JA, Ramkissoon S, Suh J, Frampton GM, Sun JX, Morley S, Spritz D, Ali S, Gay L, Erlich RL, Ross JS, Buxhaku J, Davies H, Faso V, Germain A, Glanville B, Miller VA, Stephens PJ, Janeway KA, Maris JM, Meshinchi S, Pugh TJ, Shern JF, Lipson D. Genomic profiling of a large set of diverse pediatric cancers identifies known and novel mutations across tumor spectra. Cancer Res. 2017;77(2):509–19. https://doi.org/10.1158/0008-5472.CAN-16-1106.
41. Boeva V, Louis-Brennetot C, Peltier A, Durand S, Pierre-Eugene C, Raynal V, Etchevers HC, Thomas S, Lermine A, Daudigeos-Dubus E, Geoerger B, Orth MF, Grunewald TGP, Diaz E, Ducos B, Surdez D, Carcaboso AM, Medvedeva I, Deller T, Combaret V, Lapouble E, Pierron G, Grossetete-Lalami S, Baulande S, Schleiermacher G, Barillot E, Rohrer H, Delattre O, Janoueix-Lerosey I. Heterogeneity of neuroblastoma cell identity defined by transcriptional circuitries. Nat Genet. 2017;49(9):1408–13. https://doi.org/10.1038/ng.3921.
42. Wan JCM, Massie C, Garcia-Corbacho J, Mouliere F, Brenton JD, Caldas C, Pacey S, Baird R, Rosenfeld N. Liquid biopsies come of age: towards implementation of circulating tumour DNA. Nat Rev Cancer. 2017;17(4):223–38. https://doi.org/10.1038/nrc.2017.7.
43. Murtaza M, Dawson SJ, Pogrebniak K, Rueda OM, Provenzano E, Grant J, Chin SF, Tsui DWY, Marass F, Gale D, Ali HR, Shah P, Contente-Cuomo T, Farahani H, Shumansky K, Kingsbury Z, Humphray S, Bentley D, Shah SP, Wallis M, Rosenfeld N, Caldas C. Multifocal clonal evolution characterized using circulating tumour DNA in a case of metastatic breast cancer. Nat Commun. 2015;6:8760. https://doi.org/10.1038/ncomms9760.
44. Bettegowda C, Sausen M, Leary RJ, Kinde I, Wang Y, Agrawal N, Bartlett BR, Wang H, Luber B, Alani RM, Antonarakis ES, Azad NS, Bardelli A, Brem H, Cameron JL, Lee CC, Fecher LA, Gallia GL, Gibbs P, Le D, Giuntoli RL, Goggins M, Hogarty MD, Holdhoff M, Hong SM, Jiao Y, Juhl HH, Kim JJ, Siravegna G, Laheru DA, Lauricella C, Lim M, Lipson EJ, Marie SK, Netto GJ, Oliner KS, Olivi A, Olsson L, Riggins GJ, Sartore-Bianchi A, Schmidt K, Shih M, Oba-Shinjo SM, Siena S, Theodorescu D, Tie J, Harkins TT, Veronese S, Wang TL, Weingart JD, Wolfgang CL, Wood LD, Xing D, Hruban RH, Wu J, Allen PJ, Schmidt CM, Choti MA, Velculescu VE, Kinzler KW, Vogelstein B, Papadopoulos N, Diaz LA Jr. Detection of circulating tumor DNA in early- and late-stage human malignancies. Sci Transl Med. 2014;6(224):224ra224. https://doi.org/10.1126/scitranslmed.3007094.
45. Combaret V, Iacono I, Bellini A, Brejon S, Bernard V, Marabelle A, Coze C, Pierron G, Lapouble E, Schleiermacher G, Blay JY. Detection of tumor ALK status in neuroblastoma patients using peripheral blood. Cancer Med. 2015;4(4):540–50. https://doi.org/10.1002/cam4.414.
46. Chicard M, Boyault S, Colmet Daage L, Richer W, Gentien D, Pierron G, Lapouble E, Bellini A, Clement N, Iacono I, Brejon S, Carrere M, Reyes C, Hocking T, Bernard V, Peuchmaur M, Corradini N, Faure-Conter C, Coze C, Plantaz D, Defachelles AS, Thebaud E, Gambart M, Millot F, Valteau-Couanet D, Michon J, Puisieux A, Delattre O, Combaret V, Schleiermacher G. Genomic copy number profiling using circulating free tumor DNA highlights heterogeneity in neuroblastoma. Clin Cancer Res. 2016;22(22):5564–73. https://doi.org/10.1158/1078-0432.CCR-16-0500.
47. Salazar BM, Balczewski EA, Ung CY, Zhu S. Neuroblastoma, a paradigm for big data science in pediatric oncology. Int J Mol Sci. 2016;18(1):37. https://doi.org/10.3390/ijms18010037.
48. Choi H, Sheng J, Gao D, Li F, Durrans A, Ryu S, Lee SB, Narula N, Rafii S, Elemento O, Altorki NK, Wong ST, Mittal V. Transcriptome analysis of individual stromal cell populations identifies stroma-tumor crosstalk in mouse lung cancer model. Cell Rep. 2015;10(7):1187–201. https://doi.org/10.1016/j.celrep.2015.01.040.
49. Reinartz S, Finkernagel F, Adhikary T, Rohnalter V, Schumann T, Schober Y, Nockher WA, Nist A, Stiewe T, Jansen JM, Wagner U, Muller-Brusselbach S, Muller R. A transcriptome-based global map of

signaling pathways in the ovarian cancer microenvironment associated with clinical outcome. Genome Biol. 2016;17(1):108. https://doi.org/10.1186/s13059-016-0956-6.
50. Schulte JH, Eggert A. Neuroblastoma. Crit Rev Oncog. 2015;20(3–4):245–70. https://doi.org/10.1615/critrevoncog.2015014033.
51. Pugh TJ, Morozova O, Attiyeh EF, Asgharzadeh S, Wei JS, Auclair D, Carter SL, Cibulskis K, Hanna M, Kiezun A, Kim J, Lawrence MS, Lichenstein L, McKenna A, Pedamallu CS, Ramos AH, Shefler E, Sivachenko A, Sougnez C, Stewart C, Ally A, Birol I, Chiu R, Corbett RD, Hirst M, Jackman SD, Kamoh B, Khodabakshi AH, Krzywinski M, Lo A, Moore RA, Mungall KL, Qian J, Tam A, Thiessen N, Zhao Y, Cole KA, Diamond M, Diskin SJ, Mosse YP, Wood AC, Ji L, Sposto R, Badgett T, London WB, Moyer Y, Gastier-Foster JM, Smith MA, Guidry Auvil JM, Gerhard DS, Hogarty MD, Jones SJ, Lander ES, Gabriel SB, Getz G, Seeger RC, Khan J, Marra MA, Meyerson M, Maris JM. The genetic landscape of high-risk neuroblastoma. Nat Genet. 2013;45(3):279–84. https://doi.org/10.1038/ng.2529.
52. Attiyeh EF, London WB, Mosse YP, Wang Q, Winter C, Khazi D, McGrady PW, Seeger RC, Look AT, Shimada H, Brodeur GM, Cohn SL, Matthay KK, Maris JM, Children's Oncology G. Chromosome 1p and 11q deletions and outcome in neuroblastoma. N Engl J Med. 2005;353(21):2243–53. https://doi.org/10.1056/NEJMoa052399.
53. Diskin SJ, Hou C, Glessner JT, Attiyeh EF, Laudenslager M, Bosse K, Cole K, Mosse YP, Wood A, Lynch JE, Pecor K, Diamond M, Winter C, Wang K, Kim C, Geiger EA, McGrady PW, Blakemore AI, London WB, Shaikh TH, Bradfield J, Grant SF, Li H, Devoto M, Rappaport ER, Hakonarson H, Maris JM. Copy number variation at 1q21.1 associated with neuroblastoma. Nature. 2009;459(7249):987–91. https://doi.org/10.1038/nature08035.
54. Bosse KR, Maris JM. Advances in the translational genomics of neuroblastoma: from improving risk stratification and revealing novel biology to identifying actionable genomic alterations. Cancer. 2016;122(1):20–33. https://doi.org/10.1002/cncr.29706.
55. Brodeur GM, Bagatell R. Mechanisms of neuroblastoma regression. Nat Rev Clin Oncol. 2014;11(12):704–13. https://doi.org/10.1038/nrclinonc.2014.168.
56. Sausen M, Leary RJ, Jones S, Wu J, Reynolds CP, Liu X, Blackford A, Parmigiani G, Diaz LA Jr, Papadopoulos N, Vogelstein B, Kinzler KW, Velculescu VE, Hogarty MD. Integrated genomic analyses identify ARID1A and ARID1B alterations in the childhood cancer neuroblastoma. Nat Genet. 2013;45(1):12–7. https://doi.org/10.1038/ng.2493.
57. Peifer M, Hertwig F, Roels F, Dreidax D, Gartlgruber M, Menon R, Kramer A, Roncaioli JL, Sand F, Heuckmann JM, Ikram F, Schmidt R, Ackermann S, Engesser A, Kahlert Y, Vogel W, Altmuller J, Nurnberg P, Thierry-Mieg J, Thierry-Mieg D, Mariappan A, Heynck S, Mariotti E, Henrich KO, Gloeckner C, Bosco G, Leuschner I, Schweiger MR, Savelyeva L, Watkins SC, Shao C, Bell E, Hofer T, Achter V, Lang U, Theissen J, Volland R, Saadati M, Eggert A, de Wilde B, Berthold F, Peng Z, Zhao C, Shi L, Ortmann M, Buttner R, Perner S, Hero B, Schramm A, Schulte JH, Herrmann C, O'Sullivan RJ, Westermann F, Thomas RK, Fischer M. Telomerase activation by genomic rearrangements in high-risk neuroblastoma. Nature. 2015;526(7575):700–4. https://doi.org/10.1038/nature14980.
58. Valentijn LJ, Koster J, Zwijnenburg DA, Hasselt NE, van Sluis P, Volckmann R, van Noesel MM, George RE, Tytgat GA, Molenaar JJ, Versteeg R. TERT rearrangements are frequent in neuroblastoma and identify aggressive tumors. Nat Genet. 2015;47(12):1411–4. https://doi.org/10.1038/ng.3438.
59. Cheng L, Yang T, Kuang Y, Kong B, Yu S, Shu H, Zhou H, Gu J. MicroRNA-23a promotes neuroblastoma cell metastasis by targeting CDH1. Oncol Lett. 2014;7(3):839–45. https://doi.org/10.3892/ol.2014.1794.
60. Das S, Bryan K, Buckley PG, Piskareva O, Bray IM, Foley N, Ryan J, Lynch J, Creevey L, Fay J, Prenter S, Koster J, van Sluis P, Versteeg R, Eggert A, Schulte JH, Schramm A, Mestdagh P, Vandesompele J, Speleman F, Stallings RL. Modulation of neuroblastoma disease pathogenesis by an extensive network of epigenetically regulated microRNAs. Oncogene. 2013;32(24):2927–36. https://doi.org/10.1038/onc.2012.311.
61. Ray SK. Emerging roles of microRNAs in malignant neuroblastoma. Clin Exp Pharmacol. 2013;3(126):1. https://doi.org/10.4172/2161-1459.1000126.
62. Zhang S, Wei JS, Li SQ, Badgett TC, Song YK, Agarwal S, Coarfa C, Tolman C, Hurd L, Liao H, He J, Wen X, Liu Z, Thiele CJ, Westermann F, Asgharzadeh S, Seeger RC, Maris JM, Guidry Auvil JM, Smith MA, Kolaczyk ED, Shohet J, Khan J. MYCN controls an alternative RNA splicing program in high-risk metastatic neuroblastoma. Cancer Lett. 2016;371(2):214–24. https://doi.org/10.1016/j.canlet.2015.11.045.
63. Pandey GK, Mitra S, Subhash S, Hertwig F, Kanduri M, Mishra K, Fransson S, Ganeshram A, Mondal T, Bandaru S, Ostensson M, Akyurek LM, Abrahamsson J, Pfeifer S, Larsson E, Shi L, Peng Z, Fischer M, Martinsson T, Hedborg F, Kogner P, Kanduri C. The risk-associated long noncoding RNA NBAT-1 controls neuroblastoma progression by regulating cell proliferation and neuronal differentiation. Cancer Cell. 2014;26(5):722–37. https://doi.org/10.1016/j.ccell.2014.09.014.
64. Blumrich A, Zapatka M, Brueckner LM, Zheglo D, Schwab M, Savelyeva L. The FRA2C common fragile site maps to the borders of MYCN ampli-

cons in neuroblastoma and is associated with gross chromosomal rearrangements in different cancers. Hum Mol Genet. 2011;20(8):1488–501. https://doi.org/10.1093/hmg/ddr027.
65. Alaminos M, Davalos V, Cheung NK, Gerald WL, Esteller M. Clustering of gene hypermethylation associated with clinical risk groups in neuroblastoma. J Natl Cancer Inst. 2004;96(16):1208–19. https://doi.org/10.1093/jnci/djh224.
66. Carter H, Hofree M, Ideker T. Genotype to phenotype via network analysis. Curr Opin Genet Dev. 2013;23(6):611–21. https://doi.org/10.1016/j.gde.2013.10.003.
67. Decock A, Ongenaert M, Cannoodt R, Verniers K, De Wilde B, Laureys G, Van Roy N, Berbegall AP, Bienertova-Vasku J, Bown N, Clement N, Combaret V, Haber M, Hoyoux C, Murray J, Noguera R, Pierron G, Schleiermacher G, Schulte JH, Stallings RL, Tweddle DA, Children's C, Leukaemia G, De Preter K, Speleman F, Vandesompele J. Methyl-CpG-binding domain sequencing reveals a prognostic methylation signature in neuroblastoma. Oncotarget. 2016;7(2):1960–72. https://doi.org/10.18632/oncotarget.6477.
68. Decock A, Ongenaert M, Hoebeeck J, De Preter K, Van Peer G, Van Criekinge W, Ladenstein R, Schulte JH, Noguera R, Stallings RL, Van Damme A, Laureys G, Vermeulen J, Van Maerken T, Speleman F, Vandesompele J. Genome-wide promoter methylation analysis in neuroblastoma identifies prognostic methylation biomarkers. Genome Biol. 2012;13(10):R95. https://doi.org/10.1186/gb-2012-13-10-r95.
69. Decock A, Ongenaert M, Van Criekinge W, Speleman F, Vandesompele J. DNA methylation profiling of primary neuroblastoma tumors using methyl-CpG-binding domain sequencing. Sci Data. 2016;3:160004. https://doi.org/10.1038/sdata.2016.4.
70. Gomez S, Castellano G, Mayol G, Queiros A, Martin-Subero JI, Lavarino C. DNA methylation fingerprint of neuroblastoma reveals new biological and clinical insights. Genom Data. 2015;5:360–3. https://doi.org/10.1016/j.gdata.2015.07.016.
71. Olsson M, Beck S, Kogner P, Martinsson T, Caren H. Genome-wide methylation profiling identifies novel methylated genes in neuroblastoma tumors. Epigenetics. 2016;11(1):74–84. https://doi.org/10.1080/15592294.2016.1138195.
72. Boloix A, Paris-Coderch L, Soriano A, Roma J, Gallego S, Sanchez de Toledo J, Segura MF. Novel micro RNA-based therapies for the treatment of neuroblastoma. An Pediatr (Barc). 2016;85(2):109.e101–6. https://doi.org/10.1016/j.anpedi.2015.07.016.
73. Geoerger B, Deschamps F, Puget S, Koubi-Pick V, Lacroix L, Vielh P, Varlet P, De Baere T, Bautista F, Tsambou LB, Valteau Couanet D, Ngo-camus M, Le Deley M-C, Minard-Colin V, Grill J, Brugieres L, Dufour C, Gaspar N, Vassal G, Soria J-C. Molecular screening for cancer treatment optimization (MOSCATO 01) in pediatric patients: first feasibility results of a prospective molecular stratification trial. J Clin Oncol. 2014;32(15_suppl):10050. https://doi.org/10.1200/jco.2014.32.15_suppl.10050.
74. TARGET-Neuroblastoma. https://ocg.cancer.gov/programs/target/projects/neuroblastoma.
75. Vassal G, Zwaan CM, Ashley D, Le Deley MC, Hargrave D, Blanc P, Adamson PC. New drugs for children and adolescents with cancer: the need for novel development pathways. Lancet Oncol. 2013;14(3):e117–24. https://doi.org/10.1016/S1470-2045(13)70013-5.
76. Kumar S, Mokhtari RB, Yeger H, Baruchel S. Preclinical models for pediatric solid tumor drug discovery: current trends, challenges and the scopes for improvement. Expert Opin Drug Discov. 2012;7(11):1093–106. https://doi.org/10.1517/17460441.2012.722077.
77. Houghton PJ, Morton CL, Tucker C, Payne D, Favours E, Cole C, Gorlick R, Kolb EA, Zhang W, Lock R, Carol H, Tajbakhsh M, Reynolds CP, Maris JM, Courtright J, Keir ST, Friedman HS, Stopford C, Zeidner J, Wu J, Liu T, Billups CA, Khan J, Ansher S, Zhang J, Smith MA. The pediatric preclinical testing program: description of models and early testing results. Pediatr Blood Cancer. 2007;49(7):928–40. https://doi.org/10.1002/pbc.21078.
78. Townsend EC, Murakami MA, Christodoulou A, Christie AL, Koster J, DeSouza TA, Morgan EA, Kallgren SP, Liu H, Wu SC, Plana O, Montero J, Stevenson KE, Rao P, Vadhi R, Andreeff M, Armand P, Ballen KK, Barzaghi-Rinaudo P, Cahill S, Clark RA, Cooke VG, Davids MS, DeAngelo DJ, Dorfman DM, Eaton H, Ebert BL, Etchin J, Firestone B, Fisher DC, Freedman AS, Galinsky IA, Gao H, Garcia JS, Garnache-Ottou F, Graubert TA, Gutierrez A, Halilovic E, Harris MH, Herbert ZT, Horwitz SM, Inghirami G, Intlekofer AM, Ito M, Izraeli S, Jacobsen ED, Jacobson CA, Jeay S, Jeremias I, Kelliher MA, Koch R, Konopleva M, Kopp N, Kornblau SM, Kung AL, Kupper TS, LeBoeuf NR, LaCasce AS, Lees E, Li LS, Look AT, Murakami M, Muschen M, Neuberg D, Ng SY, Odejide OO, Orkin SH, Paquette RR, Place AE, Roderick JE, Ryan JA, Sallan SE, Shoji B, Silverman LB, Soiffer RJ, Steensma DP, Stegmaier K, Stone RM, Tamburini J, Thorner AR, van Hummelen P, Wadleigh M, Wiesmann M, Weng AP, Wuerthner JU, Williams DA, Wollison BM, Lane AA, Letai A, Bertagnolli MM, Ritz J, Brown M, Long H, Aster JC, Shipp MA, Griffin JD, Weinstock DM. The public repository of xenografts enables discovery and randomized phase II-like trials in mice. Cancer Cell. 2016;30(1):183. https://doi.org/10.1016/j.ccell.2016.06.008.
79. Braekeveldt N, Wigerup C, Gisselsson D, Mohlin S, Merselius M, Beckman S, Jonson T, Borjesson A, Backman T, Tadeo I, Berbegall AP, Ora I, Navarro S, Noguera R, Pahlman S, Bexell D. Neuroblastoma

patient-derived orthotopic xenografts retain metastatic patterns and geno- and phenotypes of patient tumours. Int J Cancer. 2015;136(5):E252–61. https://doi.org/10.1002/ijc.29217.
80. Braekeveldt N, Wigerup C, Tadeo I, Beckman S, Sanden C, Jonsson J, Erjefalt JS, Berbegall AP, Borjesson A, Backman T, Ora I, Navarro S, Noguera R, Gisselsson D, Pahlman S, Bexell D. Neuroblastoma patient-derived orthotopic xenografts reflect the microenvironmental hallmarks of aggressive patient tumours. Cancer Lett. 2016;375(2):384–9. https://doi.org/10.1016/j.canlet.2016.02.046.
81. Cekanova M, Rathore K. Animal models and therapeutic molecular targets of cancer: utility and limitations. Drug Des Devel Ther. 2014;8:1911–21. https://doi.org/10.2147/DDDT.S49584.
82. Amatruda JF, Patton EE. Genetic models of cancer in zebrafish. Int Rev Cell Mol Biol. 2008;271:1–34. https://doi.org/10.1016/S1937-6448(08)01201-X.
83. Berry T, Luther W, Bhatnagar N, Jamin Y, Poon E, Sanda T, Pei D, Sharma B, Vetharoy WR, Hallsworth A, Ahmad Z, Barker K, Moreau L, Webber H, Wang W, Liu Q, Perez-Atayde A, Rodig S, Cheung NK, Raynaud F, Hallberg B, Robinson SP, Gray NS, Pearson AD, Eccles SA, Chesler L, George RE. The ALK(F1174L) mutation potentiates the oncogenic activity of MYCN in neuroblastoma. Cancer Cell. 2012;22(1):117–30. https://doi.org/10.1016/j.ccr.2012.06.001.
84. Zhu S, Lee JS, Guo F, Shin J, Perez-Atayde AR, Kutok JL, Rodig SJ, Neuberg DS, Helman D, Feng H, Stewart RA, Wang W, George RE, Kanki JP, Look AT. Activated ALK collaborates with MYCN in neuroblastoma pathogenesis. Cancer Cell. 2012;21(3):362–73. https://doi.org/10.1016/j.ccr.2012.02.010.
85. Tang Q, Abdelfattah NS, Blackburn JS, Moore JC, Martinez SA, Moore FE, Lobbardi R, Tenente IM, Ignatius MS, Berman JN, Liwski RS, Houvras Y, Langenau DM. Optimized cell transplantation using adult rag2 mutant zebrafish. Nat Methods. 2014;11(8):821–4. https://doi.org/10.1038/nmeth.3031.
86. Tang Q, Moore JC, Ignatius MS, Tenente IM, Hayes MN, Garcia EG, Torres Yordan N, Bourque C, He S, Blackburn JS, Look AT, Houvras Y, Langenau DM. Imaging tumour cell heterogeneity following cell transplantation into optically clear immune-deficient zebrafish. Nat Commun. 2016;7:10358. https://doi.org/10.1038/ncomms10358.
87. White RM, Sessa A, Burke C, Bowman T, LeBlanc J, Ceol C, Bourque C, Dovey M, Goessling W, Burns CE, Zon LI. Transparent adult zebrafish as a tool for in vivo transplantation analysis. Cell Stem Cell. 2008;2(2):183–9. https://doi.org/10.1016/j.stem.2007.11.002.
88. Zhu S, Thomas Look A. Neuroblastoma and its zebrafish model. Adv Exp Med Biol. 2016;916:451–78. https://doi.org/10.1007/978-3-319-30654-4_20.
89. White R, Rose K, Zon L. Zebrafish cancer: the state of the art and the path forward. Nat Rev Cancer. 2013;13(9):624–36. https://doi.org/10.1038/nrc3589.
90. Moreno L, Caron H, Geoerger B, Eggert A, Schleiermacher G, Brock P, Valteau-Couanet D, Chesler L, Schulte JH, De Preter K, Molenaar J, Schramm A, Eilers M, Van Maerken T, Johnsen JI, Garrett M, George SL, Tweddle DA, Kogner P, Berthold F, Koster J, Barone G, Tucker ER, Marshall L, Herold R, Sterba J, Norga K, Vassal G, Pearson AD. Accelerating drug development for neuroblastoma—new drug development strategy: an innovative therapies for children with cancer, European network for cancer research in children and adolescents and International Society of Paediatric Oncology Europe Neuroblastoma project. Expert Opin Drug Discov. 2017;12(8):801–11. https://doi.org/10.1080/17460441.2017.1340269.
91. Lopez JS, Banerji U. Combine and conquer: challenges for targeted therapy combinations in early phase trials. Nat Rev Clin Oncol. 2017;14(1):57–66. https://doi.org/10.1038/nrclinonc.2016.96.
92. Geoerger B, Schulte J, Zwaan CM, Casanova M, Fischer M, Moreno L, Trahair T, Jimenez I, Kang HJ, Pappo AS, Schafer E, Weiss BD, Healy ME, Li K, Lin T, Boral A, Pearson ADJ. Phase I study of ceritinib in pediatric patients (pts) with malignancies harboring a genetic alteration in ALK (ALK+): safety, pharmacokinetic (PK), and efficacy results. J Clin Oncol. 2015;33(15_suppl):10005. https://doi.org/10.1200/jco.2015.33.15_suppl.10005.
93. Mosse YP, Lipsitz E, Fox E, Teachey DT, Maris JM, Weigel B, Adamson PC, Ingle MA, Ahern CH, Blaney SM. Pediatric phase I trial and pharmacokinetic study of MLN8237, an investigational oral selective small-molecule inhibitor of Aurora kinase A: a children's oncology group phase I consortium study. Clin Cancer Res. 2012;18(21):6058–64. https://doi.org/10.1158/1078-0432.CCR-11-3251.
94. DuBois SG, Marachelian A, Fox E, Kudgus RA, Reid JM, Groshen S, Malvar J, Bagatell R, Wagner L, Maris JM, Hawkins R, Courtier J, Lai H, Goodarzian F, Shimada H, Czarnecki S, Tsao-Wei D, Matthay KK, Mosse YP. Phase I study of the Aurora a kinase inhibitor alisertib in combination with Irinotecan and temozolomide for patients with relapsed or refractory neuroblastoma: a NANT (new approaches to neuroblastoma therapy) trial. J Clin Oncol. 2016;34(12):1368–75. https://doi.org/10.1200/JCO.2015.65.4889.
95. Moreno L, Marshall LV, Pearson AD, Morland B, Elliott M, Campbell-Hewson Q, Makin G, Halford SE, Acton G, Ross P, Kazmi-Stokes S, Lock V, Rodriguez A, Lyons JF, Boddy AV, Griffin MJ, Yule M, Hargrave D. A phase I trial of AT9283 (a selective inhibitor of aurora kinases) in children and adolescents with solid tumors: a cancer research UK study. Clin Cancer Res. 2015;21(2):267–73. https://doi.org/10.1158/1078-0432.CCR-14-1592.

96. Novartis Pharmaceuticals. Phase I study of LDK378 in pediatric, malignancies with a genetic alteration in anaplastic lymphoma kinase (ALK) (NCT01742286). ClinicalTrials.gov. https://clinicaltrials.gov/ct2/show/NCT01742286.
97. Infarinato NR, Park JH, Krytska K, Ryles HT, Sano R, Szigety KM, Li Y, Zou HY, Lee NV, Smeal T, Lemmon MA, Mosse YP. The ALK/ROS1 inhibitor PF-06463922 overcomes primary resistance to crizotinib in ALK-driven neuroblastoma. Cancer Discov. 2016;6(1):96–107. https://doi.org/10.1158/2159-8290.CD-15-1056.
98. Guan J, Tucker ER, Wan H, Chand D, Danielson LS, Ruuth K, El Wakil A, Witek B, Jamin Y, Umapathy G, Robinson SP, Johnson TW, Smeal T, Martinsson T, Chesler L, Palmer RH, Hallberg B. The ALK inhibitor PF-06463922 is effective as a single agent in neuroblastoma driven by expression of ALK and MYCN. Dis Model Mech. 2016;9(9):941–52. https://doi.org/10.1242/dmm.024448.
99. https://clinicaltrials.gov/ct2/show/NCT03107988.
100. Fouladi M, Laningham F, Wu J, O'Shaughnessy MA, Molina K, Broniscer A, Spunt SL, Luckett I, Stewart CF, Houghton PJ, Gilbertson RJ, Furman WL. Phase I study of everolimus in pediatric patients with refractory solid tumors. J Clin Oncol. 2007;25(30):4806–12. https://doi.org/10.1200/JCO.2007.11.4017.
101. Geoerger B, Kieran MW, Grupp S, Perek D, Clancy J, Krygowski M, Ananthakrishnan R, Boni JP, Berkenblit A, Spunt SL. Phase II trial of temsirolimus in children with high-grade glioma, neuroblastoma and rhabdomyosarcoma. Eur J Cancer. 2012;48(2):253–62. https://doi.org/10.1016/j.ejca.2011.09.021.
102. Spunt SL, Grupp SA, Vik TA, Santana VM, Greenblatt DJ, Clancy J, Berkenblit A, Krygowski M, Ananthakrishnan R, Boni JP, Gilbertson RJ. Phase I study of temsirolimus in pediatric patients with recurrent/refractory solid tumors. J Clin Oncol. 2011;29(21):2933–40. https://doi.org/10.1200/JCO.2010.33.4649.
103. Gore L, Trippett TM, Katzenstein HM, Boklan J, Narendran A, Smith A, Macy ME, Rolla K, Pediatric Oncology Experimental Therapeutics Investigators C, Narashimhan N, Squillace RM, Turner CD, Haluska FG, Nieder M. A multicenter, first-in-pediatrics, phase 1, pharmacokinetic and pharmacodynamic study of ridaforolimus in patients with refractory solid tumors. Clin Cancer Res. 2013;19(13):3649–58. https://doi.org/10.1158/1078-0432.CCR-12-3166.
104. Pearson AD, Federico SM, Aerts I, Hargrave DR, DuBois SG, Iannone R, Geschwindt RD, Wang R, Haluska FG, Trippett TM, Geoerger B. A phase 1 study of oral ridaforolimus in pediatric patients with advanced solid tumors. Oncotarget. 2016;7(51):84736–47. https://doi.org/10.18632/oncotarget.12450.
105. Geoerger B, Bourdeaut F, DuBois SG, Fischer M, Geller JI, Gottardo NG, Marabelle A, Pearson ADJ, Modak S, Cash T, Robinson GW, Motta M, Matano A, Bhansali SG, Dobson JR, Parasuraman S, Chi SN. A phase I study of the CDK4/6 inhibitor Ribociclib (LEE011) in pediatric patients with malignant rhabdoid tumors, neuroblastoma, and other solid tumors. Clin Cancer Res. 2017;23(10):2433–41. https://doi.org/10.1158/1078-0432.CCR-16-2898.
106. Amoroso L, Haupt R, Garaventa A, Ponzoni M. Investigational drugs in phase II clinical trials for the treatment of neuroblastoma. Expert Opin Investig Drugs. 2017;26(11):1281–93. https://doi.org/10.1080/13543784.2017.1380625.
107. Mody R, Naranjo A, Van Ryn C, Yu AL, London WB, Shulkin BL, Parisi MT, Servaes SE, Diccianni MB, Sondel PM, Bender JG, Maris JM, Park JR, Bagatell R. Irinotecan-temozolomide with temsirolimus or dinutuximab in children with refractory or relapsed neuroblastoma (COG ANBL1221): an open-label, randomised, phase 2 trial. Lancet Oncol. 2017;18(7):946–57. https://doi.org/10.1016/S1470-2045(17)30355-8.
108. Corbacioglu S, Steinbach D, Lode HN, Gruhn B, Fruehwald M, Broeckelmann M, Suttorp M, Escherich G, Cario G, Ehlert K, Meister B, Simon T, Debatin K-M, Kuhlen M, Feddersen I. The RIST design: a molecularly targeted multimodal approach for the treatment of patients with relapsed and refractory neuroblastoma. J Clin Oncol. 2013;31(15_suppl):10017. https://doi.org/10.1200/jco.2013.31.15_suppl.10017.
109. Hutchinson RJ, Sisson JC, Shapiro B, Miser JS, Normole D, Shulkin BL, Francis IR, Zasadny K, Carey JE, Johnson JW, et al. 131-I-metaiodobenzylguanidine treatment in patients with refractory advanced neuroblastoma. Am J Clin Oncol. 1992;15(3):226–32. https://doi.org/10.1097/00000421-199206000-00009.
110. Klingebiel T, Berthold F, Treuner J, Schwabe D, Fischer M, Feine U, Maul FD, Waters W, Wehinger H, Niethammer D. Metaiodobenzylguanidine (mIBG) in treatment of 47 patients with neuroblastoma: results of the German neuroblastoma trial. Med Pediatr Oncol. 1991;19(2):84–8. https://doi.org/10.1002/mpo.2950190203.
111. Lashford LS, Lewis IJ, Fielding SL, Flower MA, Meller S, Kemshead JT, Ackery D. Phase I/II study of iodine 131 metaiodobenzylguanidine in chemoresistant neuroblastoma: a United Kingdom children's cancer study group investigation. J Clin Oncol. 1992;10(12):1889–96. https://doi.org/10.1200/JCO.1992.10.12.1889.
112. Matthay KK, Yanik G, Messina J, Quach A, Huberty J, Cheng SC, Veatch J, Goldsby R, Brophy P, Kersun LS, Hawkins RA, Maris JM. Phase II study on the effect of disease sites, age, and prior therapy on response to iodine-131-metaiodobenzylguanidine therapy in refractory neuroblastoma. J Clin Oncol.

2007;25(9):1054–60. https://doi.org/10.1200/JCO.2006.09.3484.
113. Delgado DC, Hank JA, Kolesar J, Lorentzen D, Gan J, Seo S, Kim K, Shusterman S, Gillies SD, Reisfeld RA, Yang R, Gadbaw B, DeSantes KB, London WB, Seeger RC, Maris JM, Sondel PM. Genotypes of NK cell KIR receptors, their ligands, and Fcgamma receptors in the response of neuroblastoma patients to Hu14.18-IL2 immunotherapy. Cancer Res. 2010;70(23):9554–61. https://doi.org/10.1158/0008-5472.CAN-10-2211.
114. Cheung NK, Sowers R, Vickers AJ, Cheung IY, Kushner BH, Gorlick R. FCGR2A polymorphism is correlated with clinical outcome after immunotherapy of neuroblastoma with anti-GD2 antibody and granulocyte macrophage colony-stimulating factor. J Clin Oncol. 2006;24(18):2885–90. https://doi.org/10.1200/JCO.2005.04.6011.
115. Merchant MS, Baird K, Wexler LH, Rodriguez-Galindo C, Mackall C. Ipilimumab: first results of a phase I trial in pediatric patients with advanced solid tumors. J Clin Oncol. 2012;30(15_suppl):9545. https://doi.org/10.1200/jco.2012.30.15_suppl.9545.
116. Russell HV, Strother D, Mei Z, Rill D, Popek E, Biagi E, Yvon E, Brenner M, Rousseau R. Phase I trial of vaccination with autologous neuroblastoma tumor cells genetically modified to secrete IL-2 and lymphotactin. J Immunother. 2007;30(2):227–33. https://doi.org/10.1097/01.cji.0000211335.14385.57.
117. Krishnadas DK, Shapiro T, Lucas K. Complete remission following decitabine/dendritic cell vaccine for relapsed neuroblastoma. Pediatrics. 2013;131(1):e336–41. https://doi.org/10.1542/peds.2012-0376.
118. Kanold J, Paillard C, Tchirkov A, Lang P, Kelly A, Halle P, Isfan F, Merlin E, Marabelle A, Rochette E, Demeocq F. NK cell immunotherapy for high-risk neuroblastoma relapse after haploidentical HSCT. Pediatr Blood Cancer. 2012;59(4):739–42. https://doi.org/10.1002/pbc.24030.
119. Lee DW, Barrett DM, Mackall C, Orentas R, Grupp SA. The future is now: chimeric antigen receptors as new targeted therapies for childhood cancer. Clin Cancer Res. 2012;18(10):2780–90. https://doi.org/10.1158/1078-0432.CCR-11-1920.
120. Louis CU, Savoldo B, Dotti G, Pule M, Yvon E, Myers GD, Rossig C, Russell HV, Diouf O, Liu E, Liu H, Wu MF, Gee AP, Mei Z, Rooney CM, Heslop HE, Brenner MK. Antitumor activity and long-term fate of chimeric antigen receptor-positive T cells in patients with neuroblastoma. Blood. 2011;118(23):6050–6. https://doi.org/10.1182/blood-2011-05-354449.
121. Pule MA, Savoldo B, Myers GD, Rossig C, Russell HV, Dotti G, Huls MH, Liu E, Gee AP, Mei Z, Yvon E, Weiss HL, Liu H, Rooney CM, Heslop HE, Brenner MK. Virus-specific T cells engineered to coexpress tumor-specific receptors: persistence and antitumor activity in individuals with neuroblastoma. Nat Med. 2008;14(11):1264–70. https://doi.org/10.1038/nm.1882.
122. Kunkele A, Taraseviciute A, Finn LS, Johnson AJ, Berger C, Finney O, Chang CA, Rolczynski LS, Brown C, Mgebroff S, Berger M, Park JR, Jensen MC. Preclinical assessment of CD171-directed CAR T-cell adoptive therapy for childhood neuroblastoma: CE7 epitope target safety and product manufacturing feasibility. Clin Cancer Res. 2017;23(2):466–77. https://doi.org/10.1158/1078-0432.CCR-16-0354.
123. Quintarelli C, Orlando D, Boffa I, Guercio M, Polito VA, Petretto A, Lavarello C, Sinibaldi M, Weber G, Del Bufalo F, Giorda E, Scarsella M, Petrini S, Pagliara D, Locatelli F, De Angelis B, Caruana I. Choice of costimulatory domains and of cytokines determines CAR T-cell activity in neuroblastoma. Onco Targets Ther. 2018;7(6):e1433518. https://doi.org/10.1080/2162402X.2018.1433518.
124. Crossland DL, Denning WL, Ang S, Olivares S, Mi T, Switzer K, Singh H, Huls H, Gold KS, Glisson BS, Cooper LJ, Heymach JV. Antitumor activity of CD56-chimeric antigen receptor T cells in neuroblastoma and SCLC models. Oncogene. 2018;37(27):3686–97. https://doi.org/10.1038/s41388-018-0187-2.
125. Bocca P, Di Carlo E, Caruana I, Emionite L, Cilli M, De Angelis B, Quintarelli C, Pezzolo A, Raffaghello L, Morandi F, Locatelli F, Pistoia V, Prigione I. Bevacizumab-mediated tumor vasculature remodelling improves tumor infiltration and antitumor efficacy of GD2-CAR T cells in a human neuroblastoma preclinical model. Onco Targets Ther. 2017;7(1):e1378843. https://doi.org/10.1080/2162402X.2017.1378843.
126. Li N, Fu H, Hewitt SM, Dimitrov DS, Ho M. Therapeutically targeting glypican-2 via single-domain antibody-based chimeric antigen receptors and immunotoxins in neuroblastoma. Proc Natl Acad Sci U S A. 2017;114(32):E6623–31. https://doi.org/10.1073/pnas.1706055114.
127. Walker AJ, Majzner RG, Zhang L, Wanhainen K, Long AH, Nguyen SM, Lopomo P, Vigny M, Fry TJ, Orentas RJ, Mackall CL. Tumor antigen and receptor densities regulate efficacy of a chimeric antigen receptor targeting anaplastic lymphoma kinase. Mol Ther. 2017;25(9):2189–201. https://doi.org/10.1016/j.ymthe.2017.06.008.
128. Heczey A, Louis CU, Savoldo B, Dakhova O, Durett A, Grilley B, Liu H, Wu MF, Mei Z, Gee A, Mehta B, Zhang H, Mahmood N, Tashiro H, Heslop HE, Dotti G, Rooney CM, Brenner MK. CAR T cells administered in combination with lymphodepletion and PD-1 inhibition to patients with neuroblastoma. Mol Ther. 2017;25(9):2214–24. https://doi.org/10.1016/j.ymthe.2017.05.012.

129. Paoletti X, Geoerger B, Doz F, Baruchel A, Lokiec F, Le Tourneau C. A comparative analysis of paediatric dose-finding trials of molecularly targeted agent with adults' trials. Eur J Cancer. 2013;49(10):2392–402. https://doi.org/10.1016/j.ejca.2013.02.028.
130. Moreno L, Pearson ADJ, Paoletti X, Jimenez I, Geoerger B, Kearns PR, Zwaan CM, Doz F, Baruchel A, Vormoor J, Casanova M, Pfister SM, Morland B, Vassal G, Innovative Therapies for Children with Cancer C. Early phase clinical trials of anticancer agents in children and adolescents—an ITCC perspective. Nat Rev Clin Oncol. 2017;14(8):497–507. https://doi.org/10.1038/nrclinonc.2017.59.
131. Onar-Thomas A, Xiong Z. A simulation-based comparison of the traditional method, rolling-6 design and a frequentist version of the continual reassessment method with special attention to trial duration in pediatric phase I oncology trials. Contemp Clin Trials. 2010;31(3):259–70. https://doi.org/10.1016/j.cct.2010.03.006.
132. Ensign LG, Gehan EA, Kamen DS, Thall PF. An optimal three-stage design for phase II clinical trials. Stat Med. 1994;13(17):1727–36. https://doi.org/10.1002/sim.4780131704.
133. Moroz V, Wilson JS, Kearns P, Wheatley K. Comparison of anticipated and actual control group outcomes in randomised trials in paediatric oncology provides evidence that historically controlled studies are biased in favour of the novel treatment. Trials. 2014;15:481. https://doi.org/10.1186/1745-6215-15-481.
134. Sposto R, Stram DO. A strategic view of randomized trial design in low-incidence paediatric cancer. Stat Med. 1999;18(10):1183–97. https://doi.org/10.1002/(sici)1097-0258(19990530)18:10<1183::aid-sim122>3.0.co;2-p.
135. Deley MC, Ballman KV, Marandet J, Sargent D. Taking the long view: how to design a series of phase III trials to maximize cumulative therapeutic benefit. Clin Trials. 2012;9(3):283–92. https://doi.org/10.1177/1740774512443430.
136. ADJ P, Pfister SM, Baruchel A, Bourquin JP, Casanova M, Chesler L, Doz F, Eggert A, Geoerger B, DTW J, Kearns PR, Molenaar JJ, Morland B, Schleiermacher G, Schulte JH, Vormoor J, Marshall LV, Zwaan CM, Vassal G, Executive, Biology Committees of the Innovative Therapies for Children with Cancer European C. From class waivers to precision medicine in paediatric oncology. Lancet Oncol. 2017;18(7):e394–404. https://doi.org/10.1016/S1470-2045(17)30442-4.
137. Saulnier Sholler GL, Ferguson W, Bergendahl G, Currier E, Lenox SR, Bond J, Slavik M, Roberts W, Mitchell D, Eslin D, Kraveka J, Kaplan J, Parikh N, Malempati S, Hanna G, Eugster E, Cherba D, Miller J, Webb C. A pilot trial testing the feasibility of using molecular-guided therapy in patients with recurrent neuroblastoma, Vol 3, Issue 5, p 602–612, 2012. https://doi.org/10.4236/jct.2012.35077.
138. Saulnier Sholler GL, Bond JP, Bergendahl G, Dutta A, Dragon J, Neville K, Ferguson W, Roberts W, Eslin D, Kraveka J, Kaplan J, Mitchell D, Parikh N, Merchant M, Ashikaga T, Hanna G, Lescault PJ, Siniard A, Corneveaux J, Huentelman M, Trent J. Feasibility of implementing molecular-guided therapy for the treatment of patients with relapsed or refractory neuroblastoma. Cancer Med. 2015;4(6):871–86. https://doi.org/10.1002/cam4.436.
139. Mody RJ, Wu YM, Lonigro RJ, Cao X, Roychowdhury S, Vats P, Frank KM, Prensner JR, Asangani I, Palanisamy N, Dillman JR, Rabah RM, Kunju LP, Everett J, Raymond VM, Ning Y, Su F, Wang R, Stoffel EM, Innis JW, Roberts JS, Robertson PL, Yanik G, Chamdin A, Connelly JA, Choi S, Harris AC, Kitko C, Rao RJ, Levine JE, Castle VP, Hutchinson RJ, Talpaz M, Robinson DR, Chinnaiyan AM. Integrative clinical sequencing in the management of refractory or relapsed cancer in youth. JAMA. 2015;314(9):913–25. https://doi.org/10.1001/jama.2015.10080.

14 Future Aspects of Neuroblastoma Research

Frank Westermann and Shahab Asgharzadeh

The technological advancements in omics analyses have substantially improved the molecular understanding and classification of childhood neuroblastoma. Several markers have been identified that robustly identify low-risk neuroblastomas, which may allow to adapt treatment intensity and to avoid overtreatment for truly low-risk cases. Similarly, molecular markers have been established that identify highly aggressive cases. Thus, risk prediction at the time of diagnosis is likely to come to a very high precision once all these markers are integrated into the upcoming trial protocols. Despite improvements in risk prediction, survival rate has not significantly improved over the last decade with mortality rate of over 50% in children with high-risk, metastasized disease (stage 4). We are also at the limits of toxicity in treatment of these patients with aggressive multimodal therapy, including polychemotherapy, high-dose chemotherapy with autologous stem cell rescue, surgery, irradiation, followed by immunotherapy. Current therapy mostly achieves complete remission, but poor survival is mainly due to lethal relapse resulting from therapy resistance and early metastasis already manifested at diagnosis. The only reasonable conclusion from this sobering collective experience is that our approach of treating children with high-risk neuroblastomas requires urgent rethinking the principles of treatment. There is hope in improvement of outcomes with the combination of chemotherapies with anti-GD2 antibody both in children with relapse and refractory disease, as well as those with newly diagnosed disease. While the exact mechanisms of response are not clear, emerging data suggest the activation of immune system that likely is responsible for sustained disease-free status. The challenge remains in understanding the exact mechanisms of response and resistance, and likely identification of a novel set of prognostic features. Implementation of novel combinations of immunotherapeutic approaches and better understanding of the tumor microenvironment and immune responses to these approaches should lead to improved outcomes in children with high-risk neuroblastoma.

Recent basic research studies investigating relapsed neuroblastomas have identified novel mechanisms of tumor evolution and treatment failure: (1) clonal genetic evolution resulting in the acquisition of targetable mutations and genomic alterations in oncogenic pathways and (2) the novel observation of non-genetic evolution in the form of phenotypic tumor plas-

F. Westermann (✉)
Department of Neuroblastoma Genomics, German Cancer Research Center, Heidelberg, Baden-Württemberg, Germany
e-mail: f.westermann@dkfz.de

S. Asgharzadeh
Department of Pediatrics, Children's Hospital Los Angeles, Los Angeles, CA, USA
e-mail: sasgharzadeh@chla.usc.edu

S. Asgharzadeh, F. Westermann (eds.), *Neuroblastoma*, Pediatric Oncology,
https://doi.org/10.1007/978-3-031-51292-6_14

ticity (often along normal embryonic sympathetic nervous system (SNS) (de-)differentiation trajectories) (3) diversity of tumor microenvironment and its correlation with aggressive tumors. Exploitation of newly won insights integrating concepts of tumor evolution and its microenvironment and their effects on resistance and metastasis would break ground toward completely novel concepts in personalized neuroblastoma treatment. Neuroblastomas possess considerable intratumor heterogeneity that can arise from both genetic and non-genetic variability, which appear to be not mutually exclusive. Recent evidence points to the importance of the interplay between genetic and non-genetic cancer evolution. This interplay is likely to have a significant impact on precision medicine. Precision medicine has relied, to date, on the premise that the genomic landscape would sufficiently guide therapeutic decisions. However, intratumor heterogeneity and cancer evolution have already proven major challenges for treatment. As a result, the mutation catalogs identified in bulk tumor samples have, as yet, made only a modest impact on neuroblastoma clinical medicine. Indeed, molecular therapies are often of limited clinical benefit if prediction is based on a sensitizing mutation detected by bulk sequencing of a single sample from a single time point. Driver mutations may be subclonal and resistance mechanisms can evolve rapidly in single cells. As our understanding of adaptive mechanisms used by tumor cells to evade therapies grows, it becomes increasingly apparent that a gene-centric vision at the time of first diagnosis is probably an oversimplification of the task ahead. The role and heterogeneity of tumor microenvironment must also be better characterized as emerging data in neuroblastoma and other cancers show their significant influence in promoting metastasis and protecting tumor cells from targeted therapies that likely leads to subclonal evolution. Non-genetic mechanisms of therapy resistance and early metastasis that include reactivation of embryonal stem cell features must gain similarly broad recognition in the field. Only then will we be able to design clinical trials to deal with both major sources of therapy resistance. A prerequisite to this next step of designing effective precision medicine approaches is a better understanding of how these different evolutionary driving forces work together to drive metastasis and therapy resistance in neuroblastoma.

Complementary and integrated studies are needed using innovative single-cell technologies, informative patient material and predictive model systems, ranging from cell-based in vitro systems to novel animal disease models to reach the level of cellular precision needed to understand genetic and phenotypic evolutionary processes in neuroblastoma. Additional human studies analyzing immune cell repertoire and function using technologies such as CyTOF and single-cell technologies are also needed to provide a compendium of immune alterations and activations observed for various immunotherapies. The translation of this new knowledge into clinical benefit implies rethinking therapeutic strategies. Gaining deeper insight into evolutionary and immunologic events, mechanisms and synergies may prove central to creating radically new treatment approaches considering not only individual oncogenes as targets but the evolving nature of human tumors and immune responses. In addition to opening such new avenues for future personalized treatment design, the most recent insights demonstrating that neuroblastoma cells can adopt at least two different phenotypes put all previous data into new perspective: (a) evolutionary mechanisms of resistance and relapse may strongly rely on cell plasticity since ADRN and MES cell types strongly differ in sensitivity to chemotherapy and targeted drugs; (b) mutant oncogenes and the key neuroblastoma drivers, MYCN and ALK, strongly differ in function, expression, and/or activity in cells of different type in the same tumor, making a complete re-evaluation of their function in the context of cell identity necessary; (c) expression of major immunomodulatory genes (i.e., HLA-A, B, C) strongly differs in ADRN and MES cell types, requiring the integration of cell type evaluation with immunotherapy design; and (d) both MES and ADRN cell populations need to be eliminated by appropriate combination therapies in preclinical studies, making this concept attractive to prevent neuroblastoma relapse in the clinical setting. This shift in perspective highlights the necessity to analyze both genotypic and phenotypic intratumor heterogeneity to understand how complex tumor evolutionary processes impact resistance, relapse, and metastasis so the understanding can be optimally exploited for patient benefit. These fundamental understandings will also likely aid in improving efficacy of both new approaches to immunotherapies such as cellular therapies and bispecific T cell engagers, as well as traditional antibody-based approaches and vaccine developments.

In summary, our failure to inform treatment of neuroblastoma with an understanding of embryonic SNS development and immune dysregulation has driven inefficient, often anecdotal, efforts to improve therapy. Designing effective new molecular-targeted treatments and immunotherapies for children with neuroblastomas will require a better understanding of neuroblastoma-specific dependencies that allow selective and durable killing, differentiation of neuroblastoma cells, and establishment of anti-neuroblastoma immunity.